CAPPA

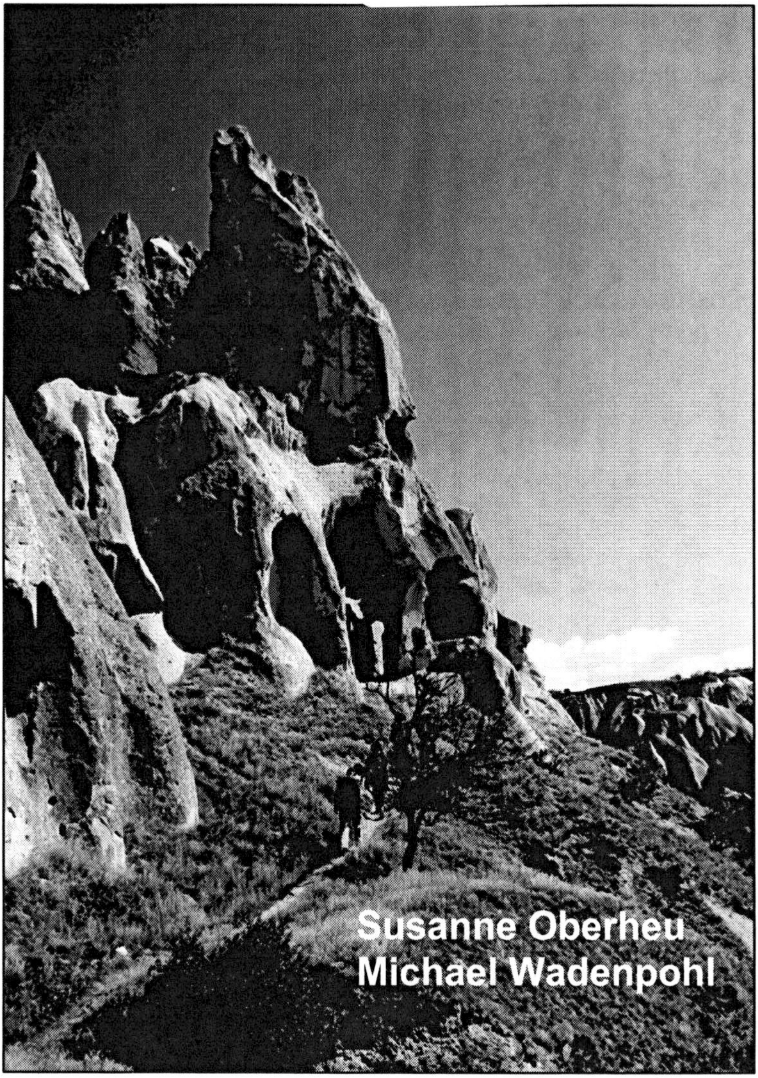

Susanne Oberheu
Michael Wadenpohl

Bibliographic information by the Deutsche Bibliothek:
This publication has been listed in the German National Bibliography (Deutsche Nationalbibliographie); detailed bibliographic data are available on the Internet at **http:/dnb.ddb.de**.

© 2010 Susanne Oberheu and Michael Wadenpohl
All rights reserved. All information without guarantee.

Production and publishing: Books on Demand GmbH,
Norderstedt

ISBN: 978-3-8391-5661-2

Texts, photos, maps and cover design
(unless otherwise mentioned):
Susanne Oberheu and Michael Wadenpohl

General map of Turkey

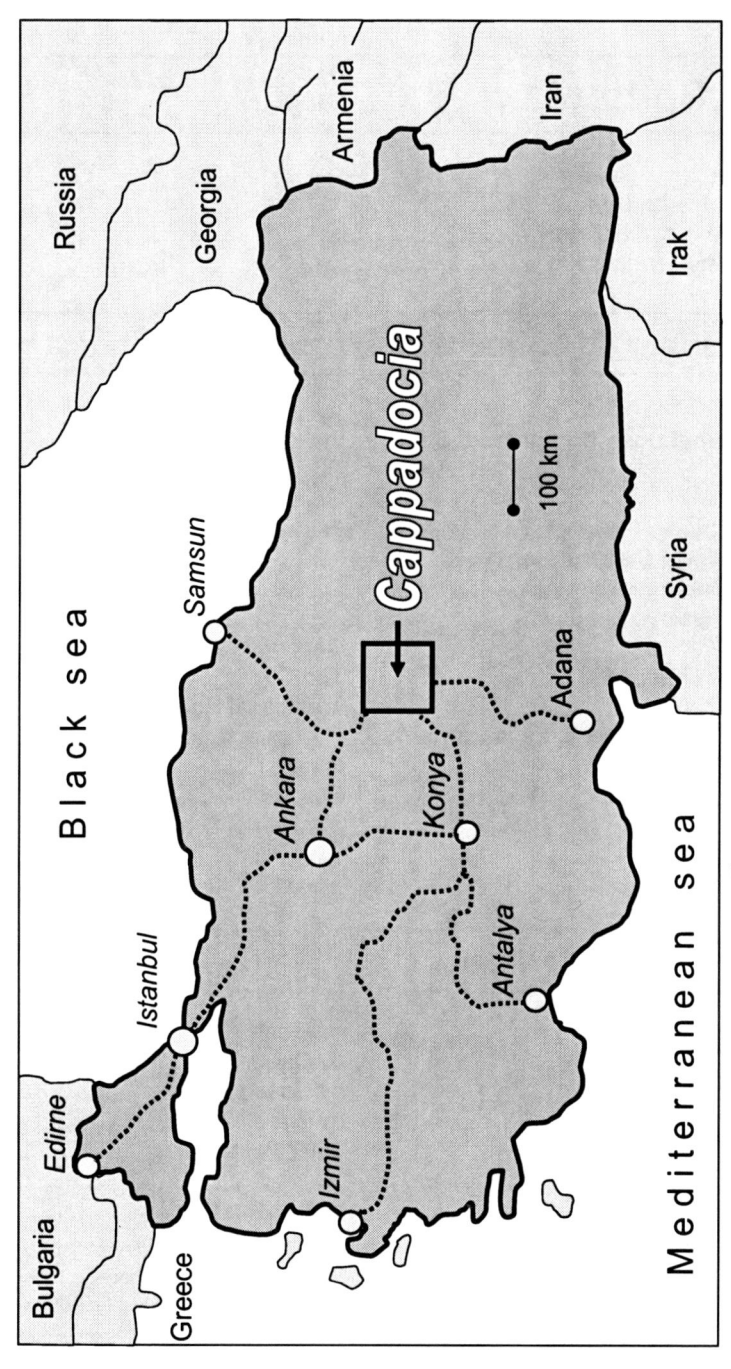

Contents

Introduktion		8
About this Book		10
The Translation		11

What You Should Know about Cappadocia

What does Cappadocia offer	In General	14
	Climate and Travelling Season	16
	Geography	18
	Flora and Fauna	20
World Cultural Heritage		24
Geologocal origin		29
History		35
	Cappadocia in Christianity	48
Architecture	The Caves	57
	Traditional Houses	65
The Country a. its Inhabitants	Politics and Administration	71
	Islam	75
	Economy	79
	Traditionel Family Life	82
Tourism		85
	Travel Offers	87

Travel Informations

How to Get There	by Plane	92
	by Car	93
	by Coach	96
	by Train	97
	other Possibilities	98
Entry Requirements		99
Through the Country	by the own Car	102
	by Motorcycle	106
	by Rented Vehicles	106
	by Long-distance Coaches	107
	By Lokal Buslines	110

Accommodations.............................	....	114
Camping...	....	116
Monetary Questions........................	....	121
Medical and Health Care................	....	123
Security...	....	125
Travelling Woman............................	....	127
Food and Drink................................	....	134
Shopping...	....	143
Exotic Services...............................	....	145
Travelling Dogs...............................	....	147
Holydays and Festivals..................	....	148
Language and Communication.......	....	150
Blunders...	....	151
Begging..	....	155
Leisure Activities............................	Walking	156
	Ballooning	158
	Cycling	163
	Swimming	164
	Horseriding	164
	Pottery	166
Taking Fotos....................................	....	167
Hamam...	....	169
Souveniers and Carpets.................	....	173
Museums..	....	179
Clothes...	....	180
Post Offices.....................................	....	181
Internet...	....	181
Electricity...	....	182
Telephone..	....	182
Taxis...	....	183
Toilets...	....	183
Garbage Problems..........................	....	185
Time..	....	186
Hitchhiking.......................................	....	186
Parking Taxes		187
Maps...	....	188
Important Adresses and Telephone Numbers..	....	188

Sights and Places

Central Cappadocia	Uçhisar...........................	192
	Göreme...........................	198
	Göreme Museum...................	205
	Çavuşin...........................	214
	Paşabağı..........................	218
	Zelve.............................	220
	Devrent Valley.....................	223
	Ürgüp.............................	224
	Ortahisar.........................	231
	Hospital Monastery................	234
	Ibrahimpaşa.......................	235
	Nevşehir..........................	236
The North	Avanos............................	239
	Özkonak..........................	248
	Bayramhacı.......................	250
	Sarıhan...........................	251
The East	Kayseri and Erciyes-Dağı.........	253
	Theodore Church..................	260
	Incesu............................	262
The Southeast....................	Sarıca Church.....................	267
	Mustafapaşa.......................	267
	Cemil	274
	Keşlik Monastery..................	275
	Taşkınpaşa........................	275
	Soğanlı Valley.....................	276
The Southwest....................	Kaymaklı..........................	281
	Derinkuyu.........................	283
The Northwest....................	Çat Valley.........................	285
	Açık Saray........................	286
	Hacıbektaş........................	288
The West.........................	Nargöl............................	294
	Gaziemir..........................	294
	Güzelyurt.........................	295
	Ihlara Canyon.....................	300
	Selime............................	303

The Little Hiking Guide

Tour 1...............	Çavuşin - Paşabağı – Zelve..............	308
Tour 2...............	Uçhisar – Pigeon Valley – Göreme.......	311
Tour 3 A.............	Çavusin – Lookout point..............	314
Tour 3 B.............	Lookout point – Güllüdere – Çavuşin....	317
Tour 3 C.............	Lookout point - Çavuşin..............	319
Tour 4...............	Uçhisar - Aşkdere – Çavuşin.............	321
Tour 5...............	Zemidere - Göreme........................	324

The Little Dictionary

Pronunciation, numbers, important words and phrases......... 327

Outline Maps

Outline Map of Central Cappadocia......................... 338
General Map of Cappadocia................................. 340

Additional Information

The Hittites.......................	......................the Lost People	37
Women and Islam...............	......................a Different View	130
Cappadocian Wine............	................the Rediscovering	140
Like Dogs and Cats..........	................Views of two Worlds	153
Cappadocian Carpets......	.........a Rare Nomad Furniture	177
Ecstasy and Asceticism...	....Early Christian Communitiys	212
The Karamanlı..................	....Caviar Trade in Cappadocia	229
Pottery by the Red River..	...............a Craft shapes a City	242
Karamustafa.....................	......a Visier has Great Projects	265
Population Exchange.......	.........a Tragedy of two Nations	270
Hacı Bektaş Veli................	.........and Anatolian Humanism	291

Introduction

"It's as if Walt Disney had ordered a Grand Canyon from Gaudi"

This is how a German "Die Zeit" magazine journalist once characterized Cappadocia, and one cannot describe the landscape more appropriately. In many travel reports you can read things like "nightcap towers", "a moon landscape" or "dunes turned to stone". Again and again fairy-chimneys and rock cones are referred to – nevertheless, the first view of this fantastic landscape will still leave most visitors speechless. Cappadocia seems to be indescribable.

If you then leave the great tourist routes and dive into the unreal silence of the numerous canyons, you will feel you have left our planet. It will become clear to you why this landscape has so often served as a background in adventure or science fiction movies.

But this planet of Cappadocia is inhabited: green and fertile gardens between barren rocks and thousands of rock-hewn dwellings betray the presence of human beings. Entire villages, underground towns, churches and monasteries perforate Cappadocias like Swiss cheese. More than 3000 years ago, the Hittites had already scratched caves into the soft tufa. The first Christians took refuge in the remote beauty of Cappadocia, decorating their churches with valuable Byzantine frescoes and making church history. Right up until the last century, Greeks settled down in Cappadocia and helped shape many villages with their beautifully decorated houses. The Seljuks from Central Asia built huge caravanserais here at this intersection of the Asian trade routes. And finally, the Islamic Turks lived side by side with their Christian neighbours for almost 500 years, cultivating the fertile valleys and living in countless cave dwellings. This is why Cappadocia is not only a World Natural Heritage, but also a World Cultural Heritage, and an unusual openness to the world can be perceived here to the present day.

In old times Cappadocia encompassed a huge area between the Taurus mountain range in the south, the Euphrates River in the east and the Kızılırmak, or Red River, in the north. Today the name – in terms of tourism - refers to a rather small area of just about a hundred and eighty square miles in the heart of Anatolia. This region, where erosion by wind, water and snow has carved one of the most impressive landscapes on earth into the soft tuff stone, is today called Cappadocia.

Even though tourism has left its marks, you will still meet people here who have not given up their old traditional way of living. It is a clash of two worlds when a farmer dressed in his jacket, Turkish trousers and peaked cap tries to steer his donkey cart laden with harvest goods past modern tourist coaches without collision, never forgetting to offer his freshly picked grapes to the visitors. Or when on the weekly market Turkish women dressed in their colourful headscarves very skilfully press their goods on casually dressed female tourists. The Cappadocians do not know any fear of contact. They observe the excesses of western culture with interest and are happy to give advice.

Here in Cappadocia, Islamic culture and tourism get on with each other. And this happens although each year more than a million tourists from all over the world invade this small region. Consequently, the tourist offer has increased a lot recently.There is something to suit all tastes – from discotheques for nightbirds to guided hiking tours for the peace-loving nature freak. Nothing remains of the small villages which were seemingly in danger of dying out completely. According to a travel report, in the 1960's there were only just three families left in Göreme, which today is thought to be the main goal of many tourists. In those days, only a narrow donkey path connected the village with the outside world. Then, near the end of the seventies, the first backpackers discovered Cappadocia. The first boarding houses were opened, and some former inhabitants who had emigrated to Europe a few years before returned home. Even today, a year like 1989 - a tourist boom year when the few boarding houses and hotels of the time were overcrowded and sleeping space on the flat roofs began to get scarce - is talked about with nostalgia.

Today, the picture has changed, unfortunately not in favour of the people living here. The number of long term holidaymakers has decreased steadily; they were replaced by day trippers from the beaches of the Turkish Mediterranean coast. "Cappadocia in two days" is today's motto.

The fact that this is not appropriate to this landscape and its inhabitants was an important reason for us to write this travel guide. We want to show that there is more to be discovered than what the tourist brochures are trying to tell us and that it is worthwhile staying here longer.

Whoever walks through Cappadocia with open eyes will not only see spectacular sights. He will not be able to resist the charm and hospitality of the country and its people. With this in mind, we wish you a pleasant journey and memorable days in Cappadocia.

A word about the structure of this travel guide

We have tried to make the information and the descriptions in this travel guide as up to date and as precise as possible. But a mistake or some misinformation can always creep in. We therefore would like to ask you to forgive us in advance, and we would be very grateful for any corrections from our
readers. On the other hand, Turkey is a country that is presently undergoing constant change so that alterations are happening all the time. All information about prices and times as well as the descriptions of the accommodation details refer to the summer of 2008. There can be dramatic changes, especially regarding accommodation and restaurants -sometimes the owner and consequently the basic concept changes, not necessarily always in a positive way.
If you should find a mistake or any outdated information in this book, please contact us via E-Mail at the following address: **avanos@gmx.de**.

This travel guide is divided into four main parts

In the first part you will find some general information about Cappadocia, but also about Turkey in general. If you want to move about safely and securely in this country, you should possess some basic knowledge in order to avoid too many faux pas. Even though tourism has not been an unknown word in Cappadocia for a long time, there are still considerable differences between the Orient and the West. If you happen to meet people not yet involved in the tourist business, this first part of the book will be especially useful to you.

In the second part the practical aspects of a journey to Cappadocia are dealt with. The individual section titles – from arrival to reservations – are explained in detail here.

In the third part the individual places and sights or other important locations are described. There you will find a detailed description of the place and information about accomodation or important utilities.
Only very rarely will you find details about restaurants or cafés. One reason for this is that we are not gourmets, but also because everybody knows that tastes can be very different. Some people like the delicate refined cuisine,

whereas others prefer large heaps of French fries and a pork chop that is bigger than the plate. But often restaurants also change their owners. Maybe the former owner took great care to run his place with commitment and devotion, while his successor only has his eye on easy profit, and thus it happens that the place goes to ruin within months. For this reason we have only mentioned those few restaurants that struck us because of their special atmosphere or their reasonable value for money. If you come upon restaurants worth recommending that have eluded us during your journey, we would be very grateful if you let us know about them.

The fourth (and last) part is of special interest to the hiking fan. Here we have searched out a number of hiking routes leading through the landscape of Cappadocia and have also provided some hiking maps for this purpose.

The travel guide is finally completed by a short dictionary containing all important words for this region of the country.

Note on the translation

The reader will realize very quickly that this travel guide is not originally from the English-speaking world. It first appeared in German in 2007. As we again and again received requests for an English edition, we decided to venture on this project in 2010. In this context we would like to cordially thank Siegfried Heppner, Susanne's former English teacher, for the excellent translation. Our thanks go also to William Burlace and Lisa van Gaardner from Melbourne, who kindly agreed to do the proofreading as native speakers.
With the distances we have retained the metric system. Firstly, out of consideration for all those readers who speak English as a second language, but also because in Turkey all distances are given in metres or kilometres. Besides, even the speedometer of your rental car will be calibrated in kilometres per hour. We have done the same with the temperature data.

Here are a few conversions between metric and Anglo-American measures:

1 mile = 1.6094 km
1 yard = 0.9144 m
1 foot = 0.3048 m

1 gallon = 4.546 litres

° Fahrenheit = ° Celsius x 1.8 + 32

We, the authors, now wish you much fun in reading this book.

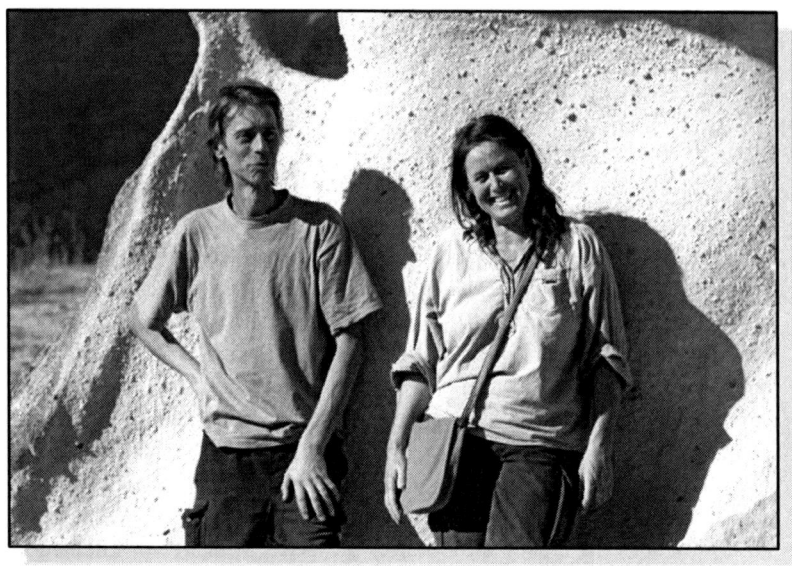

Foto: Uwe Schmitz

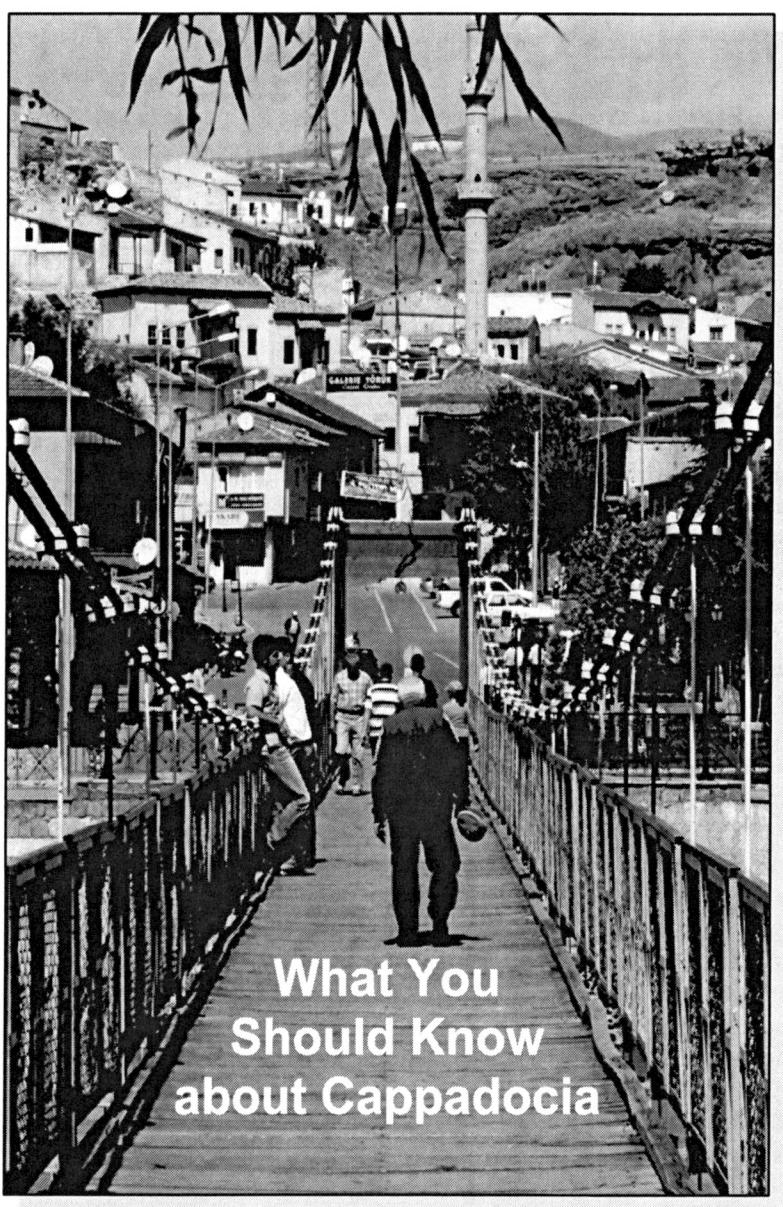

What You Should Know about Cappadocia

What does Cappadocia offer ?

First, let us reverse the question and ask: What have I got to do to be able to enjoy a trip to Cappadocia? Above all, one must not be a lazy person. Hours of sunbathing on the beach are out of the question because of the geographical position. But the shopping and leisure facilities are also limited, and a nightlife exists only sporadically. Cappadocia is an Eldorado for active holidaymakers who want to experience and discover things and who are interested in culture. You are not allowed to be footsore here. It is an advantage to be a good walker not only because of the partly difficult terrain, but also because Turkish street curbs are something special. Flexibility in an intellectual sense of the word is necessary, too. Above all, individual tourists will notice very soon that life is somewhat different here. After all, you are travelling in an Islamic country, a fact that the 'beach tourist' is very often unaware of. The cultural differences reach as far as such trite things as the somewhat unusual local bus service system. Introverted or shy people will have certain problems in finding their way in this foreign country. As always, the motto here is: ask, and you will be helped, none but the brave deserve the fair. Don't be afraid to approach people directly and openly! If you encounter people frankly and fearlessly, you will have already fulfilled the most important precondition for spending unforgettable days in Cappadocia.

But what is it that causes the special charm of this region? Two factors are important here. Firstly, there is the archaic scenery. Whoever sees it for the first time is overwhelmed at once. But it is really rewarding for those who grab their rucksack and walking shoes and wander through the many side valleys. The most incredible rock formations can be discovered during these walks – and the silence is characterized by the warbling of birds and the humming of insects. And all the time you find yourself walking through a fertile valley in which one orchard follows another. The nature lover will find everything he needs here and will also find relief from working-day stress.

The second factor is called culture. Nowhere else in the world can such a unique landscape be found, a landscape that is at the same time full of traces of great cultures. In particular, early Christianity has inscribed its name here hundreds of times. Numerous rock-cut churches and monasteries can be found on both sides of the valleys. Ornately decorated with frescoes that are

partly in excellent condition, they tempt the wanderer to leave his path, thus doubling the span of many excursions.
It is this combination of art, culture and a magnificent natural scenery that forms Cappadocia's secret.
Everywhere there are hidden corridors and corners to be discovered which deceive you into thinking that you are the first person to see them. Entire settlements can be explored, either beehive-shaped in enormous rock towers, or up to 80 metres deep down in the ground. Human beings have always made use of the soft rock to provide dwelling space for themselves in this fashion.

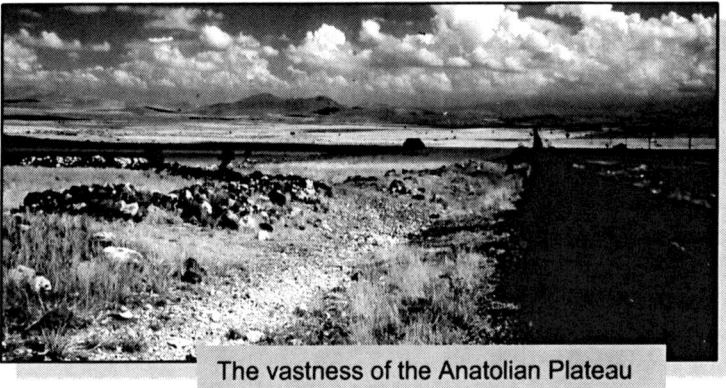
The vastness of the Anatolian Plateau

But where exactly is Cappadocia? Only a very rough definition is possible here. Indeed, there is the centre round Göreme with a diameter of 15 km, where most tourist highlights are concentrated. But there are also some more distant attractions like e.g. the Ihlara Canyon, which is no less than 90 km away. When looking at a map of Turkey, it is best to find out the southernmost point of the Kızılırmak (Red River) with the village of Avanos. Göreme is situated about 10 km to the south of it. Cappadocia is thus situated almost precisely in the centre of the Anatolian Plateau. This means that we are moving at an altitude of betweeen 900 and 1400 metres above sea level, which now leads us to our next topic.

Climate and Travelling Season

The climate can sometimes be called almost desert-like. Scorching summers alternate with icy cold winters. The main reason for this is the altitude of the region in addition to the relative dryness of the climate in general. Rainfall occurs mostly in winter and in springtime; but even then it is scarce. It is often followed by long periods of drought which can last until well into November. Also something like an Indian summer is known in Cappadocia. Daily temperatures in November then soar up to 77° F (25° C), while at night it already gets bitterly cold. Towards the end there is often a short sandstorm that heralds the first rain, and with the increasing humidity the daily temperatures sink to rock bottom. The best time for travelling is late spring and autumn. In the middle of summer, that is in July and in August, temperatures can rise to over 104°F (40° C), whereas in winter it can be as cold as minus 4°F (-20° C) - for weeks. There are even more advantages to visiting Cappadocia in the moderate seasons: in spring the landscape is covered by a magnificent sea of blossom in combination with lush green. Both will usually disappear very fast by the middle of summer. In autumn – the harvest season – the country is flooded with an endless abundance of fruit, and the colours change to red just like in other Europeancountries.

In many places a veritable microclimate can be distinguished. While in Avanos, situated at the bank of the river, you can still lie in the sun dressed in a T-shirt the whole day long if you are lucky, in Ortahisar, which is 250 m higher, you will sit on your terrace wrapped up in thick pullovers all day. Even in Avanos there is a difference of up to 40°F (5° C) between its southern slope and the new town on the opposite bank of the river.

Generally, it has to be said that Cappadocia is rather dusty. The soft wind that blows almost continuously always carries the eroded tufa dust with it. Again and again this settles down on the cars and on the furniture. If you should find a thin layer of dust in your apartment, do not panic – this is not poor cleanliness, but the past few hours' erosion. A highlight can be seen in the rare and short but heavy sandstorms. At first you will only see a yellowish hue of the sky. But then the wind begins to blow. At a speed of up to 80 km per hour, it seems to clear away the entire landscape, letting it rain down again on you. If you have been lying in the sun lightly dressed and sweating before, you will then learn how it feels to be a wienerschnitzel. Only a long shower will help after this.

Climate and travelling season

Average day and night temperatures in ° C

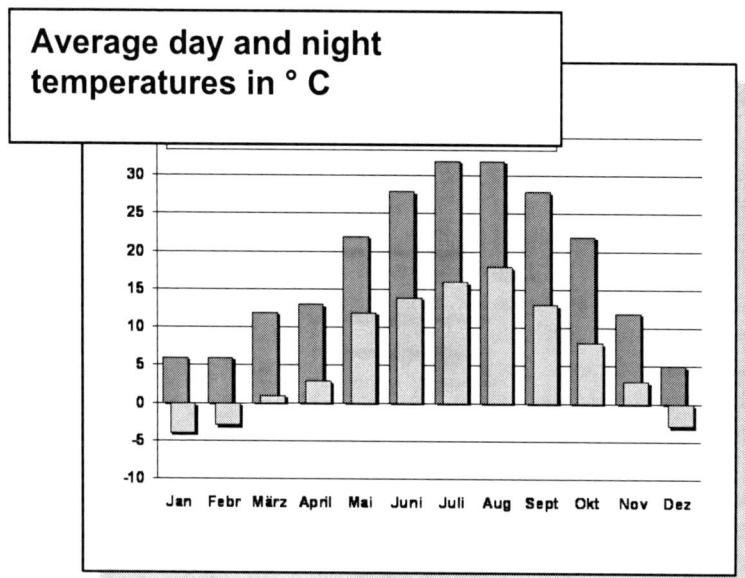

Average amount of rainfall per month in mm

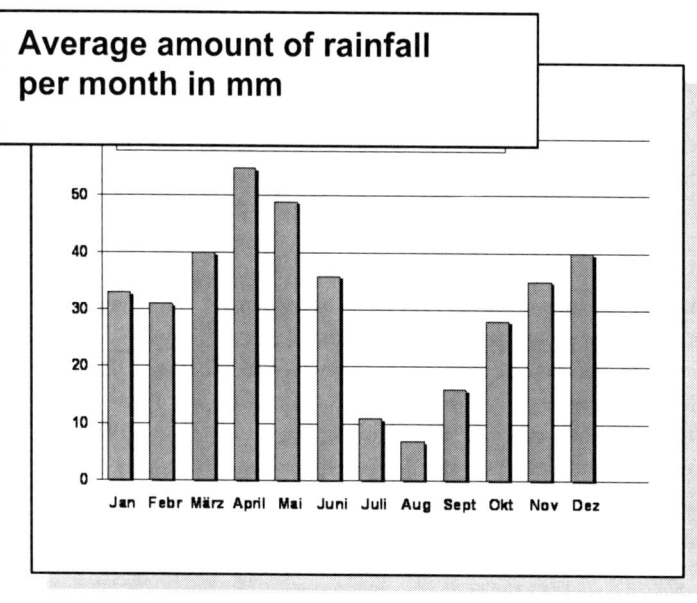

Geography

Cappadocia is situated almost exactly in the centre of the Anatolian plateau. As has been said before, it lies between 900 and 1400 m above sea level. At 300 km to the northwest there is Ankara, the capital of Turkey. The distance to Kayseri, another city of a million, is 60 km to the east, and in the south it is about 150 km to the Taurus mountains which separate the plateau from the Mediterranean Sea. Again and again the question of Cappadocia's earthquake security arises. But here we can assure you: there have not been any earthquakes for ages. Some years ago we were talking on the phone to some friends in Ankar from Avanos, when suddenly we heard screams of panic on the other end because the walls were shaking over there. We did not feel any vibrations at all. This can be explained by the fact that Cappadocia lies in the middle of the Anatolian plate. This plate is situated between the African and the northern Eurasian plate and is treated badly by both. As a result there is an extreme frequency of earthquakes on its fringes. To the north there is the Pondtian Trench which was the scene of the drama of the latest great earthquake that took 14000 lives in 1999. To the south the tectonic crevice is in the sea, close to the coast so that Adana was often afflicted too, and in the west the Aegean Sea forms the dividing line between the plates. The centre, however, is free of earth movement. This can also be proved by the discussion about a ban on heavy lorry traffic in Cappadocia. The vibrations caused by such traffic might destroy some fairy chimneys or make the boulders on top of them fall off. Well, any earthquake would have made these rocks break down long ago. Only once did the earth move here in Cappadocia, too. This was in 1939, during the great earthquake at Erzurum, 700 km from here. The town of Cavusin was damaged most severely then.

Therefore, a more humorous note is struck by the stories told by various tourist guides. The tourists are made to believe in all seriousness that the Cappadocians hang eggs next to their front doors to find out if the earth trembles. It becomes more of a sad thing, though, when TV stations take over this nonsense and present it on the screen in our living-rooms at home.

The well-informed reader will object that obviously there are volcanoes in the area. This is true, but they have been inactive for many thousands of years. The only geothermal evidence of volcanic activity are the hot springs that are to be found here and there. The largest of the volcanoes, Erciyes, is rather impressive though. It lies about 80 km to the east, south of Kayseri. With an altitude of 3920 m it is the highest mountain far and wide and its isolated position in the surrounding landscape makes it look especially gigantic. The even higher mountains of the Taurus Range can only be seen from a great distance and in good weather. The second large crater, Hassan-Dagi, is situated 90 km away, near Aksaray, with a height of 3270 m a bit lower and not so impressive, the more so because, in contrast to Erciyes, it also lacks the shape of a classical volcano.

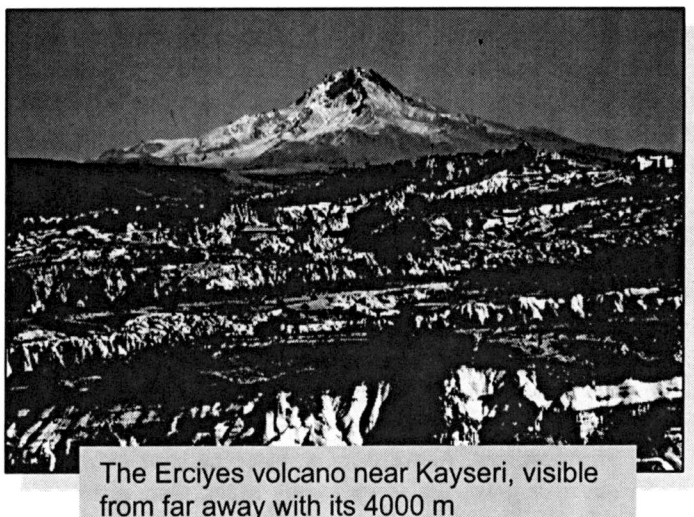

The Erciyes volcano near Kayseri, visible from far away with its 4000 m

Last but not least Kızılımak, the Red River, has to be mentioned. With its length of about 2000 km it is the longest river in Turkey. It has its source in the east, 150 km east of Sivas in the Köse mountains, then turns to the southwest towards Cappadocia, where it reaches its southernmost point, and then gradually moves to the north past Ankara and towards the Black Sea. At Avanos it does not yet look like the biggest river of the country. Especially in the summer there is so little water in it that large parts of the riverbed fall dry.

Flora and Fauna

Cappadocia's Flower World .....

Cappadocia is covered to a great extent by desertlike vegetation, and especially in autumn this looks rather bleak. While in Europe and America the forests present themselves in most beautiful colours, the largely unused land in Cappadocia is covered by a brownish grey blanket of dust from late summer onwards. The lack of rain, which has then lasted for months, makes the sparse vegetation - mostly consisting of low shrubbery - wither. Only in spring do the endless plains shine in fresh green. Vegetation is more luxuriant near the rivers or at the bottom of the valleys. East of Avanos the inhabitants have set up fruit and vegetable plantations that are irrigated with water from the river or from a well. The putt-putt of the diesel pumps can be heard for miles. The plants in the narrow valleys exist on the water that the tufa can store up for months. Now and again you can discover artificial cisterns behind narrow openings in the rock. You can distinctly hear the rock giving off the water drop by drop in them. The little orchards that extend seamlessly through the canyons have been irrigated this way for centuries. The Cappadocians grow all the things they need for their everday life in them. These are mainly tomatoes, onions, cucumbers and paprika - but also beans and peas are grown here. Above them, as a second layer of vegetation, all kinds of fruit trees grow. These are mainly apple, pear, apricot and plum trees. There are no citrus fruits, however – the Cappadocian winters are too frosty for them. Occasionally you will see walnut and mulberry trees. Where the valleys broaden a little towards their end, you will sometimes find melon or pumpkin fields.

Between the orchards there are occasionally poplar groves. They mean good profit for the farmers because they make the only building timber at hand in the area.

Numerous grapevine fields extend endlessly along the dusty plains. They even grow on the arid plateaus above the valleys, their long roots drilling deeply into the rock in order to reach the vital water.

The vine here grows under the best conditions one can imagine. Lots of sunshine, a secure water supply and frosty winters bring about grapes of unsurpassed quality here. Some kinds develop their grapes as dense as corn-cobs so that you cannot pick them off one by one. You eat them as you do the yellow corn, the delicious juice running down the corners of your mouth, malking a marvellous mess. The vines are not tied to poles as we know it, but are spread out flat on the ground, as it is impossible for them to rot on the ground due to the aridity of the Cappadocian climate.

It is a pity that many of the small orchards are no longer in use. On the one hand this is due to the difficult access to them, on the other hand fruit and vegetable prices are so low in the autumn that it is not worth the labour any more. Some years ago there was a fruit juice factory here that used to buy up the entire fruit crop of the area. Since it went bankrupt, picking the fruit has not been worth the effort for the farmers any more.

...and its Animals

The biggest wildlife animal in Cappadocia that the visitor sometimes catches sight of is the fox. One has to be very lucky, though, to encounter one of these timid creatures, in spite of the fact that the fox and its fellow, the marten, have ideal food conditions here. Millions of mice have taken over control in the dusty plains. Especially in the evening near sunset their squeaking can be heard everywhere. But do not worry, the mice avoid human contact and mostly keep away from populated areas because the cat police are on guard there – in large numbers. Occasionally rabbits hop across the plains, but they are also a rare sight because they are the main prey of the local hunters. Inside the valleys you find frogs, lizards and small harmless snakes. You will often see the so-called Greek Tortoise, which of course bears a different name here, the Turkish Tortoise. A somewhat bigger problem is contact with scorpions and the conspicuous big camel spiders. Their sting is not life-threatening, but it can spoil several days of your holidays. In any case you should see a doctor for treatment. So be careful when lifting up small rocks or when putting your hand into narrow holes! Both are nocturnal animals. Unfortunately the scorpions sometimes do not stick to the house rules and drop in for a visit instead. But do not panic! They will not jump at you and on the whole they are very lethargic. Just put a glass over the animal and slip a sheet of paper under it. Secured like that you can take it outside where it belongs. And then there are also the horror stories about an animal that is said to be a combination of the scorpion and the spider and whose dangerousness is legendary. But this is only a kind of Cappadocian werewolf used in stories to make little children panic.

22 Flora and Fauna

Wolves are rare in Cappadocia. Only in very long and cold winters do they make it from the far east to here. The Anatolian sheep dog is their greatest enemy – and this takes us to domestic animals. The Kangal, as this breed is called, is markedly bigger than the wolf. As a shepherd's dog its ears and tail are cropped, i.e. made shorter, and it is made to wear a big spiked collar. This way it is invulnerable to its enemies. When treated well, these animals weigh about 25 kgs at an age of four months and reach a shoulder height of about 60 cm. When fully grown, a shoulder height of 80 cm.

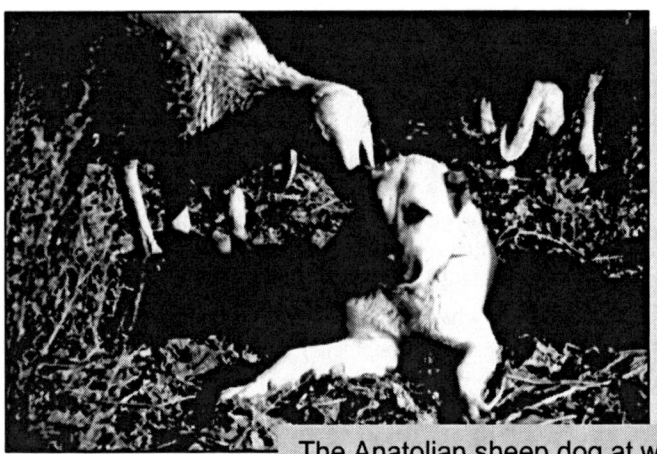
The Anatolian sheep dog at work

Is quite frequent. The animals have quite a peaceful character, but they develop an intense feeling of responsibility for their flock. Therefore you are better to avoid them when you meet them in the company of their flock of sheep. The same applies when they are on the chain. Besides this, dogs are of no great importance in the lives of Turkish people, as the dog is regarded as an impure animal by the Islamic religion. The few existing watchdogs often lead a terrible life. Badly nurtured and tied up on a much too short rope in the blazing sun, their life expectancy is mostly very short. The wealthy people have recently developed a habit of keeping a dog as a lapdog. But meeting the demands of an appropriate education about dogs seems to be far more than Turkish people can cope with.

But what does the Kangal keep watch over, by the way? Sheep, of course, because they populate the wide Anatolian grassland by the thousands. Whereas in former times Cappadocia was called 'the land of the beautiful horses', nowadays malicious tongues call it 'the land of the lambs' although sheep farming has had a long tradition here from time immemorial. Very rarely will you see a herd of cows trot through Cappadocia, because the few cows that exist are mostly kept in stables next to the houses. While some years ago donkeys could be seen roaming the village streets in spring, in pairs with a certain purpose, today the donkey and the horse have disappeared almost completely from the streets. They have become victims of motorization. However, a reverse tendency can be noticed in some villages. The exorbitant fuel prices in the country have caused the donkey and the horse to reappear in some cases.

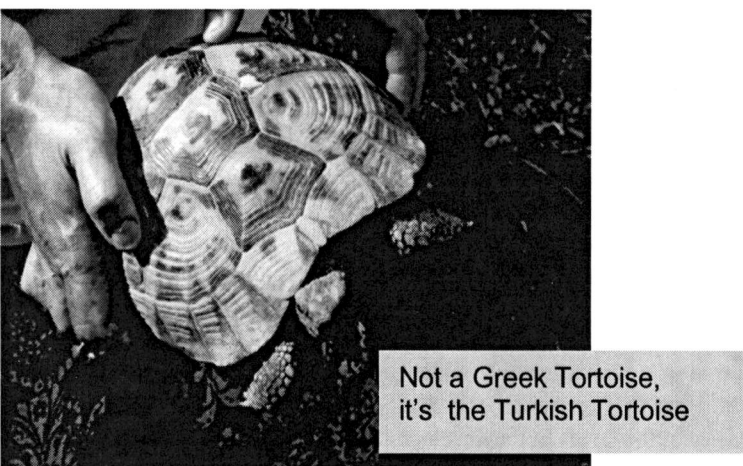

Not a Greek Tortoise, it's the Turkish Tortoise

At some tourist points camels can be found. They are not from the area, however, but have been transported here for the sake of the tourist business.
The only animals that still run about freely in the villages today are stray cats and the villagers' poultry. Hens, ducks and turkeys do not know any pens, but regardless of the bird flu they peck the ground freely and widely round the houses, looking for anything worth eating. The large turkey flocks which are driven through the streets before New Year's Day, feverishly awaiting the festive days, are especially impressive.

UNESCO World Heritage Site Göreme – Cappadocia

On bureaucratic complexities and the necessity of multiple thinking

By Andus Emge, PhD

In the year 1985 the area of the former Byzantine monastery in the Göreme valley with its many frescoed cave churches and also the central area of the unique Cappadocian landscape were included in the UNESCO world heritage list. Subsequently the Göreme Open Air Museum, which is under the care of the Ministry for Culture and Tourism, and the Göreme National Park, which is governed by the Ministry of Forests and Agriculture, were created. Thus Cappadocia is one of the very few regions in the world which have a double UNESCO classification, but at the same time it is influenced by a multitude of government authorities and commercial interests.

Above all, the rapid progress of Cappadocia's tourism has led to increasingly problematic interrelations during the past two decades. The tourist industry with its own powerful economic principles, but also the individual interests and the geographical needs of the local population have played an important part in this.

In contrast to the prevailing public opinion, UNESCO does not always play the role of a supporting and omnipresent authority. The contrary is the case here. Here in Cappadocia the highly esteemed status of World Cultural Heritage rather leads to the development of an intricate network of local and regional government regulations and control mechanisms. As a consequence the Cappadocia World Heritage is primarily seen as a product for commercial exploitation by international tourism. On the other hand this also means that the authorities in charge show practically no consideration for the econimically unimportant interests of the local population. This is indeed a paradoxical situation. On the one hand decisions by investors and the authorities are made only in their own interest and with no regard to the population, on the other hand the regional culture is, as it were, decorated with a 'folklore' ribbon and sold to the tourists as 'original' and 'traditional'.

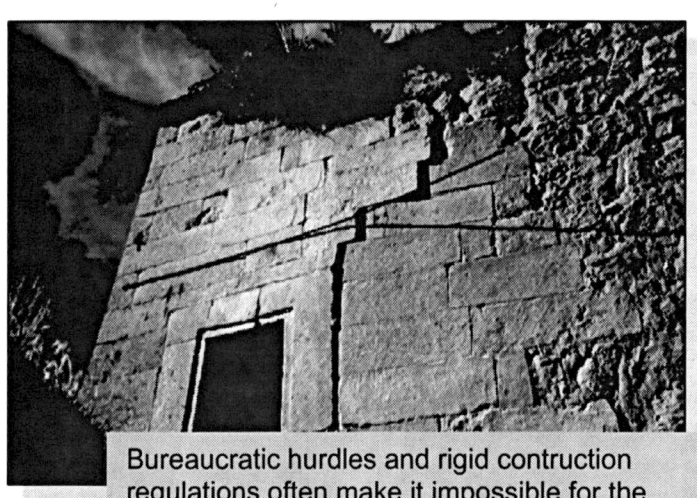
Bureaucratic hurdles and rigid contruction regulations often make it impossible for the inhabitants to maintain their homes or even refurbish them properly

A further delicate circumstance is created by the fact that even today many Cappadocians who still live in the ancient cave and rock houses are themselves part of this extraordinary historical landscape. But apart from the traditional use of their homes they have modern needs and demands, too, which often have nothing in common with the romantic tourist image. The situation is so confused that sometimes even people whose ancestors used to live in Cappadocia and its typical cave dwellings for centuries will be sentenced to prison in cases where they have altered the size of their houses or even carved new rooms from the rock. Of course this does not prevent all of them from continuing their activities inside the endless tufa of Cappadocia. Above all, investors from the field of tourism have no difficulties in including considerable fines in their long-term financial plans for the future, for example for carving a profitable luxury hotel out of the rock, as the profit will possibly be many times higher than the fine.

The intense growth of culture tourism has generally contributed to an increase in aesthetic and prestige value of the typical regional features. A cave dwelling formerly seen as primitive can almost achieve a stylish image today. This gradually encourages a more discriminating architectural view and a greater sensitivity for details and for history. The standard of refurbishing and renovation work has also risen in recent years. Sometimes this is a direct consequence of better financial support, but also of the increase of practical experience in construction work and increasingly better trained workmen. Nevertheless, the important subregional differences are often disappearing, e.g. the ones that distinguish villages of Greek origin (Mustafapaşa) from those of plain Turkish farmers (Göreme). Today the stone masons mostly come from other areas and work according to the catalogue and to the owner's wishes.

The main danger today lies in the fact that whole parts of towns or villages may be cleared or destroyed by rash and ill-considered reconstruction by means of too much money and badly informed foreign investors. The classical, sometimes shabby character of the rural villages with their donkeys and hens among the last picturesque ruins of decaying houses which were described as special cultural assets in the brochures of the eighties is disappearing in almost no time. Almost any old building in the villages of central Cappadocia is slowly turning into a small luxury boardinghouse or a small villa for newcomers.Their style and architecture are often determined mainly by the owner's taste and much less by tradition. Thus it becomes inevitable that the border to kitsch and 'Disneylandification' will be crossed, quite often even under the formally correct surveillance of the authorities.

Taking a final closer look at the politico-cultural situation of the UNESCO World Heritage Site of Göreme-Cappadocia, we firstly observe a lack of a clear concept of how the architectural and natural monuments can be protected and used at present, and secondly we see a lack of ideas about how the specific character of Cappadocia can be presented to the interested cultural tourist. It is especially this missing clarity regarding an up-to-date common concept (master-plan) that lies at the heart of the present political and economic confusions and misguided developments in this region. Mutual cooperation of all responsible persons with all different interest groups would be most welcome. Thus Cappadocia might be defined as its own 'trademark', which would also reflect the cultural and ethno-religious tolerance and variety of the past centuries. The Greek and Turkish coexistence and likewise the Armenian influence or later Islamic Sunni or Alevi settlements – all of them have fertilized Cappadocia's culture over a long period of time by their cultural amalgamation and their diversity. Only this way can a long-term development and a variety of cultural forms of expression be made possible in the sense of UNESCO.

The German Ethnologist Dr. Andus Emge has been living in Cappadocia since 1997, has written his doctor's thesis on "Living in the Caves of Göreme" here and has taken great efforts for the protection of the World Heritage Site for many years. Further information about his work can be found on the internet under: www.fairychimney.com

The UNESCO website is available under: www.unesco.org

Some critical remarks about the Göreme National Park

If you want to move about freely in the Göreme National Park, you will meet with quite a number of obstacles. Bus schedules are not on display, there are no signposts and hiking trails are not marked. No wonder, for the local tourist lobby is very powerful. Taxi drivers want to catch passengers, travel agencies want to sell their sightseeing tours and the Turkish tourist guides are not too keen on visitors moving about freely in the area without making use of their service. But those are only the lesser evils.
Turkish National Parks, like so many of the country's institutions, suffer from a lack of enforcement of the existing rules. Forest workers or even park rangers will not be found here. And that is why many of the rules and regulations for the protection of the park are not taken seriously by parts of the population. Unauthorized waste disposals and illegal buildings are quite frequent in the National Park.
The Military Policemen that you see again and again are only there for public security and do not care about waste transgressions or architectural offences.
But not only the average citizen ignores the nature preservation measures. Local authorities within the boundaries of the Park, too, have no problems in erecting modern estates on protected territory. In 2007 the commune of Uchisar, for example, did not have the slightest scruples about cutting open strips through the popular Pigeon Valley in order to install a new sewage pipe with the help of extra heavy machinery there. Nothing remained of the former enchanted gardens and shady poplar groves – apart from the fact that the smelly bilge water now seeps away somewhere in the valley area. Obviously

there had been no previous arrangement with the park administration or even UNESCO staff members.

The lack of control by the park authorities is also the reason why real crimes remain unpunished. Warning signs in front of steep slopes where the ground goes dangerously downhill e.g. are regularly removed in order to be able to offer oneself as a guide or life-saver to the tourists – for a small fee, of course. This means putting the lives of foreigners at risk in cold blood!

Unfortunately the Göreme National Park is not seen as a community project and as a chance for everybody, but is too often used only for one's own financial advantage. This is why there still are hotel owners who dispose of their waste illegally, souvenir sellers who erect shabby nissen huts in front of cave-cut churches and tourist guides that make signposts disappear. And as long as there is no park administration that vigorously enforces the legal instructions, there will always be some people who unscrupulously take advantage of the system's weak spots.

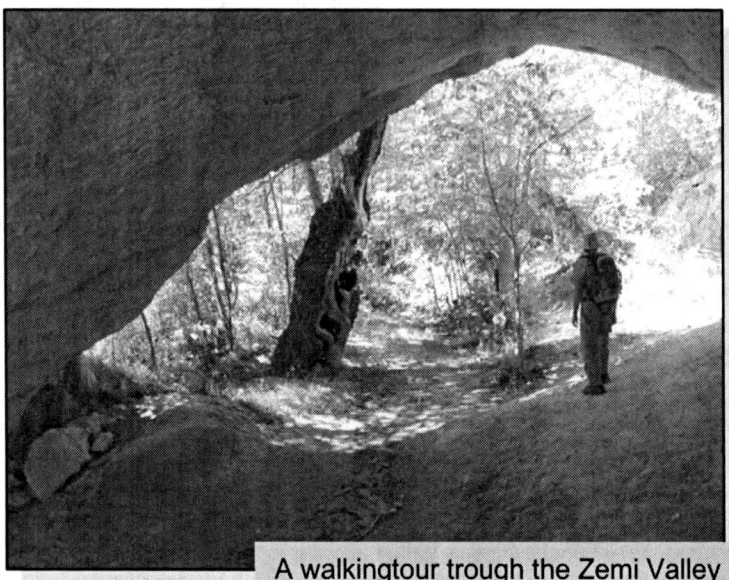

A walkingtour trough the Zemi Valley

Foto: Johann Munker

Geological origin and Volcanism

Legend has it that one day three master builders asked God for building material. Thereupon God made the volcanoes Erciyes and Hassan emit so much material that the three master builders – the wind, the rain and the snow – have been building and moulding this enchanted landscape up to the present day.

As has been mentioned in the 'Geography' chapter, no volcanic activity whatsoever can be detected in our days. But a few million years ago this was quite different. Cappadocia's spacious and thick tufa layers and the adjacent volcanoes betray intense volcanic activity in the past.
Besides, Cappadocia originally looked quite different from today. A wide landscape of rivers and lakes covered the region in which only a couple of small mountains stood out from the plains. The Sultan Marches south of the Erciyes and the great salt lake 100 km north-west of it could be the remains of those humid areas. The presence of obsidian proves the existence of a former lake system. This mineral, which was already popular for toolmaking in the stone age, is created by fast cooling masses of lava. When liquid lava gets in touch with water, it hardens into very hard, glassy rock.
A long time ago the ground burst open and volcanoes arose, throwing numerous layers of dust and ash over Cappadocia during a period of several millions of years.
Moreover, the eruptions must have been extraodinarily violent. Tufa consists of so-called pyroclastites, that is, small particles which are distributed over many miles across an area by extremely violent eruptions. In this process pyroclastic clouds must have played a crucial role. These extremely hot and explosively growing clouds are an emulsion of high temperature gases, pulverized particles or drops of magma and ash particles. The distribution of the eruption material is a proof of the fact that the tufa layers mainly consist of the remains of these murderous rolls of fire: pyroclastic clouds can move forward at a speed of several hundred miles per hour, but they are so heavy that they are seldom able to surmount greater obstacles like e.g. small mountain ranges. That is why today in the area between Kirşehir, Nigde, Aksaray and Kayseri numerous mountain tops emerge from the surrounding landscape covered by no or only a very thin layer of hardened ash.

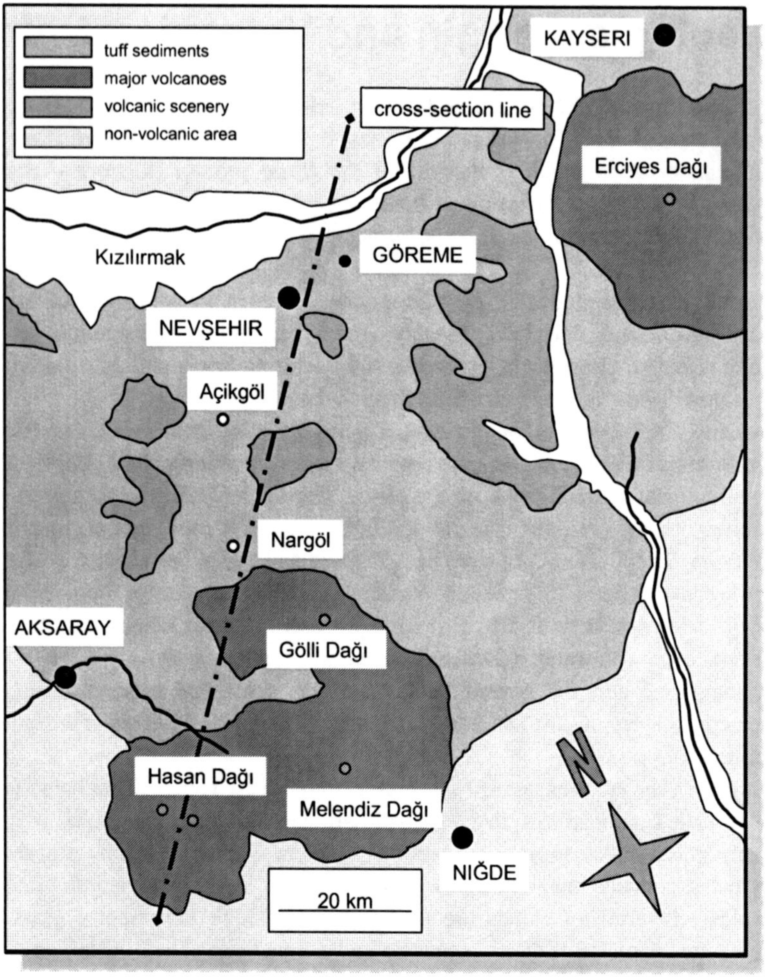

30 Geological origin

Legend:
- tuff sediments
- major volcanoes
- volcanic scenery
- non-volcanic area

Map labels: KAYSERI, cross-section line, Erciyes Dağı, Kızılırmak, GÖREME, NEVŞEHIR, Açikgöl, Nargöl, AKSARAY, Gölli Dağı, Hasan Dağı, Melendiz Dağı, NIĞDE, 20 km

Distribution off tuff sediments over Cappadocia

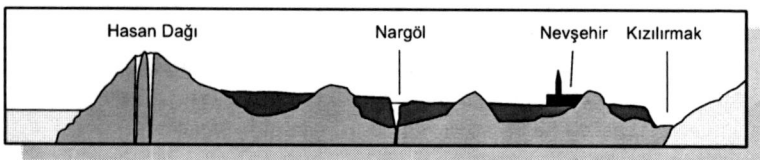

Hasan Dağı — Nargöl — Nevşehir — Kızılırmak

It is also remarkable that all high volcanic mountains are situated at the edge of the tufa area, just as though they had made an agreement to deposit their eruption material right in the middle between them (see map). But it is the little maars (small volcanic lakes) that seem to have been more decisive for the origin of the enormous tufa layers. Thus, until a few decades ago when it fell dry, there was the Acık-Göl off the road between Nevsehir and Aksaray, and near the road between Derinkuyu and Güzelyurt there is the little lake Nar-Göl. Both lie in the middle of the wide tufa landscape. Volcanic lakes are surrounded by a ring of tufa, which is another proof of extremely violent eruptions. The growing tufa cones on their edges were regularly blasted away. In short, these volcanic chimneys never had a chance to develop into mountains. All over the world most volcanoes are found on top of so-called tectonic crevices, that is at places where the continental plates rub against each other or pull at each other or are pressed against each other. But volcanism outside those friction areas, that is, in the centre of the continental plates, is also not unusual. In order to understand this phenomenon, one has to consider the movements of the tectonic plates around Asia Minor. The great African plate moves north towards the Eurasian plate. Stuck in between them is the small Anatolian plate, and this one is really stubborn. It does not in any way want to slide on top or under one of the other plates. It thinks of itself as a small wedge that is just being pushed aside to the west. But that does not work without causing problems, above all because it is not shaped like a wedge. This is why an enormous amount of pressure has to accumulate inside it before anything starts moving at all. Sometimes this is also the reason why there were – and always will be – so many devastating earthquakes in Turkey. But sometimes the pressure inside a continental plate is so great that cracks open in the central part and volcanic activity can occur there. This is what also happened in Cappadocia, and the volcanoes Erciyes Dağı, Hassan Dağı, Göllü Dağı and Melendiz Dağı were born, together with many small chimneys in between them.

Meanwhile scientists doubt, however, that Erciyes Dagi played a crucial role in the formation of the Cappadocian tufa layers. If you examine the historical buildings around the mountain more closely, you will notice that they were built of a somewhat different rock material; these rocks are much darker and harder than the ordinary tufa which was used in central Cappadocia.

At some point of time there must have occurred an eruption that distributed different rock material over Cappadocia. Maybe Erciyes rather played a protective role in this drama of nature. A much harder layer of basalt covered the masses of soft tufa, sealing them off and protecting them from erosion. Even today it can be seen from the fairy chimneys how important this protective layer was. Many meters they tower up slender into the sky, getting thinner and thinner to a minimum towards the top. On top of this instable platform there is a conic boulder of harder rock, protecting it like a cap. Whenever this protection rock slips down, the whole mighty tower disappears within a very short while.

The shaping of the present landscape started with the intrusion of the Kizilirmak river into Cappadocia. On its edges, wind and water got access to the soft underground rock layers. Little creeks and rivulets steadily ate away parts of the rock material and eroded it. Remains of old riverbeds can be found in the upper parts of the historic town centre of Avanos, about 30 m above the present riverbed. The Çakılkaya (gravel rock), a mixture of rough gravel and petrified sediments as hard as concrete, forms a protective layer of several meters on top of the soft tufa there.

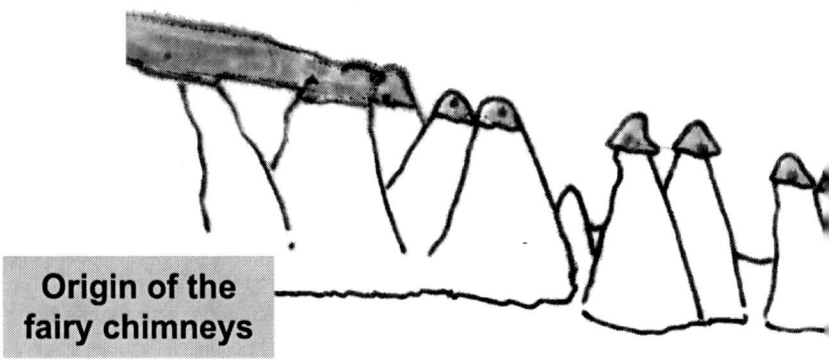

Origin of the fairy chimneys

1. Table mountain

Ash layers are compressed and petrifield into tufa.
A layer of harder rock protects the soft material completely

2. Separation

Small fissures develop in the hard protection layer and allow water to filter through, digging small canals into the rock layers. Gradually, 'chimneys' emerge from the mountain

Today, the erosion landscape has withdrawn several miles from the river. This indicates that the climate must have been more humid in former times. This is the only possible explanation for the wideness of the main valleys that extend towards the river from the south.The pathetic little streamlets that often disappear in the sand – if there is any water at all in them – do not contribute a lot to erosion. Wind and rain have taken over the main job in eroding the landscape today. The wind blows incessantly through the ravines, unrelentingly polishing the soft rock and levelling the grooves left behind by the rain. This remodelling of the landscape can be seen most impressively at Paşabağı, which lies on the road to Zelve. There the mighty fairy chimneys thrust their dark pointed caps towards the sky. South of them, there is the edge of a table mountain where the various stages of the development of new towers can be seen very well. Gradually they are carved out of the wall by wind and rain. This can rightly be called a mountain giving birth to another one.

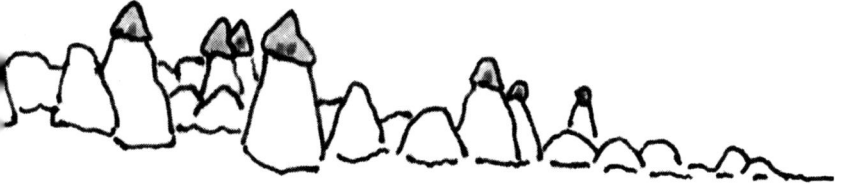

3. Group formation

The first fairy chimneys disapear, that is, are washed away by rainwater. Groups of towers remain, the members protecting each other from erosion by wind

4. Individualization

More and more protective boulders fall down so that only isolated towers remain, wich are exposed to erosion by wind without protection

5. Levelling

Without ist protective rock cap, the soft tufa is eroded completely and the area is made level

34 Geological origin

Additional building material has not been produced for a long time by the volcanoes. The first – and also the last – testimony of an eruption was left behind by the inhabitants of Çatal Höyük about 8000 years ago. They documented this last great eruption in a wall painting. But after all, Catal Höyük lies near Konya, at a distance of about 150 km from Cappadocia.

If we think in geological categories, however, the region is only taking a temporary rest that can be over again in a few thousand years.

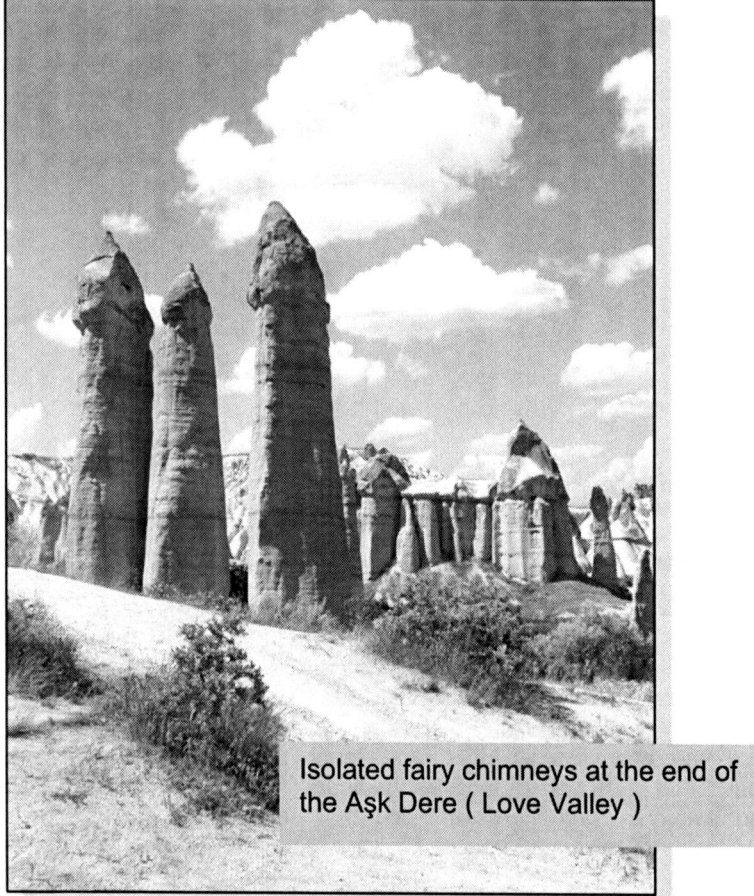

Isolated fairy chimneys at the end of the Aşk Dere (Love Valley)

Foto: Johann Munker

History

There is hardly another country in the world that can offer so much historical background as Turkey does. Many famous individuals – some perhaps quite unexpectedly – are from here. Whether it is St. Nicholas, who was a bishop in Myra, or Diogenes, who was born on the coast of the Black Sea, you will find their names everywhere. Antony and Cleopatra, too, had their love nest here. And Cappadocia was again and again conquered and ruled by a variety of nations. For thousands of years the most varied nations travelled through here and left their traces behind, among them cultures and nations that many readers will probably have never heard of before. And here, in the centre of Anatolia, at the crossroads of the great caravans and trade routes, lies Cappadocia. It would be too much for this book to describe the history of this region at length and in every detail. This chapter can only be seen as a little orientation help for the traveller interested in history. Therefore, only a rough overview of the rise and fall of powers and the consequences for Cappadocia will be given here.

8000 to 3000 BC - The Prehistoric Period

The area was populated as early as in the Neolithic age. During excavations at Aksaray and near Gülşehir archeologists found primitive crockery and tools made of bone and obsidian. The findings were especially numerous at Asıklı-Höyük near Aksaray. Several thousands of artefacts were brought to the surface there, among them low burned clay statuettes and jewelry objects made of bone. Also archaic limestone buildings were discovered during those excavations. Trade relations between Mesopotamia and the people of the eastern Mediterranean existed at a very early age, because the latter needed the hard obsidian that was found here in those days for the production of tools and farming utensils.

3000 to 1200 BC – The Bronze Age

As the name indicates, bronze gradually became dominant in the production of tools, arms and jewelry and made the hitherto popular, but softer, copper become obsolete. This led to an increase in trade with Mesopotamia. Gold, silver and copper were found in sufficient quantity in Cappadocia, but there was no tin that was necessary for the production of bronze. This was supplied by Assyrian merchants, and it was them who brought another important invention with them: writing. Today we have clay-tablets in Assyrian arrowhead writing which lay down the tax, customs and interest regulations between the merchants and the people of Cappadocia. Also tablets with marriage contracts were found in which the rights of the Anatolian women who married Assyrian merchants were attempted to secure.

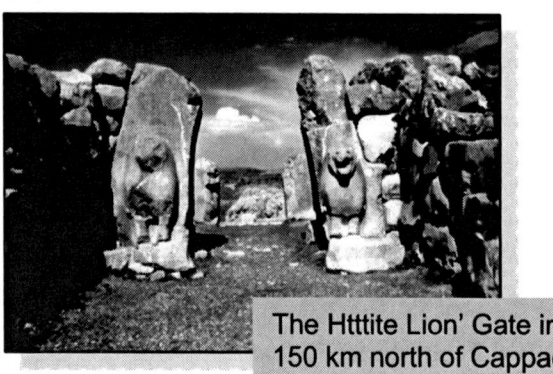

The Htttite Lion' Gate in Hattuşa, 150 km north of Cappadocia

In those days the Hatti were the dominant people, who were able to maintain their status up to about 1600 BC. In the preceding centuries, groups of indo-germanic Hittites from the Caucasus mountains had slowly but constantly been invading the area. They usurped the Hatti kingdom and founded their first capital, Kanish, near Kayseri. In the course of time the Hittites steadily increased their sphere of interest. They founded a new capital called Hattusha in the north, 150 km north of Cappadocia.

This way an empire developed which encompassed nearly all of modern Turkey and which bordered on Egypt in the south. Thus, conflicts with the southern neighbour were destined. The battle of Kadesh in Syria in the year 1285 BC has become famous. For a long time the Egyptians were believed to be the winners, because Ramses II had proclaimed himself victorious army leader at home, but today it is known that this was only an example of ancient Egyptian domestic policies. In reality, the pharaoh's troops were defeated and were only able to save their lives by hastily signing a peace treaty – by the way, the first historically documented one in human history.

The Hittites

The Lost People

A copy of the first peace treaty in the world between the Egyptians and the Hittites can be admired in the United Nations building in New York today. At that time, such treaties were more sustainable than today: the border between the Hittite and the Egyptian Empire remained stable, nobody dared to attack, and at home everyone was celebrated as the winner. Ramses II immortalized his alleged victories in domestic Karnak. And up to the 20th century he was believed by both the tourists and the scientists, because every trace was lost of the Hittites. Their mighty empire vanished around 1170 BC. Only the hieroglyphics at Karnak and some passages in the Bible still indicate that the Hittites must have existed. But who were the Hittites?

They were finally rediscovered in 1905 by German archeologists, and a Czech deciphered their language from cuneiform tablets and found out that the Hittites were Indo-Europeans.

Today, nearly 2.5 billion people belong to the Indo-European language group: almost all Eastern and Western Europeans, the Russians, the Americans, but also the Kurds and the Iranians belong to it. The Chinese, the Turks, the Arabs and the Africans for example belong to other language families.

The unknown Hittite Empire was thus one of the largest ancient Indo-European empires, and its centre was in the region of today's Cappadocia in Central Anatolia, in the north and in the south of the Kızılırmak River, which was called Marassanta by the Hittites. Inscribed clay tablets, the so-called Cappadocian tablets from today's Kültepe near Kayseri, brought a forgotten people to light again after thousands of years. 3500 years ago, Kültepe was called Nesha (Kanish) and had been the first Hittite capital and an Oriental trade centre prior to Hattuşa. Their later capital, Hattusha, is situated about 150 km north of Cappadocia.

At the same time, the Mycenaean culture was at its peak in Greece. Most likely, an exchange between cultures took place on the Anatolian coast (Troy / Miletus). Also the Lion Gate at Hattusha (about 1550 BC) is remarkably similar to the one at Mycenae (1250 BC) in Greece. The Mycenaean civilization in Greece has hitherto been regarded as the root of European culture. But 1000 years before the first traces of democracy in Greece and more than 3000 years before the first basic constitutional document in the World, the Bill of Rights (1689), the Hittites in Anatolia possessed a constitution and a binding law. Their very sophisticated and humane jurisdiction was also unique and far ahead of its time.

Could the cradle of modern European thought and feeling, according to recent findings, lie with the Hittites in Central Anatolia instead of with the Greeks?

In any case, the Hittites are the oldest known representatives of the Indo-European language family. As well, they were fond of drinking beer, were said to be very playful, and they were brilliant military strategists. Security-loving as they were, they took the gods of conquered peoples into their Pantheon, as they feared the vengeance of foreign gods. Thus their world of gods was large and numerous; the Hittites are also called the people of the 1000 gods. To them, the gods were more important than their battles, which they now and again interrupted for religious ceremonies at home.

The ruler was king, judge, priest and commander at the same time, but he was not omnipotent. Since 1500 BC he was bound by a constitution, and he had to share the powers of government with a community of officials who controlled and advised him. His wife also had her own government powers, and as High Priestess she wielded great power.

In the divine world also, women did not play a minor role:

The Supreme Goddess, Cybele, is the most famous of all goddesses. Already by 6000 BC, the mother goddess was of utmost importance next to the bull-god in Anatolia (Çatal Höyük). In the following millennia the supreme goddess, the Great Mother (Magna Mater) or Mother Goddess, as she was called, was much worshipped. The Kubaba of the Hittites, the Athena of the Greeks, the Magna Mater of the Romans and even Mary the Mother of God of the Christians can be traced back to the Anatolian Cybele. Thus, the European cultural sphere is inseparable from Anatolia.

Replicas of Hittite pottery and of the statues of the Mother Goddess found at Calal Höyük near Konya are found at the potteries of Avanos.

1200 to 585 BC – The Iron Age

In 1200 BC the Hittite empire collapsed. The Phrygean people invaded the Anatolian highlands from the west and conquered large parts of it, and in the east the Assyrians cut off parts of the Hittite empire. Only small local Hittite kingdoms remained which could keep themselves up for some centuries. The Kingdom of Tabal that encompassed the area of Kayseri, Nevşehir and Niğde is one we know of today. Its capital was near Niğde and was called Tyana (Tuwanuwa), the present Kemerhisar. Hittite language and culture remained dominant there up to the seventh century BC. After that the Cimmerians, an equestrian people from the coast of the Black Sea, descended on Anatolia and introduced a new balance of power.

585 to 334 BC – The Persians

The Mede nation from Persia drove the Cimmerians out and made Cappadocia their western province. They located their provincial government at Pteria, not far from the ancient Hittite capital of Hatusha. They enlarged the so-called King's Road, which was intended to connect the province with the Aegean coast in the west and their home country in the east. The Halys River, today's Kızılırmak, was the border in the south. The Mede Empire was attacked twice by the Lydians in the south-west, the first attack being ended by an eclipse of the sun. When Croesus, king of Lydia, planned the second attack, he had become more careful and asked the Delphian oracle for information about the possible result of the battle. The oracle's answer was in very diplomatic language: "If you cross the Halys you will destroy a large empire." Croesus misinterpreted the message and was totally defeated by the Medes so that his own kindom perished from the earth.
The Medes had also imported their own religion, the Zarathustra cult. They were especially interested in volcanoes, as their religion was a fire cult.
The influence of the Medes in central Anatolia was only ended in 334 BC by Alexander the Great and his army.

334 BC to 17 AD – Alexander the Great and the Kingdom of Cappadocia

Alexander never caught sight of Cappadocia – he marched along the south coast – but the troops he sent out had great difficulty in conquering Cappadocia. He had subjected the region, which was still unconquered then, to his general Sabiktas, which provoked the embittered resistance of the local population. The Cappadocian leader was intended to be Ariarathes, a Persian nobleman, who first, however, had to yield to the Macedonians together with his ally, King Darius. He returned in 332 BC and founded the kingdom of Cappadocia. As a talented politician and warlord, he enlarged his sphere of influence during his rule. His dynasty reigned up to 17 AD. But he himself only sat on the throne for 10 years. The Macedonian dynasty of the Seleucides kept on ruling over Anatolia and Syria for a long time, but they could only partly accomplish their wish for political power in Cappadocia. In the second century a slight urbanization of the region took place under Ariarathes V; until then, Central Anatolia had had only few cities. The Greek influence could no longer be withheld from the region, and so the language, philosophy and architecture of Greece were introduced. Nevertheless the times remained inconstant. Conflicts with the Armenians, nations from the area of the Black Sea, and first disagreements with Rome again and again threatened the stability of the empire. In the year 188 BC Cappadocia fell under the influence of Pergamos (Bergama) and became its eastern border. The confederation of the local Attalide dynasty and Rome led to intense trade relations between Cappadocia and the Roman Empire. They were interrupted again in 96 BC by the Armenian conquest of large parts of Anatolia. By this, also Cappadocia was again removed from the sphere of influence of the western superpower.

17 to 400 AD – The Roman Period

It was Emperor Tiberius who annexed Cappadocia as a province of Rome. The last King of Cappadocia had died shortly before, and so the Romans took advantage of the power vacuum. The province was very important to Rome because the major trade routes to the east, from where Rome received spices, cloth and oil, went through it. In the following years the Romans frequently changed the function of the individual provinces and procurates. In 113 Emperor Trajanus again altered the provincial borders and proclaimed

Cappadocia a troop marshalling area against the Parthians who had become increasingly dangerous in the east. But, in spite of that, the region did not remain free from short raids by other powers. Zenobia, Arab queen from the oasis of Palmyra in Syria, rose against Rome and could only be defeated shortly before reaching what today is Ankara. Soon after this, the Sassannites from Iran invaded Central Anatolia and temporarily conquered Cappadocia, too. In connection with the Roman occupation, Roman culture was introduced in Anatolia. The towns were enlarged and equipped with the modern achievements of powerful Rome. Libraries, public baths and schools became part of public life, but also the defensive power of the cities was improved.

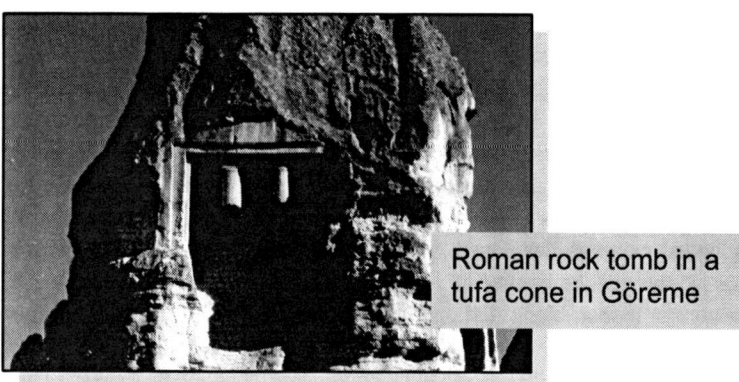

Roman rock tomb in a tufa cone in Göreme

Very early the first Christians travelled through Asia Minor. St. Paul the preacher's travels have become well-known. There is actually no proof of his visit to Cappadocia, but it is highly probable that he came through here on his way to the Galatians in the north-west of Cappadocia. In general the Christian communities remained rather small, as they were prosecuted by Rome as rebellious sects. On the whole, a chaotic mixture of religions prevailed. In addition to the official Roman gods there still existed the Persian fire cult and the belief in the ancient Greek gods to whom animals were offered. Even the old cult of Cybele, the adoration of a godess of fertility from the Hittite aera, had managed to survive well into this period. In the beginning the young Christian communities were having a very hard time facing this religious diversity. Under the Roman emperor Diocletian the religious persecution of Christians reached its climax – not only in

Cappadocia. Many Christians were killed because of their religion, among them St. Hieronymus, who had been born here in Göreme. He was the first person who is said to have taken refuge in the solitude of a secluded tufa cave. But the young religion could not be stopped, and Kayseri became a centre of Christian theology.

Scholar Alexander of Caisareia and his fellow-believer Firmilian became famous theological authorities, and here was also the starting point of the later Armenian Church. One of the most famous Christian saints was from Cappadocia as well, St. George, also known as St. George the dragon-killer. Although he was a Roman army officer he distinguished himself by his courageous defence of the Christian community. But his downright criticism of Emperor Diocletian and the prosecution of Christians cost him his life in the year 303 AD. Only ten years later the new emperor Constantine proclaimed the Christian belief state religion. Now things turned the other way round and the other religious groups, the so-called pagan cults, became victims of harassment by the Christians. In the year 363 the temple of the godess Fortuna in Kayseri was destroyed. Its destruction was the final act of the destruction of pagan cults and rites in Cappadocia. But also within the Christian religion the first tensions between the diverging groups of theological exegesis developed. While the orthodox school of thought was based on the godlike quality of Jesus Christ, the Arianists believed Jesus to be a normal human being that could not be equated with God. The tensions became so strong that Emperor Valens divided the province of Cappadocia into two parts in 371. The orthodox community consolidated itself in the north, whereas the Arianic belief was taught near Niğde, in the new province of Cappadocia Secunda. In the Great Synod of Constantinople in 381 the orthodox section prevailed.

Some of the most ardent supporters of this theological theory of of the essential unity of God, Christ and the Holy Ghost came from Cappadocia. The bishop of Kayseri, Basileos the Great, and his younger brother, Gregory of Nyssa, who was head of a community near Nevşehir, belonged to them. The Greek theologian Gregory of Naciance, who worked near the Ihlara valley and who later on managed to become Archbishop of Constantinople, was the third of them. They belonged to the most ardent supporters of the so-called Nicaean Confession of Faith.

400 to 1071 AD – The Byzantine Period

After the death of Emperor Theodosius the Great the disintegration of the Roman Empire into two parts began. Constantinople became the capital of the newly founded East Roman Empire. But also the divisison of the church into an east Roman orthodox and a west Roman Church under papal influence became foreseeable at that time. The previous decades of exterior quietness may have also been a reason for the numerous religious tensions in Cappadocia. But in the fifth and sixth century the deceitful peace was over. Like the rest of Europe, Asia Minor was struck by the "scourge of humanity". The Huns descended on the Anatolian Plateau, leaving destroyed and plundered towns behind. This onslaught, but perhaps also the subsequent hostile invasions of other powers were the reasons which caused the Christians to retreat to the inaccessible valleys of Göreme. In the following centuries the majority of the monasteries and churches were carved from the rock. Especially the monasteries were built under defensive aspects. They were often high up in the rocks and only accessible by ladders and equipped with escape tunnels. The connections between the different storeys consisted of vertical tunnels that could only be passed with ladders and could be excellently defended.

In the sixth century once again a dynasty of Armenian rulers reigned in Cappadocia and temporarily introduced the Armenian Orthodox Church. In 611 Kayseri fell into the hands of the Persian troops of the Sassanides for a couple of years. Twelve years later, the Byzantine emperor Heraclius managed to drive the enemy troops away again and to restore the country to its former borders. But the peace in the country was not going to last long. A new powerful enemy was lining up on the eastern border. Centuries of regular raids by Arab conquerors followed. In the year 636 the Byzantine army was badly defeated by them, and in 647 for the first time an Islamic-Arab army on horseback stood in front of the gates of Christian Cappadocia. But the Sassanides also attempted another attack, which was able to be averted, however. Those permanent raids from outside contributed to a considerable loss of power of Constantinople, as a population living in constant fear and insecurity is no longer able to fulfill a country's economic demands. Systematic farming was no longer possible, craftsmanship in the towns could hardly exist under these conditions and the most important trade routes were interrupted again and again. The attacks continued well into the

9th century. Only in 863 Emperor Michael III was able to defeat the Arab armies so massively that they finally gave up further conquests in the west.
Those troubled times did not keep the different Christian movements from quarrelling with each other.
During the years between 726 and 842 the great iconoclastic controversy broke out, which finally reached a climax in Leon III's ban on images, which was probably strongly influenced by the Islamic verdict against pictorial representation of Allah and his prophet, Mohamet. More and more opponents of iconoclasm settled among the rocks of Göreme. Lots of ancient religious paintings were destroyed and replaced by simple ornamental design in those days. The art of iconographic painting survived, however, and was continued secretly. Later on it prevailed and flourished again. In 1054 a final schism inside the church took place. The Greek Orthodox church with their patriarch established itself in Constantinople and the Roman Catholic one with its pope in Rome.

1071 to 1400 – the Seljuk Period

At about this time the Seljuks, a Central Asian Turk nation, conquered Anatolia. Before that, they had successfully conquered Mesopotamia and advanced up to Jerusalem. It was they who brought Islam to Cappadocia. In contrast to the Arabs, who spread their religion all over the world with fire and sword, the new rulers gave themselves the appearance of great tolerance. Christians were allowed to continue practicing their religion without restrictions. Only a special tax for non-muslims was imposed on them. The Seljuks developed a unique architectural style that can still be admired today. Under their guidance many caravanserais were built which spread all over Cappadocia from east to west. Those mighty bulwarks were erected at a day's journey from each other in order to protect the travellers against gangs of street robbers. Konya, Sivas and Kayseri were chosen as their centres.
They created new Osmanic schools and orders, of which the Order of the Whirling Dervish at Konya has remained active until today and is rather well-known.
Christianity in Cappadocia flourished once again until the end of the Seljuk rule in the year 1243, and many new churches were built. Christian military

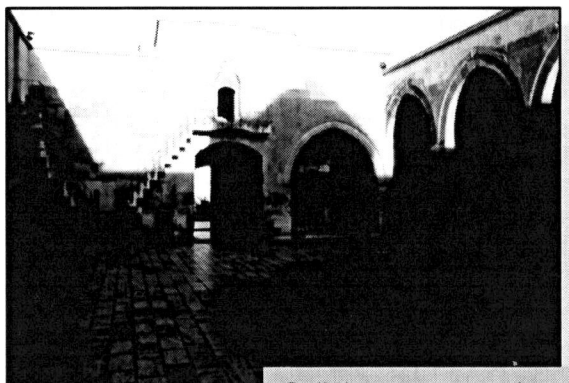
Seljuk caravanserai near Avanos

officers served in the sultan's army and climbed up to important government positions. The Mongols put an end to all that, and the Christian influence gradually lost more and more of its importance in Cappadocia. Many monks left the country and founded new communities in the west, outside the Islamic sphere of influence. After the withdrawal of the Mongols, Anatolia disintegrated into many tiny Turkmen miniature emirates.

1400 to 1918 – The Ottoman Period

Among these small emirates the one of Osman I especially distinguished itself. By clever policies, but also as an ingenious military leader, Osman I managed to unite most Turkmens under his reign. It cannot be said exactly when Cappadocia fell under Ottoman rule. They gradually enlarged their sphere of influence, spread towards Europe and finally conquered Constantinople in 1453, where they sealed the fate of the East Roman Empire.

Not much was noticed of all these conquests in Cappadocia under the Ottoman reign, and for several centuries there was to be peace in the region. As a consequence, people did not have to hide in their caves any more and began to settle on the plateau as well. Nomadism was gradually replaced and house building became increasingly important. It was only in the 17th century that Cappadocia became unsafe again. But this time the enemy came from within.

Probably some kind of unfair tax policy or repressions by local rulers were the reasons, as there is no other explanation why a gang of up to 1000 robbers could develop. This group, known as the 'felt feet', even put a fortified city like Kayseri into difficulty. They had got the name 'felt feet' because they used to wrap their feet in pieces of felt cloth in order to be able to sneak up to their victims unheard.

Until 1918, Cappadocia remained untouched by almost all events in the world. Not until after the capitulation of the Ottoman Empire and the resulting occupation by the Entente nations did – if only for a short period – foreign rulers come into the country again.

1918 to Today – The Republic of Turkey

The remainder of the Turkish state was divided up into occupied zones (like Germany in 1945). But the winners exercised their power only in the big cities of the country. With the armies worn out by the Great War, total control also of the small villages was impossible.

In 1919, Greece launched its attack on the Turkish Aegean coast in an attempt to create a so-called 'Great Greece' (Megali Hellas). During this they penetrated far into the country. Their hatred of the Turks had previously been stirred up by four centuries of Ottoman occupation of Greece. In spite of the dissolution and disarmament of the Turkish army, organized resistance against the occupiers developed very quickly. From the beginning, General Mustafa Kemal Pasa was one of the most important leaders of the resistance. In the beginning of 1921, the Greek invasion was stopped under his leadership, and in September 1922 Izmir, the last Greek stronghold in Asia Minor, fell into the hands of the Turkish army again. This success enabled the Turkish liberators to put weight to their demand for unity and self-government of the Turkish state. In Lausanne they succeeded in remodelling the capitulation treaty of Sèvres.

In 1923, the sultanate was abolished and a Turkish Republic was proclaimed. Mustafa Kemal became its first president, who later was given the title of honour, "Atatürk" (Father of all Turks).

One part of the agreement with the victorious powers of World War I consisted in the relocation of the Greek minority to their home country and the resettlement of the local Turkish population to Anatolia. Thus, in 1923 a great population exchange took place in the course of which 1.7 million Greeks, who had mostly lived in peace with the Turks, were forced to leave

Asia Minor. Cappadocia was also subjected to this. Many local villages had had Greek names, and villages like Mustafapaşa, formerly Sinasos, still show traces of the culture and Christian religion of the Greeks before 1923.

But also the Turkish population had to put up with great changes. The new republic under Kemal Atatürk started to reform the country and to orient itself towards the west in great strides. Ankara was selected as the new capital. The most far-reaching reform projects were the separation of state and religion, the introduction of women's suffrage and the abolition of polygamy, the adaptation of the Christian Calendar and the replacement of the Arabic by the Latin alphabet. All these reform projects were completed only very slowly in traditional and rural Cappadocia, as they were not understood by the population or were contradictory to the century-old ways of thinking.

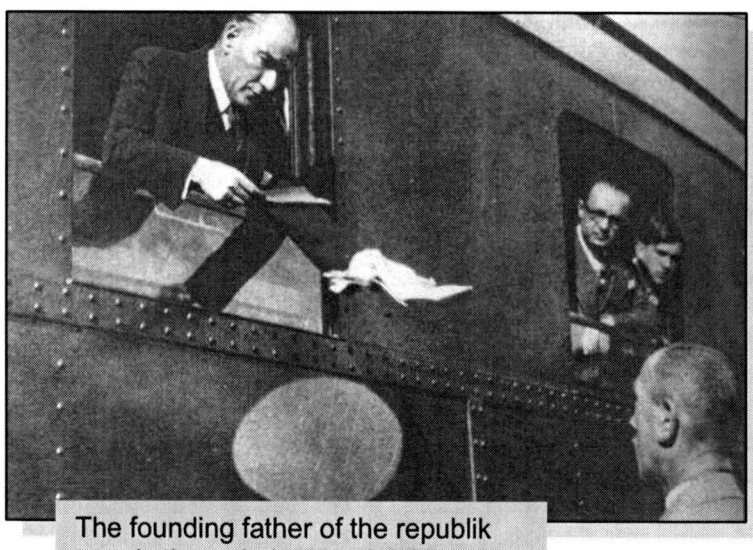

The founding father of the republik travels through the country

Foto: originator unknown

Cappadocia in Christianity

From the outset, Cappadocia was one of the centres of spreading Christianity. Apart from the Palestinian Caesarea, the Cappadocian Caesarea (present-day Kayseri) was the point of origin of an orthodoxy, the so-called "true faith", which developed during the first centuries after Christ. Here, too, there had been disputes about the nature of the true faith from the beginning. Cappadocia was literally divided among the followers of different faith groups.
In the Roman Empire, which Cappadocia was part of, Christians were still persecuted and tortured with unbelievable cruelty during the first centuries after Christ. The regime was inexorable; Jewish uprisings were brutally suppressed, people were abducted and murdered. During that time, an unheard-of message started to spread from Jerusalem towards Asia Minor and also to Cappadocia: the only God does not exist exclusively for the chosen community of the Jews (who had previously been the only ones who practiced monotheism), but for everybody, and all people are equal before God. Moreover, this God is not punishing and chastising such as with the Jews and in the Old Testament, but gracious and merciful. This was an incredible idea in that cruel time, an idea that could have validity beyond the borders of Jewish Palestine. Paul was the most successful missionary of this new idea, which first gained acceptance in present Turkey, in Asia Minor, that is, also in Cappadocia. His passionate appeal was first addressed to all Jewish communities: "Man would be released from all sin without his own effort; neither commandments, nor temples, nor rituals would be necessary in order to gain God's mercy, and this would apply to all people, not only to the chosen people of the Jews". He even regarded circumcision as unnecessary. This was incredible and revolutionary, and it captured the imagination of many people who suffered under the yoke of the Romans in that terrible time. The first ideas of what could be meant by this culminated in bizarre forms of self-chastisement. In Syria, a certain Simeon settled down on the top of a pillar for 30 years and preached his view of a godly life. In Cappadocia, one of his disciples in contrast moved as a hermit into a rather comfortable cave dwelling, which even included rock-carved furniture: the Simeon Tower in Paşabağı.
Cappadocia, which is only a few hundred kilometres away from Syria and Palestine, was an ideal area of retreat for religious contemplation from the

beginning. Here, too, the first Christians meditated on alternatives to the traditional concept of God and of their lives inside their rock-carved hermitages. They were still doing this on their own, as hermits, avoiding the people who brought so much suffering in those times, seeking the solitude and the presence of God in the unspoiled nature, free from all rules and rulers. Cappadocia provided ideal conditions for this: no houses had to be built, there was fresh water and fertile valleys in abundance, you were protected from cold and heat by the caves, and the labyrinth of the Cappadocian erosion landscape promised protection from imperial sabre-rattling. The government left you in peace, at least for the time being.

But the Christain communities were growing. Meanwhile, the hermits were sitting closely together in their caves in the valleys. They joined together in groups. The development of a pure doctrine, according to which everybody would have to live after all known rules had been renounced, gradually began to take shape. But who was this Jesus? Was he a new prophet or God himself? Those who believed in his resurrection, which was absolutely unacceptable to devoted Jews, called themselves Christians. A belief in resurrection had until then only existed in Egyptian mythology, which was hated by the Jews because of their own history. Questions of Christianity were debated controversially and passionately. In the process, different ways of thinking developed between the Orient and the West: while the idea of monotheism had been deeply rooted in the Near East for more than 1000 years, Western culture was based on Roman and Hellenistic ideas. The individual was more important in the West, in Greek democracy the individual person was responsible for his doings, human beings could turn into gods and vice versa; the world of the gods was very similar to that of the humans: they could be corrupt, evil, sly, but also in love, they were losers or heroes and had to accomplish certain tasks. In contrast, the powerful God of the Jews, whose name one was forbidden to pronounce and whose face one was forbidden to see, could not be grasped by human beings. His creatures were delivered to the Invisible One for better or worse, and one could only hope for mercy for one's own life by submitting completely to this God's commandments.

Thus, the question whether Jesus was a God became immaterial to most people in the East. Arianism, which considered Jesus a messenger of God, but by no means a God himself, had many supporters in the Orient and also in Cappadocia.

Thus the so-called nature of Jesus was debated in the first Christian Councils, where the Cappadocian bishops had significant influence. Emperor Constantine, who had appointed Byzantium on the Bosporus as the new capital of the Roman Empire, came into personal contact with the new doctrine: his mother, who had been the simple ex-wife of a landlord before becoming the mother of an emperor, urged her coronated son to accept the new religion. The message of salvation of this new religion, however much it would be altered in the ensuing centuries, at that period mainly reached the minorities, the suppressed, the disadvantaged, the poor and the women, who could not expect great mercy in the old world in those days.

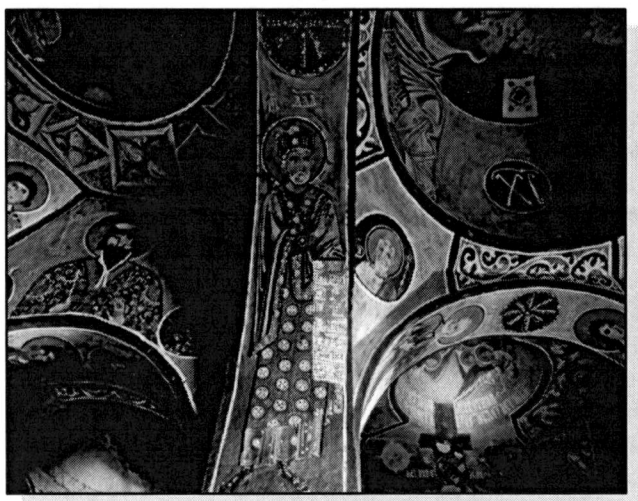

Apart from the religious details, monotheism had a unique, politically highly explosive attraction to Emperor Constantine: it confronted Greek and Roman polytheism with the idea of one single God, just as there could only be one emperor. This was an intelligent move in a time when emperors came and went in the Roman Empire and when they were attempting to establish anti-emperors in Rome. Thus, a religious idea which particularly intended to give hope to the suppressed, became a new instrument of absolutist claims to power. After the Constantinian shift, when Christianity gained support instead of prosecution, the first Ecclesiastic Councils took place. They were meant to give the new faith a fixed order and clear guidance at last; a universal, mandatory doctrine for everyone, which excluded, however, all those who were not of that opinion. Thus, the hoped-for salvation and forgiveness of sins, the key sentence of the new faith, got its first restrictions only 300 years after Christ. Although until then, Christianity had to be regarded as an Oriental religion based on the Jewish faith and although all Church Councils used to take place in Oriental Asia Minor, the Western European way of thinking gradually began to prevail.

In the meantime, the storm of the Huns had raged in Europe and had triggered a mass migration, which finally culminated in the destruction of Rome by the Vandals. Byzantine Asia Minor had remained largely spared and it experienced a time of prosperity; the Hagia Sophia was built as the largest cathedral in Christianity. After the assassination of the last Roman Emperor, Rome in fact had ceased to exist as a centre of power. The Goths were ruling Europe from Ravenna. Constantinople had become the new Rome, and its citizens continued calling themselves citizens of the Roman Empire.

Only the bishop's see had remained in Rome, but it exerted a significant influence on the Councils. The bishop of Rome even claimed a preferential position among all Christian bishops as a descendant of St. Peter, who had been executed in Rome, but this claim was rejected. But in all Councils the doctrine of the Trinity, which was postulated by the future catholics in Rome, was widely supported, also by the Metropolitan of Caesarea in Cappadocia, bishop Basil, as well as by his brother, bishop Gregory of Nyssa, and by the Archbishop of Constantinople himself, Gregory of Nazianzus, who was also from Cappadocia. It can be said that these three Cappadocian Fathers of the Church were instrumental in the new development.

This doctrine of the Trinity was a clear rejection of Arianism: God, Jesus Christ and the Holy Ghost were believed to be coessentially united in Jesus. At that time the Christian Creed originated, which is spoken in Orthodox, Catholic and Protestant churches until today: *"Jesus Christ, God's only Son, who was conceived of the Holy Spirit, born of the Virgin Mary…was made man…and ascended into heaven…"*.

This so-called consubstantitality of Jesus was the first dogma of the new Christian Church; 10 years later, nearly 400 years after the birth of Christ, this so-called Orthodox form of Christianity became the new state religion. Dissenters were persecuted, and this time Christians were hiding from Christians in the rough terrain of the Cappadocian cave world. In the council of Chalcedon (451 AD) it was moreover established that the resurrected Jesus

Christ was human and divine at the same time (doctrine of the two natures). This was again a clear rejection of the one unspeakable, unapproachable and humanly undetectable God of the Orient, and also a rejection of the so-called Monophysites, who regarded Jesus as being purely divine. The monophysite way of thinking has only survived in Syria and in Egypt (Coptic Church) until today.

This now was the universal doctrine, which was called Catholicism. The bishop of Rome called himself the Catholic Pope in a Europe dominated by the pagan Teutons. Finally the Pope also gained political power when he crowned Charlemagne as Emperor in 800 AD and thus was superior to him, at the same time denying allegiance to the emperor in Constantinople. The Byzantine bishops called themselves orthodox and were still subject to the instructions of the emperor at Byzantium. The Orthodox bishops spoke Greek, the Catholic ones spoke Latin. The relationship was marked by misunderstandings and disagreement. They finally culminated in the excommunication of the Greek Orthodox Metropolitan of Constantinople by the Roman Pope in 1054 (the Great Schism). The looting and destruction of Constantinople by the Catholic Crusaders 150 years later is the infamous climax of this schism – with disastrous consequences for Christianity: it was those destructions, from which Constantinople would never recover, which provided the conditions for the capture of the city by the Turkish Ottomans in 1453. And that meant the end of the 1,000-year-old Christian Byzantine Empire.

The steadily increasing power of the Roman Catholic Church was also theologically supported by the church father Augustine from Northern Africa. His doctrine of the original sin, which everyone has inside himself from birth, and the resulting submission to the Catholic Church as the only way to salvation was declared the generally accepted doctrine by the Council of Ephesus in 431 AD.

Thus Jesus' liberation movement was exploited by the new rulers. Dissenters were again subjected to persecution and torture, almost as in the Roman times. The Caves in Cappadocia did not remain idle.

The frightened Christians of Cappadocia, however, suffered the greatest persecution because of a new and totally unexpected directive of the Byzantine emperor. The monks and nuns who had by now joined together in monastic communities in Cappadocia were carving more and more churches and monastic complexes from the soft volcanic tuff. They worshipped their saints and martyrs and decorated their churches with so-called icons: sacred images that showed saints, martyrs or scenes from the life of Jesus. They were meant to help the viewer to take a look into the hereafter in order to be closer to God. But Emperor Leon III now announced a ban on icons: the so-called iconoclastic schism raged in the entire Byzantine Empire as the last gasp of the Eastern view of a God who is inexpressible and undescribable in his greatness ("Thou shalt not make unto thee any graven image"). Emperor Leon III was a Syrian, and was under the influence of a great new religious power which had been conquering the East since the 7th century: Islam was spreading with unprecedented rapidity, weakening the Byzantine Empire. Arabia, Egypt and Northern Africa immediately fell to the Islamic conquerors. Many Eastern Christians converted to Islam voluntarily, as it came closer to their view of an omnipotent God and his prophets than the complicated trinity and consubstantiality of the Christian Orthodox doctrine. Leon III was also an Oriental, and his ban on images took action with the violence of an oriental despot: relentless persecution, arrests, executions and torture covered the Byzantine rump state of Asia Minor, today's Turkey. Cappadocia experienced its worst period. This interference with the contemplative life of Cappadocia was worse than the regular robberies by the Islamic Arabs. Only a few icons have survived this period.

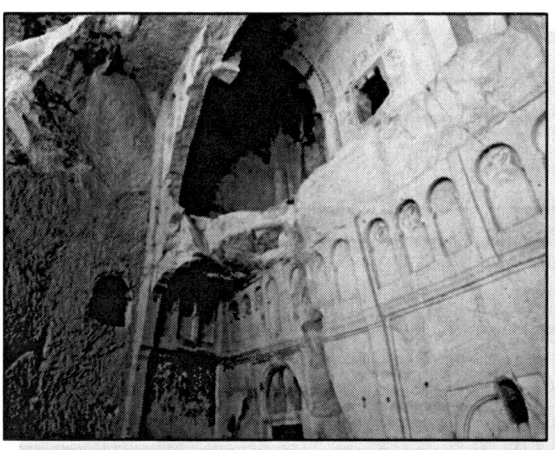

Instead of the colourful pictures of saints and frescoes, simple ornaments painted with ferric oxide began to appear on the walls of the churches in Cappadocia and in the whole Byzantine Empire. As can be guessed from some 11th century churches in the Göreme Open Air Museum, this did not always happen by force. The iconoclastic period, which is described as incredibly brutal, lasted more than a hundred years and finally came to an end in 843. The strong urge for visual presentation had won. But supporters of iconoclasm still managed to hold their ground for centuries in Cappadocia, as can be seen from numerous ornamental paintings from the 11th and the 12th centuries.

Some of the finest church frescoes, which have survived almost 1000 years unscathed, can be admired in the Kiranlik Church in the Göreme Open Air Museum. You should try to enter these small rock-carved churches alone and quietly in order to be able to expose yourself to the effect of the sacred pictures. The church walls are painted all over in the most beautiful colours in fresco technique. After entering the nave one instinctively looks straight towards the apse, in whose vault Christ, the saviour and ruler of the world, looks down from heaven. The nave is also domed, and out of the dome Jesus looks down on the viewer as if from the next world. The arcades, arches and walls show scenes from the life of Jesus. Additionally, saints and bishops and almost always Gabriel and Michael the archangels are standing next to Jesus right and left. In the Cappadocian churches, the local saints appear in addition to the images of Jesus typical of Orthodox Christianity: St. George the dragon slayer is said to have been a Cappadocian. In addition, Emperor Constantine and his mother Helena and also bishop Basil of Caesarea are revered in almost all the images. Like Christian icons, Byzantine frescoes are not works of art, but sacred images which are meant to build a bridge between this world and the hereafter. Often miraculous effects are ascribed to them. The style of painting and the layout are strictly regulated, and artistic freedoms were not wanted. Byzantine frescoes have not changed in almost 1,000 years: the figures look seriously and motionlessly into the viewer's face. Hardly a movement betrays life; the figures seem to float. Saints, angels and notables are mostly depicted in a flat, two-dimensional style and without any illusionary perspective; they seem to step off the wall into the room of the church. No worldly reality was intended to be reproduced or simulated in this way. The representations were not meant to inform the viewer, either, they were to be experienced as a transcendent spiritual reality of the afterlife. Therefore, these frescoes are not wall decoration, but part of a room which was intended to put the believers in a state of closeness to God.

The Christian basilica with its apses, cupolas, vaults, naves, transepts, narthex and atrium remained the unchanged basic religious architectural form in the East for almost 1000 years. The first churches frequently had a well in which the Christians were supposed to clean themselves before the worship service, which is only usual among Muslims today. In fact, the mosque as the Islamic temple eventually emerged from the Christian basilica.

The idea of the dome and the vault as a representation of the heavens, as much detached from the earthly things as possible, finally reached its actual implementation and perfection in the construction of the Hagia Sophia in Constantinople in 537 AD. A dome of gigantic proportions, over 30 metres in diameter, perforated by 40 windows, seems to float above the nave, idealizing the bright vault of heaven with its golden mosaics. The Hagia Sophia remained the unmatched model for all religious buildings for centuries. The fact that the Ottomans were able to convert it into a mosque with only a few accessories corresponds to the common concept of a house of God.

The precious mosaics were plastered over, however. Typically of the East, a figurative representation is not allowed in Islam. Today, however, they are exposed again by the Turkish Government.

The Cappadocian churches, which were carved into the rock with their pillars and arcades supporting a dome, had always remained faithful to the universal principles of church building. The central cupola hall, a Byzantine specialty, is strongly represented in Cappadocia, too. The Cappadocian frescoes, today frequently exposed to the weather and to destruction, often correspond to the highest Byzantine standard. Apart from local fresco painters, artists from Constantinople must also have worked here.

However, Cappadocia was soon cut off from the Christian Byzantine Empire: the Turkmen Seljuks had defeated the Byzantines at Manzikert in 1071 and extended their domain far beyond Cappadocia. They founded their capital in Konya, which was 250 km away. Now the Christians in Cappadocia were cut off from their motherland, but they remained unharmed by the Islamic Seljuks. The Seljuks built roads, caravanserais and schools, and the Christians participated in the rising prosperity. In the following centuries, the most beautiful frescoes were created, and the monastic communities were enlarged. Crusaders are believed to have passed by on their way to Jerusalem and seem to have stayed: some cave churches are more in line with the Catholic nave church than with the Byzantine domed basilica.

There were also connections between the Cappadocian Christians and the monastic communities on Mount Athos in Greece. From there, a spirituality developed in the 12th century, which had great appeal for the monks in their caves: calm, quiet, solitude, serenity and peace were supposed to be achieved through various acts of penance, prayer and meditation, called Hesychasm. This transcendent peace was to be achieved by the frequent repetition of certain formulas like the Jesus prayer with one's eyes on one's navel (omphaloskepsis, navel contemplation). At the same time, very similar exercises of meditation were done by Islamic monks in nearby Konya: the so-called dervishes wanted to achieve the same spiritual experience by repetitious gyration.

Cappadocia became a retreat area for Christian and Islamic mystics, who had many things in common. The endless recitation of surahs from the Koran corresponds to the Jesus Prayer. Prayer chains like the Catholic rosary, the Orthodox "Komboskini" (prayer rope) or the Islamic "Tasbih" help with this. Through asceticism, prayers and meditation, spirituality was to be experienced. Where else but in the fantastic landscape of Cappadocia would this have been possible? Thus, Christians and Muslims with different beliefs found a common homeland in the bizarre tufa landscape of Cappadocia. But this paradise was under threat once again: the Mongols looted Kayseri and also attacked Cappadocia. For the last time, the people took refuge in the underground towns, which had many times povided shelter for them. Finally the Mongols launched the fall of the Seljuk Empire. In their place, the Turkmen Ottomans entered the scene.

The Christian Orthodox monastic communities gradually dwindled away in the following 500 years of the Ottoman Empire, perhaps also because of a lack of incentives from the Christian world. Christian Constantinople had become Islamic Istanbul, and the Roman Catholic Church in Rome was not much interested in the scattered Orthodox Christians in Asia Minor. The last of them had to leave their home country in 1923: the military assault on Turkey by the Greeks in 1919 caused the new Turkish leader, Ataturk, to expel all Greek Orthodox Christians from the country. Since then, the Christian churches and communities have been deserted.

Thus, Christianity in Cappadocia has a history of almost two thousand years: the history of Christianity is also the history of Cappadocia. And Christianity finally inspired Islam, in which many Christian ideas lived on. The Islamic Hacı Bektaş order founded its monastery here, and its humanism had great influence on the entire Islamic world; but it was rooted in the ideas of Persian mysticism, Greek philosophy and the Christian doctrine of salvation.

Architecture

The Caves

The hollowing out of the Cappadocian rock landscape by humans probably began 3500 years ago, in the Hittite era, though there is no definite proof of this. The first written proof of life below the surface of the earth is given by the writings of the Greek writer Xenophon who reports a relocation of Hellenes to underground towns in the 4th century BC. Excavation was later used most intensely by the Christians between the 3rd and the 13th century, who carved hundreds of churches out of the rock in addition to normal dwellings.

Up to the present day, 'creation by excavation' in Cappadocia has not ceased, and long corridors are still carved into the rocks near Ortahisar and the neighbouring villages in order to make use of the natural coolness inside the mountains for storing tropical fruit and potatoes.

Monasteries, Churches and Hermitages

St. Hieronymus is said to have been the first to use the quietness and seclusion of the valleys near Göreme for living as a hermit. As this happened during the time of the persecution of Christians, it can be concluded that he was not the only one to seek refuge there. But those pious men were still a long way from carving churches out of rock. The loud noise of hammering for the excavation of churches was not heard in the valleys until the 9th to the 11th century. The majority of the circa 100 churches discovered to date were created during that period. While the hermits were at first doomed to isolation, they later turned this ascetic way of living into a philosophy. After all, even the purification of Jesus had taken place in the solitude of the desert. The Simeon Tower in Pasabagi is a very nice example of such a hermitage. It is a combination of a small chapel at the base of the fairy chimney and an almost inaccessible dwelling just below the peak.

At some point of time the hermits began to form religious and monastic communities. This in all probability was influenced by the frequent attacks of foreign armies. They were only able to defend their lives in a community of like-minded individuals and in fortified dwellings. Thus the monastic structures developed which, as they were situated high up in the rocks and distributed over several stories, were very difficult to conquer. Here, too, like everywhere in Cappadocia where people were forced to hide from aggressors, the well-known circular cover stones are to be found, that is, round discs of rock that look like millstones. They are up to 2 m in diameter and weigh tons.They have a notch at the top and at the bottom by which they can be rolled in front of the entrance to securely block it. There is a hole in the centre through which you could watch what was going on in front of the entrance and through which now and again a lance could be pushed unexpectedly.The various stories were connected by vertical shafts that possessed small recessed grips in their side walls. Heavy loads had to be pulled up with ropes, as the hands were not free to hold things, nor for using weapons. On the other hand it was an easy game for the defenders, as they could excellently defend the shafts from above by means of long, pointed spears. A shaft of this kind can also be seen in the Simeon Tower. The monasteries were equipped with everything that was necessary for the self-sufficient existence of the communities: kitchens, stables, refectories and even a wine press were part of the basic equipment, and of course there had to be a chapel.

With the end of the attacks by Arabic armies on horseback in the 10th century, the era of church building began. Their inside was built in the same way as if they stood in an open field. Pillars were carved out of the rock as though they had to support a large heavy cupola. The number of missing or destroyed pillars today shows that, in fact, the opposite is true. But somehow a Christian church was simply unthinkable without pillars. Thus church rooms of various sizes were built inside the rocks of Cappadocia: small prayer rooms in which up to four pillars seem to support a tiny dome and large naves vaulted by a huge barrel vault. A great variety of architectural styles can be distinguished: from the cruciform layout of a basilica or the tripartite Romance cathedral to the plain flat roof building, everything can be found. But one thing is common in all these churches: the sacred rooms were equipped with an apse and a small altar. And particularly devout individuals were buried under the church floor, which can be seen from the many tombholes even to the present day. However, some churches were also given up or new ones were build or carved out in the vicinity, and the old ones were used as a necropolis only.

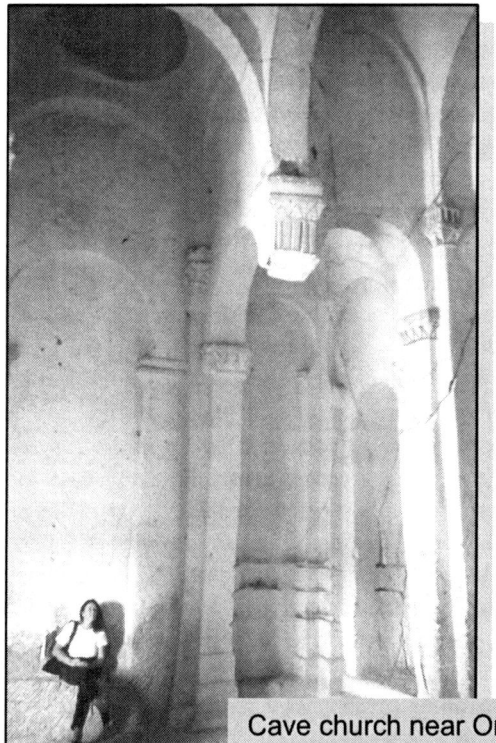

Cave church near Ortahisar – static turned to ornament

But what is most fascinating about all those houses of God is their wall paintings and frescoes, which are almost thousand years old and sometimes in excellent condition. The brilliance of the colours in some of the churches is breathtaking.They shine down strongly and richly from the ceilings and the walls and re-tell the Passion of Christ in all details. Three types of paintings can be distinguished. In the oldest period the figures were painted directly on the rock. In the following period the iconoclastic conflict broke out, officially permitting little more than plain ornamentation. In those days many old paintings were covered with plaster in order to paint them over with the new ornaments and to make them disappear for good. The iconoclastic quarrel ended with the victory of the colourful and richly ornamented frescoes which formed the climax of religious painting in Cappadocia. These pictures are painted on a layer of plaster and differ strongly from the rather earthen-coloured paintings of the early period. Tones of deep blue and purple appear in them, and the various motifs also become more and more subtle. The Tokalı church in the Göreme museum valley is an excellent example of this. In the 13th century this great Christian artistry came to a sudden end due to the Mongolian invasion of Anatolia.

Cave Dwellings and Underground Cities

The biggest and most frequented underground settlements of the region are in Derinkuyu and Kaymaklı. They were driven vertically into the ground in many stories. Basically each town or village here in Cappadocia had its own hidden subterranean defence fortress. It often consisted of horizontal rooms carved out of the rock which were connected by an intricate system of tunnels. Ortahisar and Uchisar have a conspicuously different layout. In times of trouble the inhabitants of these settlements withdrew into the huge rock formations towering far above the landscape. In whatever manner these refuge fortresses were designed, all of them had one thing in common: they are situated within the natural rock, underground, have good ventilation and their own water supply, and they are hard to conquer.These four basic criteria are typical of an underground town in Cappadocia. You can identify those defence fortresses by the rolling coverstones that safely lock up the entrances, because doors that can only be opened from inside can have no other function but to keep away intruders. For that purpose, some underground towns developed various defence techniques. Some coverstones are equipped with narrow side chambers with small openings.Through them the defenders had a good view of what was going on directly in front of the entrance and were able to act accordingly. Any aggressor who stayed directly in front of a coverstone was in mortal danger. In Özkonak there are even little oriels above the entrances through which intruders could be showered with hot water or hot oil.

The shelters were provided with everything a village community needed to survive. It can be presumed that some of them were even used permanently. The stables were mostly situated near the entrance to keep the animals there every day. It would also be an absurd idea that the corn or oil mills existed in two versions, one on the surface for times of peace and another one inside the mountain. Similarly, it would also have made sense to store the food supplies below the ground, because thus the supply for the besieged would have been secured in case of an attack. However, it seems improbable that the people should have lived in the deep caves also in times of peace. They probably lived in some individual dwellings in various places.

The stables can be easily identified by the feeding cribs carved out of the walls. There is often a hole drilled through the edge for tying up the animals. Consequently, these rooms are very large in order to
provide room for as many animals as possible. Behind them are the storerooms, which can be identified by circular hollows in the floor in which large earthenware jars were put. Often a mill and a wine press were connected with them. The wine press consisted of a bowl in which the people crushed the grapes with their bare feet. After this, the must flowed through a hole in the deepest point of the bowl and then into a jar prepared for it. Even deeper inside the mountain there followed the emergency rooms for the people in which one had to find one's way in confined spaces. An assembly room or, as in Derinkuyu, a chapel also belonged to this section.

However, some descriptions and statements propagated in local publications or by travel guides must be taken with a grain of salt. Large numbers seem to be very popular here. Tens of thousands are supposed to have found refuge in those settlements – for several months. There are said to exist more than 200 subterranean towns, which allegedly were all connected with each other. But whoever visits the caves and tunnels with a large tourist group will notice very soon that all this is improbable and exaggerated. Soon after a busload of visitors has entered the rooms, the fresh air and the coolness are gone; the air turns stuffy and the temperature rises rapidly. Now, imagine hundreds of scared people in a panic hurrying through the narrow corridors. The warmth of the oil lamps and torches adds to the rising temperature, and more and more oxygen is taken from the air. After a day at most the rooms will be filled with the stench of human excrement and this will make life below the ground a torture, while from above the screams of a wild and merciless battle for life and death come down to the imprisoned people.

The stories about miles and miles of connecting tunnels between the settlements also belong to the sphere of legend. The oxygen rate in them would drop so low after a few hundred meters that the people inside would inevitably suffocate.

If you now consider the low population density in Cappadocia at that time, you will instantly understand how exaggerated those numbers are with which many a tourist guide tries to impress his listeners.

62 Architecture

The life of the people in times of peace can be studied in the open air museum at Zelve. The caves in this village were inhabited up to the 1950s, and there are more or less no buildings above ground. In all caves you will find small niches or shelves carved into the walls. They contained the few utensils a family needed for its everyday life. There was no furniture as we know it today, because the people were still strongly influenced by the nomadic way of life. Everything a family clan possessed could be packed up and taken to a safe place in almost no time. Beds, seats or work desks were partly carved out of the walls together with the caves themselves; but most inhabitants were content with living on blankets and carpets on the floor.

Lighting was provided by narrow wall openings or by oil lamps. Doors and windows were made very narrow in order to be able to defend the caves more easily, but also to make heating more effective. On the whole the caves proved to be good shelters against extremely low temperatures. No matter how cold or warm it may be outside, inside them there is always a temperature of about 50° F (12° C). In winter the openings were closed against the cold with shutters or with thick cloth. The heating system consisted of an open charcoal bowl (mangal). In it the glowing wood used for cooking food was used, as glowing charcoal does not produce any smoke. Food, however, had to be prepared over a fire which was outside the caves under a rock ledge, as the rooms did not have any chimneys.

Even today many caves are used as storerooms for the harvest or for food because of their constant temperature, and a certain influence of cave structures can also be found in the subsequent traditional architecture of houses.

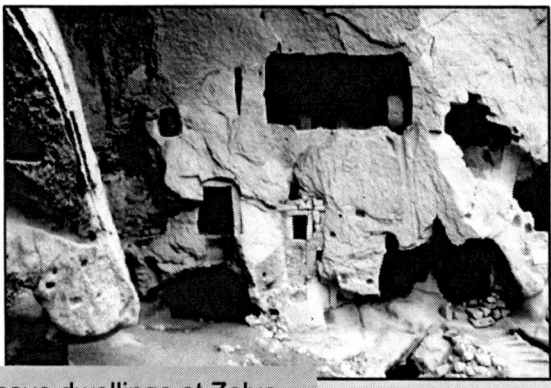
Decayed cave dwellings at Zelve

Pigeon Houses

The infertile soil of the Cappadocian plateau supported the keeping of a special breed of animals. To improve it a special fertilizing method with bird-droppings was necessary. That is why in the middle of the 19th century breeding pigeons became an important instrument of agriculture. Many old churches and monasteries were now used as pigeon houses by walling up the doors and windows, leaving only narrow loop-holes for the birds. Just a single entrance near the ground was closed with a wooden door, through which the inside of the pigeon house was entered once a year in order to take the dung out. Rows of small niches were carved into the walls of the rooms for the birds to build their nests in them, and, if necessary, additional wooden perchs were installed across the rooms. This system can be seen very well in some pigeon houses whose front walls have broken down. Where the construction is still intact, only the walled-up former openings are visible, which are decorated with colourful painted images. These decorations have been created by local artists in the style of contemporary Islamic painting and were supposed to guarantee the owner a rich harvest. Today, in an era of chemical fertilizers, breeding pigeons is more or less of no importance any longer, and flocks of pigeons are not often seen any more.

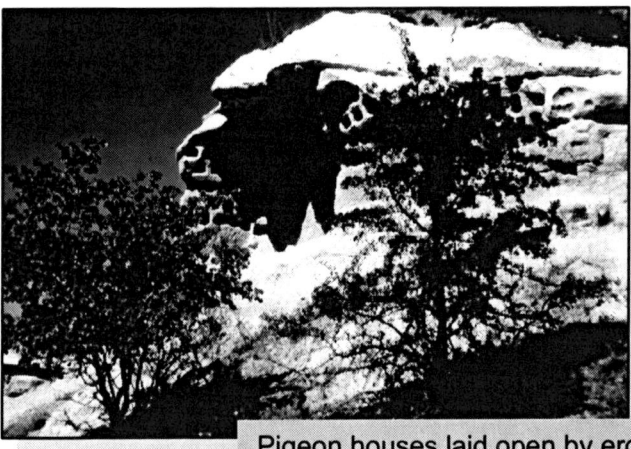
Pigeon houses laid open by erosion

Irrigation Canals

They were meant to simplify the irrigation of the fruit and vegetable gardens in the narrow side valleys, but also to transport the valuable water to the fields at the mouth of the valley without much loss. The small water-channels that originally existed were much lower than the gardens and often oozed away among the boulders after half the distance. The canals were also constructed hidden among the rocks and were wide enough for comfortably walking in them. In the upper part of the valley the little river was chanelled into such a canal and was then led slowly down the valley. Great care was taken to let the water flow above the level of the gardens. Narrow openings in the rock walls that could be closed now allowed systematic and comfortable irrigation. The tedious work of bailing water from the rivulets low in the ground had come to an end. Today large parts of the underground canals have been laid open by erosion and their course is easily discernible.

Present Modern Use of the Caves

The newest large caves were carved in the 20th century. In this era of modern agriculture, huge underground storehouses were built in some parts of Cappadocia. The natural coolness of those caves is used alternatively for storing potatoes and citrus fruits from the coastal area. Almost the complete lemon crop of the country is stored here in spring and then distributed to marketplaces all over the country in the following six months. In autumn they are replaced by the potato crop to secure Turkey's supply with potatoes also in winter. There are hundreds of such storage complexes in Cappadocia. The smaller and older storehouses have rather narrow entrances and have been carved out by hand. Here the fruits have to be unloaded from the lorry and are then carried inside by the bag. The newer complexes are many times larger and were carved into the rock by modern machinery. Their entrances are equipped with huge steel doors that are easily wide enough for lorries. The largest store complex is near the village of Kavak and comprises an area of 10,000 square metres. Here the trucks move around the whole camp area on a U-shaped track and are unloaded by movable conveyor belts. The individual storerooms which are separated by steel screens lie on both sides of the track and their size is about 8 x 15 m. If you happen to see a storehouse that is being filled, do not hesitate to walk inside and have a look. The early capitalist working conditions are worth seeing.

Some years ago, a small group of mostly non-Turkish architects, sociologists and ethnologists came together with the aim of bringing new life to the caves of Cappadocia. They tried to demonstrate with maps and models how the climatic advantages of a cave dwelling can be combined with the conveniences of a modern apartment. Unfortunately, there has been no pilot project of this, as the state forbids carving new cave dwellings out of the rock in Cappadocia.

Traditional Architecture and Living

The history of architecture in Cappadocia does not go back very far. This region was not urbanized much except for large cities like Nevsehir and Kayseri. The few village communities between them consisted of little more than a conglomeration of cave dwellings. Many centuries of invasions by foreign powers had taught the people of Cappadocia to construct very unobtrusive dwellings. The soft tufa offered an almost ideal chance to make whole villages disappear under the ground or behind walls of rock. Not until as late as in the Ottoman era did the Cappadocians begin to build normal houses, as the Ottomans were the last who claimed the region as their property, and under their rule an era of peace began which has lasted up to the present day.

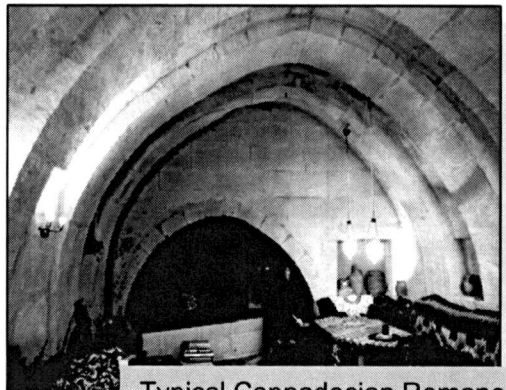
Typical Cappadocian Romanesque Construktion

They did not build complete houses at first, as the fear of sudden attacks disappeared very slowly. At first only very simple walls for defense purposes were built in front of the caves. Very gradually the inhabitants began to trust the peace and began to build houses in front of their caves. Later on, walls were erected round the house and the cave entrance to create a courtyard (avlu). This isolation from the neighbourhood can be found everywhere in the Islamic world. An additional first floor did not appear before the 19th century. In the course of time a group of small buildings around a courtyard developed in front of every cave, which were later united into a complex. The old caves lost their function as living-rooms and were only used as storerooms or as stables for livestock.

The Material

Tufa is a material that can be handled really well. It can easily be cut out of the walls of a quarry and afterwards be sawed into suitable sizes. Delivered in blocks of about 30 x 60 cm and a thickness of about 20 cm, it is excellently suited for building walls and can be made into a suitable size with very simple tools. However, a block like this weighs about 40 kg and more. The rock only begins to harden completely after some time of contact with the outside air. Tufa has good heat-insulating qualities. Rooms built of this material can be heated up to a comfortable temperature with a simple stove in no time. The thicker the walls are, the longer the warmth will persist. There are friends of ours who heat their bathroom in winter with the ignition flame of the gas warm water boiler. Only the moderate hardness of this kind of rock is a disadvantage, as the basic walls of the groud floor have to be built very thick. One thing that the tufa does not like at all is water. Because of its porosity and the high percentage of chalk it absorbs water like a sponge. During this the chalk increases in volume and causes the rock to become soft and to disintegrate quickly. As hard as it may be to imagine: the destruction of many old housing areas was closely related to the introduction of running water in pipe systems. The absence of a sewage system, the freezing of the water pipes in winter and the lavish use of water, which was initially free, caused the gradual breakdown of whole town quarters.

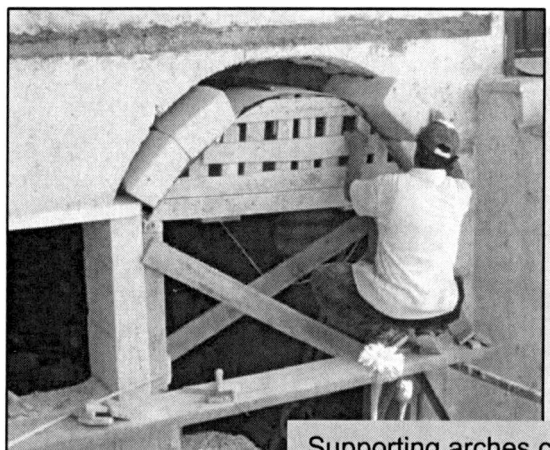

Supporting arches can also be built in afterwards

Construction Technique

As has been said above, the load-bearing capacity of tufa is much less than with other types of rock, therefore the walls of the ground floor are always very thick. Especially the basic walls of the typically Cappadocian flat-roofed-vaulted houses, where enormous horizontal weights rest on the walls, are sometimes up to 1 m in diameter. We do not know when this construction technique was first introduced. But as wood has always been very rare as a building material in the region, it can be presumed that this technique was made use of at a very early time.

First several round arches are masoned across the length of the room (1). They are so close to each other that after this the space between them can be closed with a second layer of blocks (2) and the vaulted ceiling is completed. Here, too, we see the economic use of wood as a valuable building material. If in case of a uniform long vault the complete ceiling has to be boarded with wood, with the Cappadocian technique only a small scaffold for one single arch is necessary. Afterwards the side walls (3) are continued to a little more than the height of the vault, and the resulting hollow space is filled up with soil (5), until a flat roof has been created. The thick layer of soil mixed with lime prevents the scarce rain from seeping through. These flat roofs have always been very popular as sitting or working platforms on which you were able to dry fruit and vegetables or hang up the washing and which allowed easy cleaning.

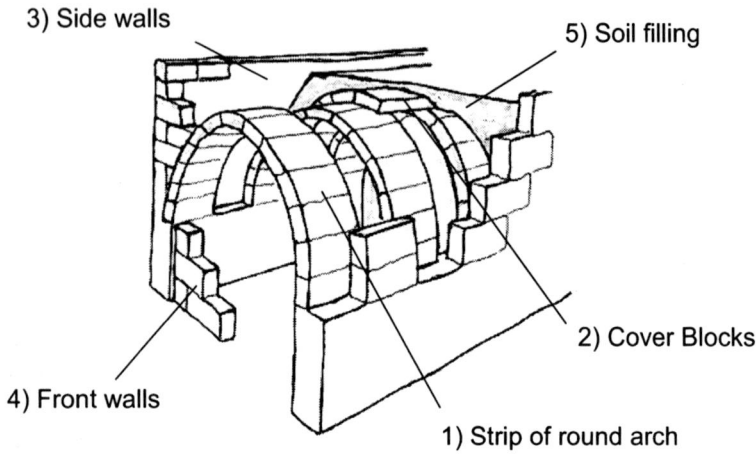

3) Side walls
5) Soil filling
2) Cover Blocks
4) Front walls
1) Strip of round arch

The addition of more stories is from later periods. Their construction is simpler. Here, the walls are thinner for reasons of weight; sometimes they are only one brick in diameter. The ceiling rests on simple round poplar logs covered with flat tufa slabs. Sometimes ornamented wooden ceilings have been put in. The flat roof of the first floor is not rainproof, however, so that a wooden frame that was covered with tiles always had to be built over it. The larger windows, which often face to the south and allow the warm sunshine to come in, are typical of the first floor. The introduction of these windows is closely connected with the beginning of the industrial production of window panes. In earlier times the windows and doors were made as narrow as possible, as they could be closed by only a wooden shutter or a piece of thick cloth.

Floor Plan

The inner courtyard (avlu) with its entrance is always the centre of the traditional Cappadocian house. There is no main door from the street directly

Architecture 67

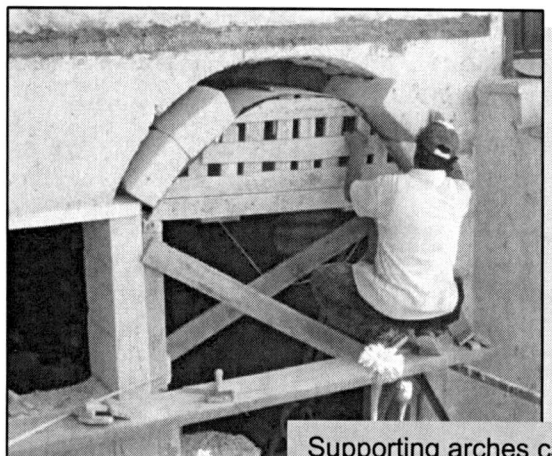

into the house. The rooms are distributed round the courtyard in irregular order on several floors. There are no connecting rooms and all rooms are accessible from the courtyard. If you are looking for the toilet you will always find it near the outer wall near the entrance, built separately and always at the greatest possible distance to the living area. It consists of a hole leading into a small chamber below it. The latter has a trap door towards the street through which it can be emptied.

Right up to the present day, all housework is done in the courtyard, weather permitting. For this purpose often an open covered porch was built. In many cases this porch (çardak) has also been built with a vaulted roof, as it is opposite the entrance on the ground floor. It provides shade in the summer and keeps the rain off in winter. In old houses you will also always find the cooking pit (tandir) here. It is a simple ceramic bowl that was dug into the ground and in which the fire was burning. When the fire had gone out, the remaining heat of the bowl was used for baking bread. Besides, there are workrooms and storerooms on the ground floor and sometimes also a room for receiving visitors in winter. A stone staircase in the courtyard leads up to the first floor, to the family's private chambers and to the roof terrace. It is quite interesting that the different areas of the house can reflect the degree of welcome of the guest. An unwelcome visitor is dealt with in front of the courtyard door. A short, friendly exchange of news mostly takes place in the entrance, and welcome guests may sit down inside the courtyard or even in the reception room. This area of the house is called the Selamlik. The upper and mostly very private rooms are called Haremlik and are taboo for visitors.

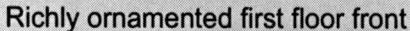
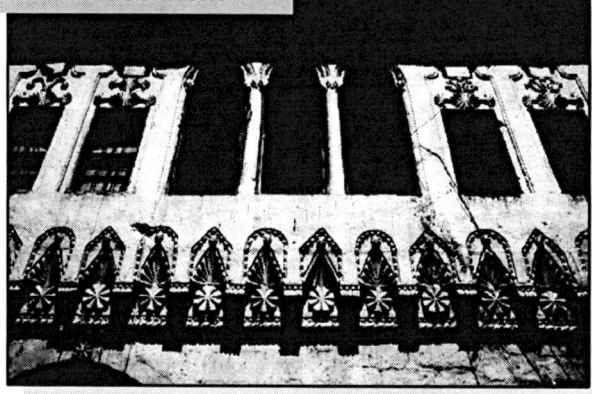

Richly ornamented first floor front

The Traditional Livingroom

In the old days furniture was a rare thing in a normal household. One used to live on the floor of a room furnished with thick carpets and cushions. In our present modern times corner seating units or plain bedsteads are gradually invading the livingrooms. Those rooms are the central point of every house. This is where you sleep, eat and also spend the rest of the day. Especially in winter, when the courtyard cannot be used because of the cold, the life of the family takes place in this room. For that purpose the furniture of the room has to be constantly changed, however. The small table round which the family assembles on the floor for their meals is cleared away right after the meal is over. The beds, which consist of simple light-weight matresses, are spread out every evening and put away again in the morning. Thus the furniture is continuously adapted to the changing needs. Even the stove disappears in one of the numerous store rooms in spring. The entrance to this 'living-room' (in the true sense of the word) is mostly at the side in one corner of the room. In the entrance section the floor is somewhat lower than in the rest of the room, and this is called Sekıaltı. This is where you have to take off your shoes, if not before. In the main wall opposite the windows there is a niche about the size of a wardrobe. This is the Yüklük, where the beds are kept during the day. This so-called closet can be closed by wooden doors, but mostly there is only a curtain. Various other small carved openings can be found in the walls. As the walls are often very thick, they prevent the room from being blocked up by cupboards and shelves. In the orifices there are utensils for everyday use that have to be at hand quickly. The walls of the whole room are lined with seats, of which the seat opposite the door is decorated most beautifully and is meant for the head of the household. This seat is often also a little higher. If this place is part of the Selamlik area, the seats to the right and to the left of the patriarch are for the guests. The family members of lower rank, like women and small children, are always seated near the door, which makes their way to the kitchen much shorter. Last but not least it has to be said that this traditional form of family life continues also in western style apartments, though not always in every detail. Even though all the furniture may have been bought from a Swedish warehouse chain, the head of the family will still be seated in a way that he can keep a watchful eye on the living-room door; just as if everybody was sitting in a Turkomen round tent that might be attacked by an enemy family clan any moment.

The Country and its Inhabitants

Politics and Administration

About 70 million Turks share an area of almost 780,000 km². Statistically this is 90 inhabitants per km². In reality, however, this looks quite different. Large parts of the Anatolian highlands and the eastern part of the country are extremely sparsely populated. On the other hand, the big cities are almost bursting at the seams. Decades of drift to the cities and a high birth rate are the reasons for the fact that meanwhile also smaller towns have a million inhabitants or more. Kayseri, which had just 168,000 inhabitants in 1970, can serve as a good example here. Especially the improvement of medical care since the proclamation of the Republic in 1923 caused the rate of infant mortality to decline steadily and presented the nation with a considerable population increase. In 1927, there were only just 13.6 million Turkish citizens. The largest cities of the country are Istanbul, Ankara and Izmir with several million inhabitants each – and with the urban problems related to this. Ankara has been the capital since 1923, when it was only an unimportant small town. The founding father of the Republic of Turkey, Mustafa Kemal Atatürk, greatly distrusted the old sultan's capital of Istanbul and its power structures. Thus Ankara experienced a fast growth and increased to 3 million inhabitants. From here the country is governed in a centralist manner. When dealing with authorities, you are informed again and again that the file has been sent to Ankara for decision. The Turkish state is subdivided into more than 80 governors' provinces, but they deal primarily with matters of administration. Political decisions are the privilege of the capital.

Every five years a new parliament is elected in Turkey. This again elects the President with a two-thirds majority, who in turn appoints the Prime Minister (Chancellor). On the Prime Minister's suggestion, the President afterwards appoints the ministers. The president is elected for seven years and is only allowed to stay in office for one legal period. In Turkish parliamentary elections, there is a 10 % threshold, which sometimes leads to peculiar results. Thus, the moderately religious AK party gained the absolute majority in parliament in the 2003 election although it had only 34% of the country's votes. All this sounds very democratic, but there is one snag to the whole system: since the military coup in 1980, in addition to the parliament there have been regular assemblies of the National Security Council, which selects its own members and consists mostly of members of the armed forces. It has the right to overrule the ministers' or the parliament's decisions. This council regards itself as a guardian of Atatürk's instructions and prevents anything that is contradictory to them.

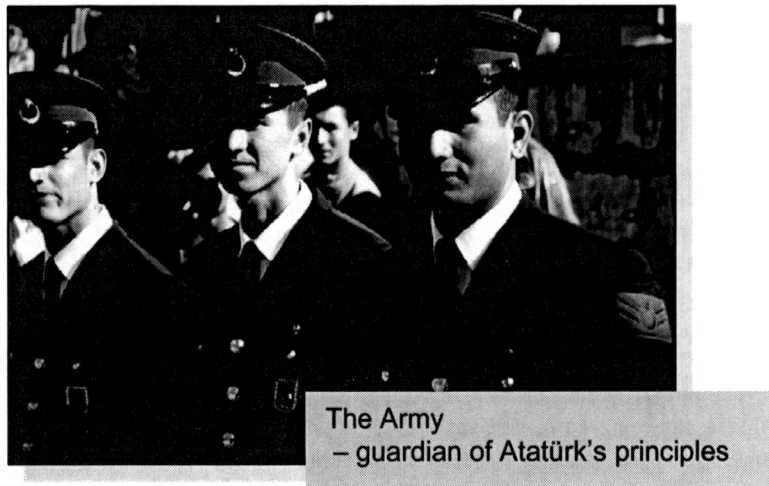

The Army
– guardian of Atatürk's principles

This way the influence of the military on the country and on the government is still strong. But this is not necessarily regarded as a disadvantage by the population. In spite of the 1980 coup d'état and its brutal consequences the military enjoys a good reputation among the people. General compulsory military service is not exactly popular, but its necessity is in no way disputed by the population. For the simple recruit compulsory military service means the beginning of 24 months of bitter hardships, far away from his home, his family and friends, exposed to the arbitrariness of his superiors and provided with a monthly pay that is just enough to buy some packs of cigarettes. Military service in Turkey can also easily turn into war experience, as has been shown by the years of conflict with the PKK in the eastern part of the country. On the other hand, the armed forces have guaranteed the adherence to the democratic rules in the past. Thus in 1960 they made a military coup against the former Menderes government, which was on the point of destroying the basic rights of the population, and commissioned a new and

Politics and Administration 73

progressive constitution to be made. In the middle of the nineties another coup was avoided altogether. When the army "parked" their tanks in front of the barracks, this was enough to make the government under Prime Minister Erbakan return to reason and to prevent him from leaving the path of democracy.

Turkey with its military forces of about 700,000 has been a member of NATO since 1952 and was an important listening post for the USA in the Cold War.The country's importance for the USA became obvious again in the 1963 Cuba crisis. The deployment of American nuclear Jupiter rockets on the border of the Soviet Union had been the original cause of this extremely dangerous situation. Even today the country is covered by a dense network of NATO or US institutions. The US Airforce base at Incirlik near Adana, which played an important role in the Iraq wars, is probably the most well-known among them.

In general, Turkey is very much oriented towards the West and vehemently presses for full membership in the EU. Turkey has great scepticism towards its eastern neighbours. The only nation with which Turkey has normal relations is Georgia.The borders to this north-eastern neighbour are open and can be crossed without any problems.

The relations to Armenia are characterized by tension. This can be traced back to the genocide against the Armenians in 1915, which Turkey has been unable to admit up to the present day. Direct entry into Armenia via Turkey is not possible. The border to Iran is open, but the secular republic looks with distrust at the Islamic theocratic state. Relations with Iraq have always been troubled, as the country has been an area of retreat of the Kurdish rebels for decades. Especially after the overthrow of Saddam Hussein and the formation of a de facto independent Kurdish region, Turkey has been keeping more than a watchful eye on the northern part of Iraq. Neither can the relations to Syria be called really happy. One reason for this is the cession of the Hatay (Antakya) region to Turkey in 1938. France as the former colonial power gave this strip of southern coastal area to Turkey as a present in connection with the treaty of friendship between Turkey and France. To the present day Syria has refused to acknowledge this cession of territory. The water policies of Turkey, that is, the damming of the Euphrates river, did not help to relax the situation, either. But relations with Greece have improved substantially during the past few years. The macabre aspect is that a disaster like the devastating earthquake of 1999 with more than 14,000 victims had to hit Turkey first. Greek support forces were the first foreigners on site to help rescue the many persons buried alive and thus finally brought the two hostile nations closer to each other. Turkey cannot warm to Bulgaria either. This has something to do with the Turk minority which has lived in the south-east of Bulgaria since the Ottoman time and which is not accepted well there. On the whole, the relations to the neighboring countries cannot be called really friendly, which is probably also an explanation for the high number of Turkish armed forces in general.

Finally, the country's really good relations to Israel should be mentioned, which are not exactly typical of an Islamic country. Turkey supplies Israel with large quantities of drinking water by tankships, maintains military contact and is engaged in brisk trade with this Jewish state, which is otherwise quite isolated in the region.

The country's urge towards the EU has led to great efforts of democratic reform. Even though this is caused by the strict European membership conditions, first steps in this direction have been taken. But the abolition of the death penalty, the reform of the judicial system and several alterations of the constitution must not hide the fact that there is still a long way to go towards Europe. Unfortunately, bureaucratic despotism and abuse of office are still widespread. Of course, a change in people's minds cannot be brought about by prescription of law.

As mentioned above, Turkey is subdivided into administrative provinces (il).The central area of Cappadocia belongs to the province of Nevşehir, and the governor's (vali) seat is in the capital of the same name. The provinces are numbered in alphabetical order, and Nevsehir is the fiftieth district. This can be seen from the number plates of the cars. All numbers of cars registered here start with 50 and all postal codes here begin with 50 as well. Some more distant Cappadocian tourist attractions belong to other provinces, however. The Soganli valley and the town of Inescu already fall under the jurisdiction of Kayseri (38), the area around the Göllü-Dağı belongs to Niğde (51) and the Ihlara valley belongs to the district of Aksaray (68). Do not wonder why a town whose name begins with an A has got number 68, as at the beginning of the Republic there were only 67 provinces. All higher numbers were caused by subsequent regional reorganizations.

The provinces are subdivided into districts (ilçe) which comprise one small town plus several villages. The next smaller units are the town communes (şehir) and the villages (köy). All settlements with more than 2000 inhabitants possess a town hall (belediye) that is supervised by a mayor (başkan) and the local council. Medium towns are subdivided into municipal districts (mahalle), in which a municipal director is the direct contact for the inhabitants' problems. From here, the citizens' inquiries, requests and issues begin their sluggish way through the channels of bureaucracy, and the red tape is not any faster in Turkey than elsewhere in the world.

Islam

98 % of the Turkish population are adherents of Islam. More than 900 years ago, the Seljuks introduced it to Anatolia. From the beginning Islam presented itself as a tolerant religion here in Turkey; thus through all the centuries peaceful coexistence of Muslims and Christians was possible. From the beginning of the Ottoman Empire to the inauguration of the Republic of Turkey, both the secular and the religious leadership were exercised by the Sultan in Istanbul. In 1924 the caliphate, i.e. the spiritual leadership, was abolished by the National Assembly. This kind of separation of state and religion had been absolutely unimaginable to many Muslims until then. In 1928, Islam even lost its status as a state religion. But this was no problem to the majority of the population, as their religious feelings were very down-to-earth. The hard-working Anatolian farmer believes in Allah and his commandments, but is very flexible in following the religious rules and prescriptions. For example, the Islamic ban on alcohol and gambling is not taken too seriously here in Turkey.

Islam is the youngest of the three great monotheistic religions. Muslims, i.e. adherents of Islam, believe in Allah as the sole and omnipotent God and in his commandments which he has revealed through the mouth of his prophet, Mohammad. Mohammad is the last of a long row of prophets which also include Abraham (Ibrahim), Moses (Musa) and Jesus (Isa).

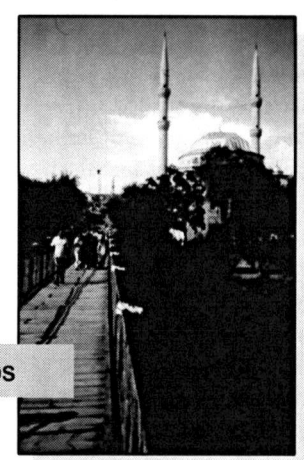

The great mosque of Avanos

Thus the narrations of the Old and the New Testament become parts of Islamic religious belief. Christianity has a special role for the Muslims, as it can claim at least part of the Godly truth for itself. Islam is based on five principal duties which every faithful Muslim has to obey:

1. The statement of faith in the sole and omnipotent God, Allah
2. Observation of the five prayer times per day and the obligatory prayer formulas
3. Observation of the fasting rules during the fasting month of Ramasan
4. The giving of alms to the poor
5. The pilgrimage to Mekka (hajj) that every devoted Muslim is supposed to make at least once in his lifetime.

The confession of faith alone is sufficient to be or become a Muslim. As soon as it is recited in the presence of witnesses and the prayer leader of the mosque, the Imam, the person is a member of the Muslim community.

The believer is expected to pray five times a day facing the Kaaba in Mecca. The ritual and the words are prescribed in every detail. Among others, washing, which has to be done before praying, belongs to the ritual. For this purpose, there are washing facilities at all mosques, where the visitor has to clean his hands, feet and face before entering the prayer room. However, the prayer can also take place within one's own four walls. If you meet a Muslim who is praying, do not disturb him or her. And if you enter a shop at prayer time, be a little patient, as the shop owner might be in a back room absorbed in prayer. The times of prayer are called out loudly and distinctly from the minarets everywhere.

The fasting month of Ramasan poses a special challenge. During this month the believers are forbidden to eat, drink or even smoke between sunrise and sunset. If the month of Ramasan falls on June, i.e. the time of the longest days of the year, it is especially hard for the believers. This Islamic month corresponds to the moon calendar and therefore shifts forward 11 days every year. During this time the tourist can buy a meal also in the daytime, but it is advisable not to seat oneself too ostentatively at the roadside (front) tables. The atmosphere among the local people is not so good during this time, as a majority of Turkish people are addicted to nicotine and are suffering from serious withdrawal symptoms.

At sunset the whole nation finally assembles in restaurants or at the private dinner table. Now everything that had to be done without is made up for. This is also the moment when every Turkish town seems to sink into sudden hibernation. The croaking of frogs, the chirp of crickets and the rustling of leaves become audible then, and you believe to hear the clatter of thousands of forks and knives in the distance. In the early morning, at least two hours before sunrise, the peace is over. A drummer rudely rouses the believers from their sleep so that they can have a good bite to eat for the day before the sun rises. Unfortunately, the tourist is not always exempted from this awakening method. The end of the fasting month is sweetened by the subsequent three days of sugar festival (Şeker Bayramı). There is high life in these three days, the children are overfed with sweets, and many a head of the family has one too many from the bottle. Such holidays are often used for family outings, among others to Cappadocia. You will find the exact dates of the religious festivals in the chapter on "holidays and festivities" p. 148.

The giving of alms to the needy has a long tradition in Islam. Because of this, begging as a profession has an importance that must not be underestimated in Islamic countries. Especially the old and the handicapped must be supported for religious reasons. Occasionally this even leads to the fact that persons who live alone are taken care of by their neighbourhood. More information is available to the reader in the chapter on "begging" p.155.

Once in the lifetime of a devoted Muslim the pilgrimage to Mecca should be made. This happens in the last month of the Islamic calendar. The "Kurban Bayrami" (festival of sacrifice, Eid-ul-Adha) is the climax of the pilgrimage month and the most important Muslim holiday. This festival goes back to the biblical story of Abraham who was told to offer his son, Isaac, as a sacrifice to God. As God refrained from the sacrifice, Abraham finally killed a sheep out of gratitude. Thus it happens that on this festive day millions of sheep in the whole Islamic world have to lose their lives.

A Muslim who returns from the hajj to Mecca from then on enjoys a high status inside his community and is entitled to add the name hajji (hacı) to his name. A hajji can be identified by his small circular head covering, at least if he is a man.

80% of Turks belong to the Sunni religious community and thus are adherents of the "Sunna". They believe in the caliphs as the rightful successors of Muhammad. The remaining Muslims of the country call themselves Alevi and belong to the Shi'a community. They question the successorship of the 4th caliph after Mohammad and regard his son-in-law,

Ali, as the rightful successor. But Ali and his sons were killed in the course of this power struggle and have since then been regarded as martyrs. But the Alevis do not have much in common with their conservative fellow Muslims in conservative Shiite Iran. They have no prayer rules, do not observe the Ramasan fasting month, have no mosques and are allowed to drink alcoholic liquors. Besides, they practise some ceremonies and rituals from the pre-Islamic time of the Turk nations. All this has made them victims of persecution by the so-called orthodox believers. (p.291)

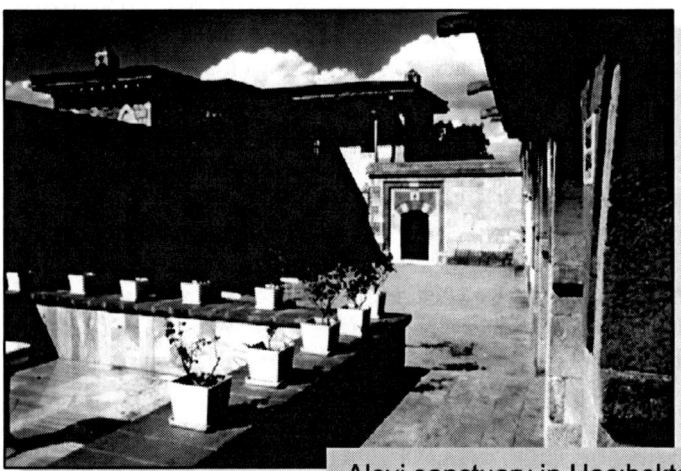

Alevi sanctuary in Hacıbektaş

In general, Islam in Turkey is rather down-to-earth. Orthodox Imams who agitate the masses against the government are rare here. On the one hand this is of course due to the government's tough line against enemies of Kemalism; on the other hand the separation of state and church is firmly anchored in the population meanwhile.

A visit in a mosque is no problem for us Christians. There are only some rules you should follow. Always wear long-sleeved shirts and long trousers whenever you enter a mosque. Women are obliged to cover their hair with a scarf - and, please, take off your shoes at the entrance! Non-Muslims are regarded as disturbing only at prayer times. Apart from that, the tourist will encounter Islam as a tolerant religion on his voyage through Cappadocia.

Economy

Contrary to many opinions, Turkey has not been a developing country any more for a long time. It is a so-called emerging nation that normally comes up with 6 to 9 per cent of economic growth per year and could be called a 'little tiger', as the aspiring Asian nations were called in the past. That the country has not advanced even further is an inheritance from the Ottoman Empire. When Atatürk proclaimed the Republic more than 80 years ago, he could not fall back on any industry or system of entrepreneurs. All technologies had hitherto been purchased from the Western superpowers. Atatürk wanted to liberate his country from this state of dependence and started to found state-owned business companies. This way, Turkey's economy was subjected to state control for almost 50 years. The state interfered with price and payment policies and developed so-called five year plans in order to gain as much economic self-sufficiency as possible. Turkey's own economy was defended against foreign products by high protective duties. Even today the customs authorities demand up to 100% of duty (on the replacement value) if you import a second-hand car.

Towards the end of the seventies, the country was no longer able to pay back its external debts. The International Monetary Fund (IMF) helped Turkey out, not without imposing conditions, however. Thus an economic liberalization has been going through Turkish politics for some decades. A gradual privatization of state-owned companies and the abolition of trade barriers are parts of it.

Travellers who reach Turkey via Rumania or Bulgaria will notice how modern and technologically advanced the country is today. Even though those countries have been members of the EU since January 2007, the new members and the "little tiger on the Bosporus" are still worlds and decades apart.

The Turkish economy is divided into three great sectors: agriculture, industry and services. The importance of the agricultural sector has been declining in recent years. In fact more than 40% of the population work in agriculture, but they produce only 15% of the GNP. Industry, however, produces twice as much with only half as many people working. The services sector is a steadily growing economic sector. The constantly rising numbers of foreign visitors are the reason for this. Tourism has become an important economic factor for Turkey.

In Cappadocia agriculture and tourism are the key sources of income. There is industry only in the Kayseri area and on the edge of Avanos in the form of brickyards. Instead, there are many small handicraft enterprises in the small towns.They are mostly situated outside the town centres in so-called industrial estates (sanai) and often only consist of the owner and one or two assistants. There is a strong urge towards economic independence, and everybody tries to avoid being wage-dependent, if possible. With minimum wages and absence of social standards, this is not surprising. Trade gives the same impression: here, too, everybody tries to build up his own little shop. And those who cannot afford their own shopping premises roam the streets of the towns with a handcart or with a vendor's tray. Vacant shopping premises are a rarity in Cappadocia.

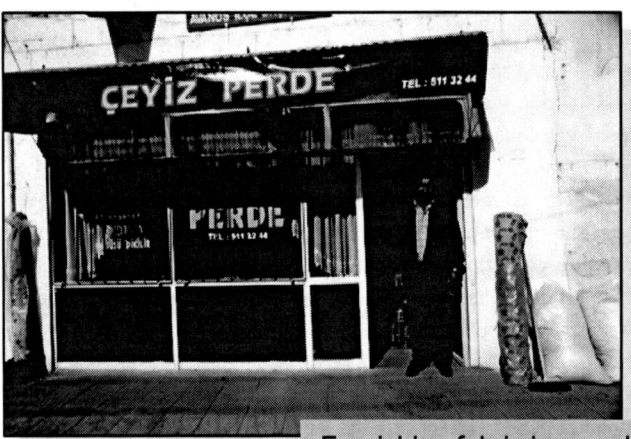

Furnishing fabric is on sale here

Agriculture is on the decline in Cappadocia, too, as the small farm businesses are hardly able to feed a family any more. One reason is the Turkish law of heritage which prescribes that all brothers and sisters inherit a share of the same size, so that the farm businesses become smaller and smaller. On the other hand, farms like that cannot keep up with the big suppliers from the coast to whom completely different means of production are available. Thus, the tomato crop for example grows throughout the whole year in greenhouses in the coastal region, whereas in Cappadocia the red vegetables are harvested only once a year. During the harvest period the market is literally flooded with tomatoes, which makes prices sink to rock bottom. The only profitable thing is the cultivation of grapes and of potatoes. The grapes are accepted gladly by the press houses of the region and the pressed wine is sold in the entire country. Potatoes are grown far and wide all over Cappadocia . The central storage facilities are an important reason for this. Near Ortahisar, Kavak and some other towns there are huge underground storerooms with a constant temperature of 40° F (4°C). The potato crop is put into storage in them in the autumn and then gradually put on the market all over Turkey in the following months. But the potato production has risen to such an extent in recent years that the ground water level around Cappadocia has become extremely low. The small fields or shady gardens in the valleys of the Cappadocian erosion landscape are only for private consumption or serve as a small extra income when the surplus production can be sold on the local markets.

Tourism is the main source of income in the region and offers the most attractive jobs. The chances of earning money are best here, as you need not work yourself to death, workplaces are clean and unrestricted contact with – in Turkish eyes – casually dressed female tourists is guaranteed. Whoever has found a job or even been able to start a business here has made it. But also here the gold rush has come to an end. The number of long-term visitors has decreased and the big tourist companies who transport their tourists to Cappadocia from the coast for two days dictate the prices. Thus, the fight for tourists is carried out with more and more grim determination and it is going to be hard for newcomers to set foot into other people's marked territories.

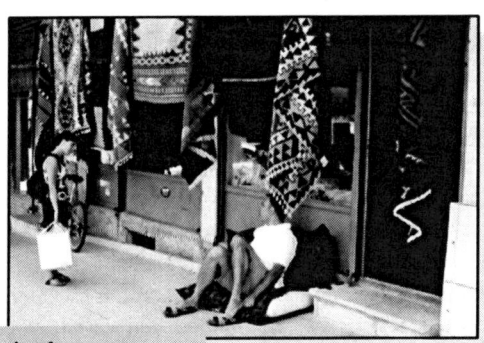

Carpet shop in Avanos

Daily Life in the Family

In spite of tourism, life in Cappadocia is still very much influenced by tradition. The extended family is the decisive centre of everything. Even though the first signs of disintegration are becoming visible, it is still usual that several generations live together under the same roof. The family structure is strictly hierarchical. Usually the husband, father or grandfather is the head of the family. It is his duty to make the decisions related to the welfare of the family. At an older age the patron transfers the privilege to make decisions to his oldest son or at least discusses things with his sons. The women do not participate in the process and are expected to accept the patriarch's decisions.

This is the image that is in the mind of the normal citizen of the Western world. All this might be approximately true, but it is the subtleties that matter here. By old tradition the husband always plays the boss. But in the background the women are busy shaping and influencing the decision-making processes according to their wishes, and they have lots of opportunities to do so. You will notice how many men are busy outside the house during the day and how seldom you meet women crowding the streets just to pass the time. During the daytime, the spheres of sojourn are clearly defined. The wife looks after the house and takes care of the children, whereas the husband has to care for the family income. This of course cannot be done at home, so that he is absent all day long and the women have their realm to themselves. Many household chores are done in community by the women so that relatives, acquaintences or neighbours come together for this purpose. On these occasions there is a lot of discussion and gossip and many practical constraints in family matters are created this way. A Turkish husband who happened to return home unexpectedly would not be able to stand all this for very long and would try to find a plausible excuse for leaving again fast. The power of those women's meetings must not be underestimated. Traditionally, this is the place where the children's marriage partners are first discussed, but quite often they get right down to brass tacks there: problems with husbands, their decisions or their shortcomings are discussed quite frankly in those intimate circles.

When in the evening the husband is sitting together with his family, worn out with the day's work, well-aimed and carefully considered information is dispensed that will lead things in the right direction. Later, the head of the family will announce "his" decision of the matter without the slightest suspicion that he has been thoroughly manipulated. Or does he perhaps suspect something? You see, being a patriarch in Turkey is not as easy as people like us tend to believe...

Bringing up the children is the wife's obligation. Only after the male offspring is out of the woods, at six or seven, does the patriarch take care of them in order to make "real" men out of them. But it can be doubted that this is going to be successful if Mum still laces her fourteen-year-old little darling's shoes for him. At that age, a marriage partner is gradually started being looked for. Not by the young man, of course, but by the family. But such stories seldom end in a so-called forced marriage today. In large areas of society the young people have their own ideas today and the partner for life is only given the parents' blessings by them. The idea of the forced marriage mainly survives only in the remote villages of east Anatolia and, unfortunately, in the minds of Turkish families who have emigrated to foreign countries.

At least those young men who have been thouroughly spoilt by their parents will have a hard time in the future. The county's young women are presently developing a very independent way of thinking within which there is no room for a life as the husband's servant any more.

It is still the husband's duty to provide financial support for the family, however, although the women basically do not care how he manages to do this. Life as a daily labourer is unfortunately still very common here in this country. Turkey's high unemployment rate is the reason why early in the morning many tired-looking and relatively disoriented young men in working clothes assemble in the central square of the town or village. Here they are waiting for a chance to get hold of one of the rare one-day jobs. And if this does not work, the next teahouse is mostly not far away. But coming home without money in the evening means bringing a lot of fuel for conflicts into the marital harmony.

A lot could be written about this topic, as family structures here in Cappadocia begin to soften and the usual prejudiced image that used to exist in our Western minds has often become inaccurate long ago. But perhaps some readers had an experience of 'déjà vu' while reading this chapter and some passages of this text may have appeared familiar to him or her.

Just a couple of sentences about the non-familiar surroundings, i.e. the neighbourhood. Neighbourly help is taken very seriously here. Wives especially do their bigger household chores together with their neighbours. Thus, there are breadbaking or laundry days which are carried out by several housewives living closely together. Of course, petty squabbles between families occur here, too, but it has to be really bad if a family will be excluded from this community. In this case the conflict or the disgrace is mostly so important that the family will move away from the town quarter. An intensified neighbourly relation can develop with one's direct next-door neighbour, the "kapıkomsu". The relation to this person is mostly very close and almost like to a family member. You go to your neighbour when serious problems have occurred or when you were having a row at home. But of course the kapikomsu cannot always be your best friend because, as we all know, friends can be chosen freely.

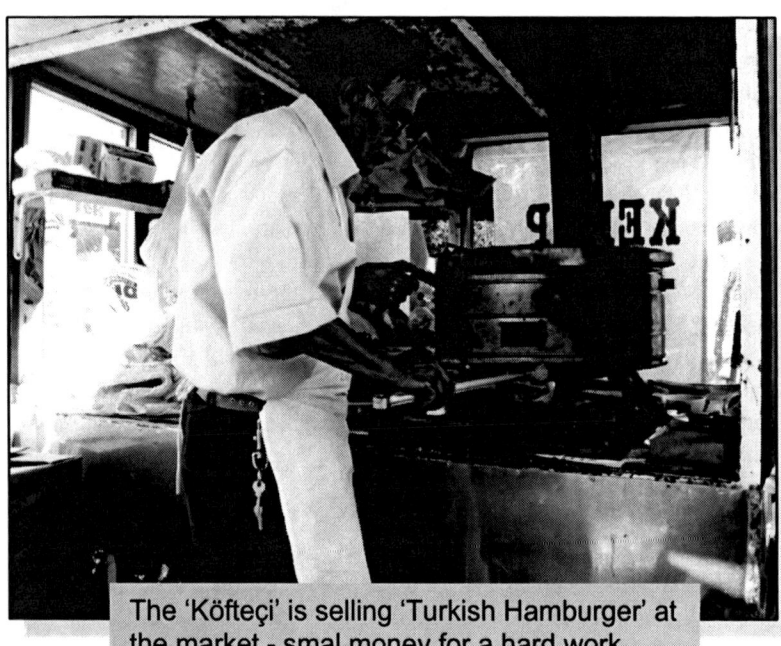

The 'Köfteçi' is selling 'Turkish Hamburger' at the market - smal money for a hard work

Tourism

About 35 years ago Turkey was treated as an absolute insiders' tip among backpackers.Travelling to a country that was socio-culturally so different from Western and Central European habits was thought to be most daring and adventurous. Besides, the miles of empty beaches, romantic fishing villages and the wide, endless, intact natural landscape were very alluring. Those returning to the places of their youthful adventures will be greatly disappointed. In the places where you used to sit together all night long with other youthful adventure-seekers from all over the world, drinking all night long and swimming in the sea in the silence of the natural landscape – today there is often a stylish disco for Yuppies, surrounded by gigantic hotel complexes and bathed in the traffic noises of a four-lane freeway.
Cappadocia has not been hit quite as hard as that. Of course, many things have changed here, too, but the region has been more or less exempt from the excesses of the Turkish Riviera. Here, too, it was the backpackers who discovered Cappadocia in the mid seventies. Without any bars and boardinghouses yet, only equipped with a teahouse and plain family accomodation, they took part in family life as the first foreigners. But, as it happens with secret insiders' tips for travellers, there soon was nothing secret about Cappadocia any longer, and more and more young people invaded the villages. The village of Göreme was the special aim of this invasion. The motto was, "We are going to Göreme", Cappadocia was not yet talked about. As Turkish people are very inventive and good businessmen, guesthouses and bed and breakfast places shot up like mushrooms. People found out very quickly how easily you can turn old cave storerooms and stables into small accommodations for modest tourists – and make good money with them. The climax came in the summer of 1989. All guesthouses were booked out to the last corner. Up to six people shared one room and even the places to sleep on the roof terraces began to get scarce. But Cappadocia was never to experience such a boom again. For one reason, the travellers' expectations had changed and secondly, air traffic prices were falling rapidly, making much more exotic destinations accessible. And thus the number of people who spent their holidays here for a longer time decreased year after year. But the Cappadocians themselves, too, contributed to the decrease. Some of them were seduced into fleecing the tourists like sheep with the smallest possible effort. This led to a number of unpleasant occurrences, which of course

became instantly known in the community of backpackers. The unfamiliar ways of behaviour towards female tourists, who sometimes appeared quite unconventional under Anatolian conditions, repeatedly caused a lot of excitement. Turkish men were merciless in chatting up young women, no matter whether a boyfriend or a husband happened to be sitting next to them. But the naivety of many tourists was also not entirely blameless in that matter. What the Cappadocians did not notice, however, was the change that only became apparent very gradually. Increasingly, a different type of tourist began to appear. This type was no longer content with the simple and sometimes unacceptable conditions of the existing accomodations.
They demanded clean beds, shower facilities in all rooms and a higher standard. Many guesthouse
owners did not understand the world any more, as the goose with golden eggs, the tourist, had been content with their accomodations for years. Thus, not all of those who lived on tourism managed to accomplish a change. And quite a few who had hitherto been able to earn good money by tourism did not avoid sliding into disaster.Today the majority of the cheap and low-standard guest houses have disappeared and hotels and private boardinghouses have managed to adapt to the more critical demands of the visitors from the West.

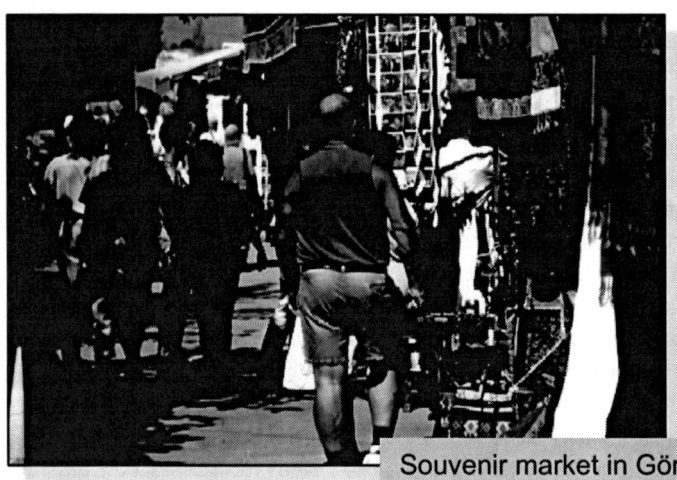

Souvenir market in Göreme

In the mid nineties, organized tourist business discovered Cappadocia. The number of tourist beds had increased without any limit on the coast and companies began to organize trips to the inner country. Apart from such bus excursions to Pamukkale and Konya, Cappadocia came into the companies' view. Accomodation for those 2 or 3 days' trips became necessary. Thus several large hotel complexes developed that were adapted to the special needs of short–term visitors. Their architecture was not always advantageous for the environment, as here, too, some wealthy Turkish people had been attracted by fast and easy money. And not a few of them became victims of miscalculation, as you can see from some half-finished buildings that have been offered for sale unsuccessfully for years. The trend towards the short-term visit in Cappadocia has continued up to the present day.Thus, up to a million visitors are counted every year. But many of those who have been here are toying with the idea of coming back to this fascinating landscape for a longer visit. Many of them did not know how to do this, as the information available to single travellers has been rather scarce. On the whole, apart from the tourist strongholds on the coast, Turkey has remained a strange and unknown country to many people.

Those who were here years ago as young persons can come back to Cappadocia without any problem. Things have changed, but you will be spared the shock of the coastal region here. 30 years of tourism have left their traces behind but they have not been able to destroy the charm of the landscape and the hospitality of the people.

Travel offers

For Cappadocia they exist like the sand of the sea: from VIP trips including a helicopter tour across the region and beluga caviar in the room at decent offers of over $1400 - to trips at a price of only a few hundred dollars, or even offers of a trip for free.

Yes, you are not mistaken: to Cappadocia for free! If you subscribed to a magazine and forgot to tick the box about passing on your data to others, and if you work in an academic profession, you will sooner or later hold such an offer in your hands. Big Turkish carpet companies buy customer lists in Europe and elsewhere and target potential customers by mail. It is perfectly clear how such a journey will be paid for afterwards.

88 Tourism

But also journeys which are offered for less than $900 or $1100 for 8 days must be treated with great care. Turkey, and especially Cappadocia, has not been a cheap travelling country any longer for years. Prices have risen considerably in the past 5 years.

With the following "translation" from a full-page advertisement we would like to demonstrate to you in what way an inexpensive holiday offer can nevertheless be profitable for a travel contractor. This 8 day's journey was offered under the title of "Fascinating Cappadocia" for $420 in 2008. Here is the description of the journey - and what will be waiting for you in reality:

1. Day: Journey to airport. Flight to Antalya. Welcome and transfer to hotel at the turkish Riviera	The first and the last day do not count, they are always travelling days. But – didnt't we want to go to Cappadocia, 800 km away from here
2. Day: town of the dancing dervishes. Trip to the former capital of the Seljuk empire, Konya. Near Aksaray you will visit the famous caravanserai of Sultanhane and the Mevlana Museum	You are still 300 km from Cappadocia, although you have been sitting in the coach all day. The Mevlana Museum is in Konya, not in Aksaray, and there are no real dancing dervishes on display here, either.
3. Day: The moon landscape of Cappadocia. Trip to the famous moon landscape and to the underground city of Kaymaklı. Sightseeing trip to Göreme with its many rock-carved churches	Arrived at last! But those 2 sights do not take the whole day. Will we be sitting on the bus again for 6 hours, or in one of Göreme's numberless souvenir shops
4. Day: The moon landscape of Cappadocia including a walk. Trip to the Valley of the Monks. Walk to the Zelve Valley. Visit of 3 different valleys and easy walk to the White Valley. Afterwards, visit to a carpet factory.	Aha, now the cat is out of the bag: moving around among various sights cannot be called a 'walk', as they are all within a radius of only 1 km. You will spend half a day in a carpet shop.
5. Day: Cappadocia – Antalya. Continuation of journey along the picturesque natural landscape of the Turkish Riviera	Amazing. We would call it a premature return trip. Again you are sitting on the bus for 12 hours, doing another 1000 km. You are looking at a landscape covered by giant hotels. Seaview is very rare

6. Day: Perge – Turkish Riviera. Trip to the famous ancient city of Perge. Followed by a visit to a typical turkish market and a waterfall as well as a jeweller's center. Opportunity to take part in a Turkish fashion show.	Perge, too is far away from Cappadocia. The writers have omitted the word 'super' in front of 'market',as this typical market is frequented by tourists only. And it is quite clear,too, what you are supposed to do in a jewellers shop.
7. Day: Day off for individual activitis or excursion (optional)	Oops, the travel agency is running out of ideas. Does this mean an excursion to another department store chain?
8. Day: Return flight to your home country	

Conclusion: you are in the most beautiful landscape of Cappacdocia for 1.5 days at a maximum. For the rest of the time you are sitting on the bus, travelling more than 2000 km, or you are somewhere else in the country. This is a pure sales promotion trip.

Above all it happens quite often that the tour guide does not get a dime for his work from his agency. He earns his money by taking the visitors to special shops with which he has arranged a certain fee beforehand.

It should be quite clear to any traveller that such a journey for $420 basically *has* to be sponsored by somebody. In any case, it is no cheap bargain. And the products offered must be over-priced to pay back the contractor's expenses.

A price from $1100 upwards for an 8 days' trip to Cappadocia can be regarded as a serious offer. But sometimes the meals and entrance fees are not included so that the real costs are over $1400. As mentioned, a serious journey to Cappadocia cannot be bought at a discount price.

So, before booking a journey to wonderful Cappadocia, please read the respective offer carefully.

Finally, a little bit of advertising for ourselves: We, the authors, arrange trips to Cappadocia, too, in the summer months. You will find group trips and creativity courses for groups of max. 8 persons, and individual offers for max. 4 participants on offer under **www. kappadokya-travel.com** on the internet.

Place for your own notices:

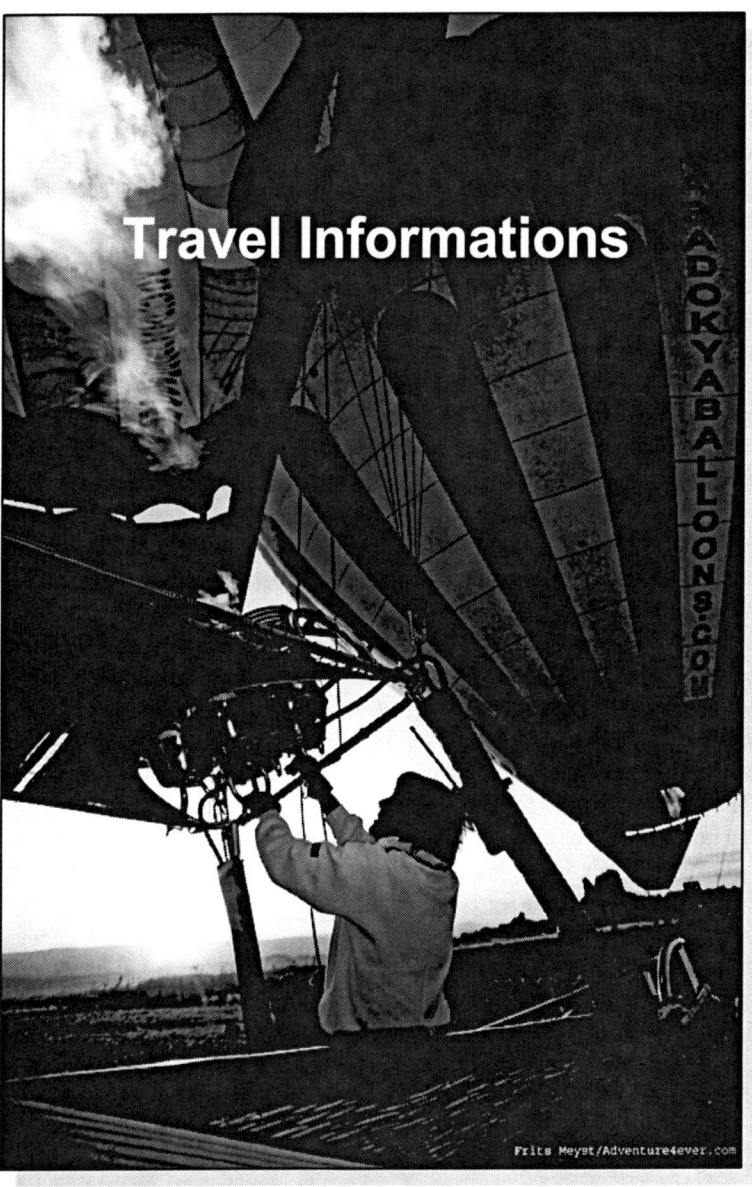

Foto: Kapadokya-Balloons

How to Get There

By Plane

Flying is the fastest and most comfortable way of getting to Cappadocia. Cappadocia even has its own airport near Gülsehir, but as this is only a few years old, it is not served very often yet and therefore is no real alternative. The nearest airport with scheduled services is in Kayseri, about 70 km from Cappadocia. Turkish Airlines THY (Türk Hava Yolari) serves Kayseri with 4 daily flights from Istanbul. Also from European cities there are daily services to Kayseri. If those direct flights should appear even cheaper to you at first sight, you are fatally wrong. The time of departure and arrival is often in the middle of the night. When the plane lands in Turkey at 3.00 a.m., the visitor will be lying in his bed not before 2 hours later, at 5.00 a.m. at the least. You can imagine vividly what the next day of your holiday will be like then. The complete costs of such flights are not entirely lower, either. At this time of the night there is no public transport available in both countries, which makes you depend on expensive taxi services.

Turkish Airways' scheduled flights via Istanbul are arranged in a way that you can take off in Europe at noon and arrive in Cappadocia in the evening. (For comparison: The flight from Kennedy Airport N.Y. departs at 12.20 and takes 11.5 hours to Istanbul.) The time taken changing planes in Istanbul mostly does not exceed 2.5 hours. The inexpensive transfer service that is offered by the airline for its flights is another advantage. This service is arranged by the "Argeus" travel agency on commission of THY and can be booked from your home via the internet. You can get to any hotel inside Cappadocia fast and safe for 15 TL per person with it.

If you do not want to use this transfer because you are flying with another airline you can take a taxi to the central bus terminal (Otogar) at 30 TL and from there change to the long-distance coach to Cappadocia, for another 10 TL. But remember: the last one leaves at 8.30 p.m. from Kayseri. Often booking the transfer service with your hotel or guest house can also be useful. Of course you can also reach Cappadocia from any other airport in Turkey by long-distance coach, but 10 to 13 hours of travelling time is not for everybody. This option is only recommended for those of you who want to combine the Cappadocia trip with a beach holiday at the seaside.

Nevertheless, we want to mention one variation for the friends of public transport. It simply seems appropriate to combine a trip to Cappadocia with several days in Istanbul. There are inexpensive night trains with sleeping cars form Istanbul to Kayseri. This journey is about 60 TL per person. You take the modern subway from Istanbul airport, change to the tramway at the "Aksaray" terminus and after crossing the Galata bridge reach the ferry terminal at Karaköy. From here you go by ferryboat to Haydarpaşa, the eastern station on the Asian shore.

Flight prices are different according to the season (vacations/holidays), where you start from and how early you book your trip. There is not much use hoping for last minute offers, on the contrary, early bookers are more likely to have price advantages.

Turkish Airline website with flight schedule: **www.thy.com**
Travel agency in Cappadocia for transfer
to and from Kayseri airport: **www.argeus.com.tr**

By Car

The following variations have one thing in common: they take time. If your holidays are shorter than 4 weeks, you should go by plane in any case. On all our journeys to Turkey we needed 4 days to get from North Germany to Cappadocia, without driving by night however. Only once did we do the distance from Düsseldorf to Avanos (3400 km), through former Yugoslavia, in 52 hours; this, however, nonstop in a VW bus and with 5 people, all of whom had a driving licence. 3 people were always asleep in the back, while in the front one was keeping the driver awake; drivers were exchanged every four hours. A strain like that is not recommended as, at least on the way back, all the effect of the holidays will be gone. Even though the greater part of the route has been enlarged into a motorway today, you should not take the reports of some of our Turkish fellow citizens seriously. They keep telling you that they have done the route in 2 days.

Three main routes lead into Turkey. On the first you travel through Hungaria (resp. Austria and Croatia), Serbia and Bulgaria, thus following the former Yugoslavian 'Autoput'.

As an alternative there is the sea route across the Adariatic Sea by the rather inexpensive Greek ferryboats that shuttle back and forth between Italy and Greece.
From Venice, Ancona and Brindisi the ships leave for Igoumenitsa in the north of Greece. We have always found the departure from Venice best. The price is almost the same as from Ancona and it saves you 300 km of driving. But you do not save any money, time or gas by using the ferry. The overland route across the Balkan peninsula is just as long as travelling via northern Greece. The ferryboat just gives you the opportunity to relax a bit in the middle of the way. On arriving in Venice or Ancona, after many hours of driving, a break of about 20 hours on board a rather luxurious ship is waiting for you. These ferries are equipped with almost every possible luxury, almost like cruise ships.

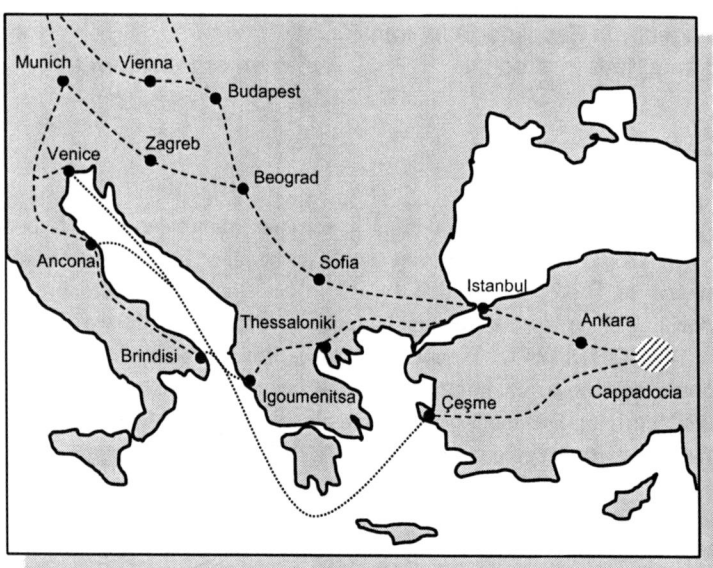

And there is a special highlight for all drivers of camping vehicles and minibuses; camping on deck. This means that you can spend the night in your own bed. Your vehicle will even get an electric hook-up of its own. However, this is only possible between May and December. These passages are offered by SUPERFAST-LINES, ANEK-LINES and MINOAN-LINES. Advance reservation is only recommended during the high travel season, that is, at Easter and in July and August. During the rest of the year you should book your passage on site to remain flexible and to be free to change your travelling plans at any time. If the ferryboat should be booked out in spite of everything, there will be another one next day. After all, a romantic night in Venice has its own charm, too. If you book the return journey as well, it will be cheaper by 30%, and you do not have to give an exact return date. Just enter "Open date" as your date of return.

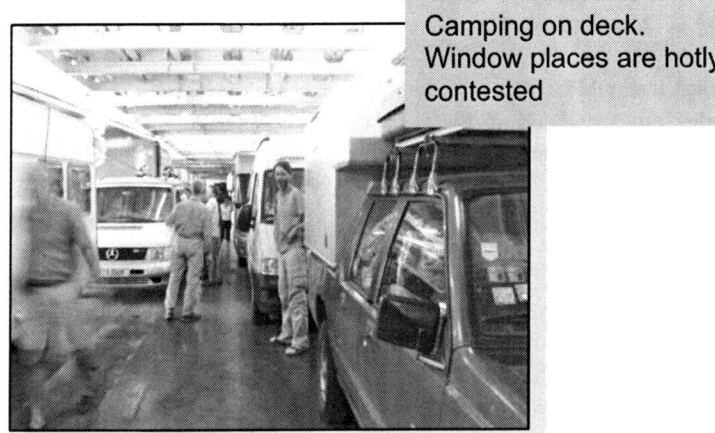

Camping on deck. Window places are hotly contested

The days when afterwards you had to crawl through northern Greece on windy, mountain pass roads behind queues of lorries for hours will soon be over. The Greeks are momentarily busy building a through motorway between Igoumenitsa and the Turkish border. But we will not put our hand into the fire for its completion date. After all, the planned route already appeared on our first map of Greece from 1980...

There is another ferry connection from Brindisi in the south of Italy to the seaside resort of Cesme near Izmir on the west coast of Turkey. The advantage is that Italian motorways are only sparsely frequented and can be used safely by night also. Additionally, they become cheaper the longer you drive on them. You pay about 20€ toll for the distance from the Brenner Pass to Venice, whereas to Brindisi it is only about 60€. After one and a half days of relaxing on board the ferry you arrive at Cesme by MARMARA-LINE and have still only got about 800 km of driving on comfortable roads ahead of

96 Travel Infomations

you. This ferry costs a bit more, however, and it only operates during the summer, and camping on deck is not possible.

The route via former Yugoslavia is open again meanwhile and the 'Autoput' of past times has lost its horror. The former concrete panel road with the typical rattle of its expansion joints has almost completely been replaced by motorways or ultra-modern roads.

For those who have a lot of time at their disposal, we should like to recommend the 'Eastern Bloc' route. Here you can plunge into another century while crossing Romania and Bulgaria - just to see how modern Turkey is. A serious warning notice: Watch out for free-roaming domestic pigs!

However, it should be clear to everybody that not all Eastern European transit countries are members of EU, and therefore cross-border controls can accordingly be strict, and the Euro has not been introduced in most of those countries.

Superfast-Ferries: www.superfast.com
Marmara-Lines: www.marmaralines.com
Minoan-Lines: www.minoan.gr
Anek-Lines: www.anek.gr

By Coach

TOURING company offers bus services to all big cities in Europe, among them to Istanbul. The passengers are picked up by various coaches all over Europe and are taken to Munich, where they have to change to a Turkish coach. The price is about $180 for one direction plus $40 for the ferrry from Italy to Greece. The journey can become a torture for people taller than 6 ft however, as the seats have been built for small sturdyTurkish people, and two and a half days on ergonomically unsuitable seats will make you get off the bus in Istanbul on all fours. We also must warn you of cut-price offers, as their safety standards are unsatisfactory and they can only be recommended to people who love long delays at the border. With tourist coaches however, the luggage will only seldom be checked and the customs officials mostly content themselves with a passport control on board of the coach.

Eurolines German Touring GmbH: www.touring.de

By Train

Gone are the days when the Istanbul Express departed from Munich. It fell victim to the war in Yugoslavia, as well as its counterpart, the Hellas Express, which went from Dortmund to Athens. There is no direct railway connection between middle Europe and Turkey any more.

One is overwhelmed by nostalgic memories of past times: we were young, we were keen on travelling, and the demands were moderate. Three days in a compartment of six, the luggage was tucked away under the seats, three people were thus able to sleep on those enlarged seats, two more unrolled their sandy camping mats and disappeared on the luggage racks.

Those who want to have railway romantics of such kind ought to travel via Eastern Europe. There are through carriages from Poland to Istanbul, and on their way through all Eastern European capitals they are gradually combined to form the Balkan Express. This means: long times of waiting, endless docking and undocking, and guaranteed delays of ten hours and more.

Cross-border trains to Turkey (Istanbul):

1. Balkan-Express	Belgrade (Serbia)	daily 7.50 am	(24h)
2. Bosfor-Express	Bucharest (Romania)	daily 12.00 am	(20h)
3. Dostluk-Express	Thessaloniki (Greece)	daily 7.40 pm	(13h)
4. Transasia-Express	Teheran (Iran)	Wednesday 8.00 pm	(67h)
5. Toros-Express	Aleppo (Syria)	Tuesday 7.20 am	(16h)

For wealthy people there is the variation of the sleeper car train. It runs from Villach, Austria, to Endirne, the first big city behind the Turkish border. Sleeping cars and couchette coaches are available. But more than $1800 for a return ticket for a family of four and a motorcar is quite a lot of money.

Travelling by train inside Turkey is a more appealing idea. There are regular night trains from Istanbul to the east of the country, which stop at Kayseri, with sleeper cabins for 2 persons available to the traveller. There is always a restaurant car in the middle of the train where the passenger is served typical local meals at reasonable prices. While you are still enjoying one of the many sugar-sweet Turkish desserts, your train attendant has already prepared the beds. However, the train needs 18 hours to Cappadocia so that there is enough time to put yourself in the right mood for the Anatolian highlands.

A famous webside about the
travelling by train worldwide: **www.seat61.com**

Turkish Public Railway: **www.tcdd.gov.tr**

Optima-Tours, car sleeper trains: **www.optimatours.de**

For people who love extravagance,
or if money is unimportant: **www.orient-express.at**

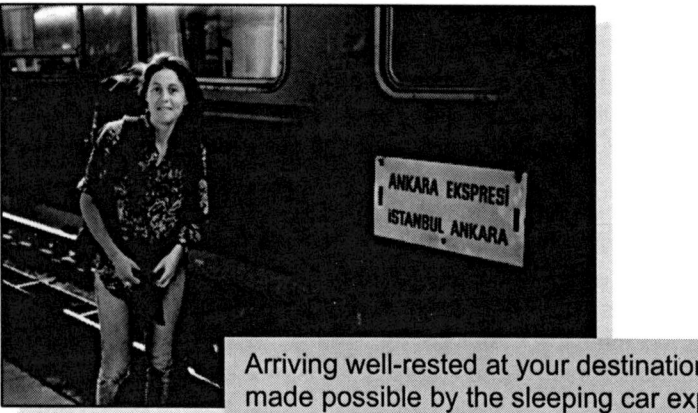

Arriving well-rested at your destination is made possible by the sleeping car express

Other Possibilities

There are no limits for those. On our journeys we have even met people who were travelling by bicycle. Most of them, however, were on their way through to more distant destinations. But we have also met people who had come hitchhiking from Europe or who were travelling on foot. Dealing with the problems of this method of traveling would however go beyond the scope of this book.Therefore we can only advise you to get suitable information from respective technical literature or from specialized magazines. Information is also available from related hiking or cycling clubs.

Entry Requirements

Entry requirements vary. For example, when entering without a vehicle, German citizens only need an ID card that must be valid for at least three months. Children need a children's ID card. This enables you to stay in the country for up to three months without a visa.

Travellers from other European nations are partly subject to different regulations. Travellers from Austria for example have to have a passport and must buy a visa for $20 at the airport. Persons from the Netherlands only have to show their 'Identiteitscard' and pay $15 for their entry permit.

Please ask for information about the entry requirements valid for your nationality prior to your journey!

Those who enter the country by private car must be able to produce a passport. Additionally, a green international insurance card for your vehicle is required, which your insurance company will send you for free. Besides, a national driver's licence and a registration certificate are sufficient. A "Carnet de Passage" is not necessary for Turkey. By all means you should have photocopies of those documents with you and keep them stored separately. If the originals should be lost, they are very helpful for the consulates in replacing them.

On your arrival in the customs building, the police will first check your passports and affix their stamps in them. Then it is the customs officials' turn. They mostly show very little to absolutely no interest
in the cargo of tourist vehicles. Finally, the data of your car are registered in the computer and the owner's passport gets another stamp with a serial number and the date on which you have to take the car out of the country again written in it. Please notice that you are only allowed to leave the car inside the country for a maximum of **180** days. Each extra day will cost you a fortune in penalty fees.

Dogs must have an international vaccination certificate, with a vaccination against rabies attested in it. The vaccination must have been made at least 11 days before the entry, and it must also be valid for at least 3 months. Additionally, an official veterinary certificate of health must be shown which – believe it or not – must not be older than **24 hours**. Those who enter the country by plane may be able to cope with this, but car drivers will be in a bad fix now. If you know your entry date in advance, just ask your official veterinary to predate the certificate. Most veterinaries will understand this. We have entered Turkey with our dog many times, and practical reality was always completely different. Only once did a customs official ask for the vaccination certificate. He soon noticed that he could not make sense of it and very politely asked us about the dog's name, which was written distinctly on the cover. He gave us back the document, remarking that this was indeed a charming animal, and wished us a good journey. Apart from that, no customs official has ever shown any interest in the dog in all those years.

By the way, microchipping will be compulsory for your four-legged darling in EU countries from 2011 onwards.

What is one allowed to bring into the country? Basically, all items that are meant for personal use, except illegal drugs, of course. Camping articles, camera equipment, a video camera or a laptop computer do not pose a problem. With professional electronical equipment things are a little bit different, however. It can be brought into the country, but everything is registered in the passport and has to be shown again on leaving the country.

Hunting weapons can be brought into the country, but the necessary permit must be applied for at the Turkish Consulate before starting the journey.

Again and again there are people who toy with the idea of exporting their vehicle to Turkey and then refinancing the holiday costs with the revenue of the sale. TheTurkish customs authorities put a powerful stop to such ideas and intentions. Firstly, the vehicle must not be older then 6 years, and secondly, the customs authority collects 100% of duty (on the basis of the value as new). There cannot thus be any question of profit any more.

Presents for friends at a value of $420 ($205 for children under 15) may be brought into the country duty-free. Please always have the sales receipts with you. Foreign and Turkish currencies may be brought into the country at an unlimited amount and taken out up to a value of $9000. But you should be able to produce exchange vouchers for the amounts carried with you in Turkish Lira on demand of the customs officials.

What should be observed when leaving the country

You should under no circumstances allow yourself to be induced to take illegal drugs out of the country. The penalties for this are extremely harsh and always consist of a stay of several years at the expense of the State of Turkey. Turkish prisons are notorious for their exorbitant luxuries: running water on the walls, fresh air through missing window panes, which is especially nice in the winter, and an excellent entertainment program presented by 40 fellow prisoners in one prison cell are part of the standard procedure.

The export of antiques is also a ticklish subject. Press reports about so-called robbers of antique stones probably have helped to sensitize you to a certain degree. Here again, arrest warrants were imposed. Directly inside the Archeological Museum of Nevsehir there is an outpost of the Turkish Antiquities Authority. If in doubt, ask for information there and make them write out an export permit. Finally, a last tip: not everything that you are allowed to export from Turkey is also permitted to be imported into your home country. Especially the guidelines for the protection of exotic animals and plants are to be observed here. For further questions, please contact the WWF or a customs official of your confidence.

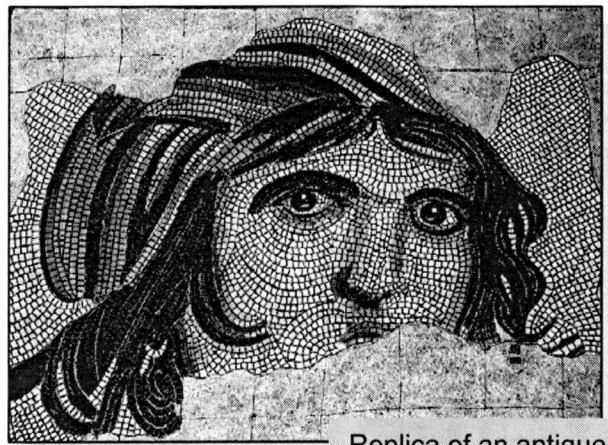
Replica of an antique mosaic

Through the country

By Car

When we first travelled to Turkey in the mid 1980s, we were among the fastest travellers on the road with our old VW bus, as they had only started building up a local car industry in the country some years before. You were always overtaking old Russian motorcycles, rickety Fiat remakes and lorries which shifted into first gear on even the smallest slope, transforming their surplus energy into loud noise right away. This has been over for a long time. Here, too, the Japanese are capturing the market. And whenever we roll along obediently on a Turkish country road at the prescribed speed of 90 km/h (55 mph) today, we feel like a moving traffic block. The country's boom of the past few years can be seen from the masses of motor vehicles on the roads. And these are not only inexpensive compact cars; there are also lots and lots of luxury cars that join the throng on the roads.

The rising numbers of new registrations have led to a rapid deterioration of secondhand car prices. Now, especially the young and inexperienced Turkish drivers buy an old and rusty Murat or Tofas of domestic production. Often they cannot afford the maintenance of such cars, and so all they do is make their own town quarters unsafe with them. For many of those young people the power of the car's stereo equipment seems to be more important than the roadworthiness of the car itself - a trend which fortunately is on the decline in the rest of Europe. But the technical control board of Turkey, which has been in existence since 2008, is busy finishing off those old rust-buckets.

All Turkish drivers are impatient in front of traffic lights. As soon as the lights have started changing from red to 'light' green, you will hear a massive chorus of horns behind you.

Meanwhile, Turkey has an excellent road network, whose ordinary roads are being enlarged to four lanes at the moment. Motorway construction is making rapid progress in the whole country. Motorways can be identified by their green roadsigns and their design is European standard or even better. Road construction has meanwhile become one of Turkey's export hits.

Things are more difficult with the little side roads, as they are found in Cappadocia. Due to the annual frost there are always lots of large potholes. Careful driving is highly recommended especially in spring, as the road construction and maintenance authorities (Karayolari) are not able to repair all side roads immediately. But in the summer everything has been mended again, and in the course of the years the roads look as if thousands of differently coloured carpets have been spread out on them. The relative instability of the roadbed of those roads is a more severe problem for the critical European (or American) driver. The road seems to be permanently moving, it seems to camber and to wrinkle up like a badly laid carpet. A preliminary check of the car's shock absorbers is called for here. Roads marked in red and yellow on your roadmap can be used well without restriction. You should avoid those in white, except if you are the proud owner of an SUV and have the appropriate driving experience.

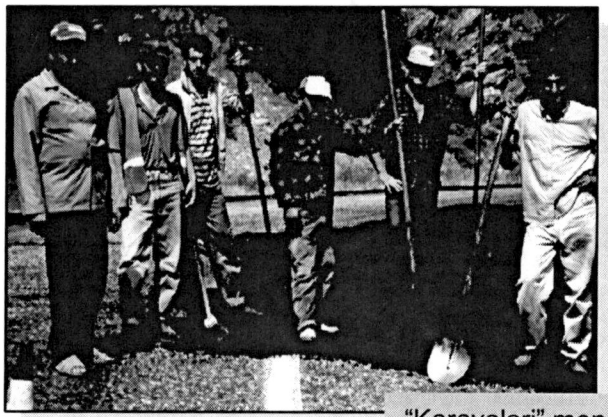

"Karayolari" men at work

Apart from that, the same traffic regulations apply as in your home country. The speed limit is 50 km/h in built-up areas, 90 on normal roads and 130 km/h on motorways. There is an absolute ban on alcohol for drivers in Turkey. Even though foreigners are never checked here in Cappadocia, they should avoid consuming alcoholic drinks or should restrict themselves to one glass of beer or wine.

There is also mandatory seat belt wearing, requirement to wear a helmet and to have two breakdown triangles on board. All these things seem to be completely unknown to the Turkish driver. He does not even possess a single warning triangle in most cases. A substitute for that is a heap of stones in front of his car, which raises the suspicion it is rather a protective wall for his own car than a warning for others. Those piles of stones are not taken away afterwards, either, but are left behind as excellent barricades on the roads for weeks after.

Another warning is necessary against unlighted horse-drawn vehicles or unlighted trailers or tractors at night. On the whole one should be very careful at night, as again and again even big animals cross the roads, not to mention people who have had one too many from the Raki bottle.

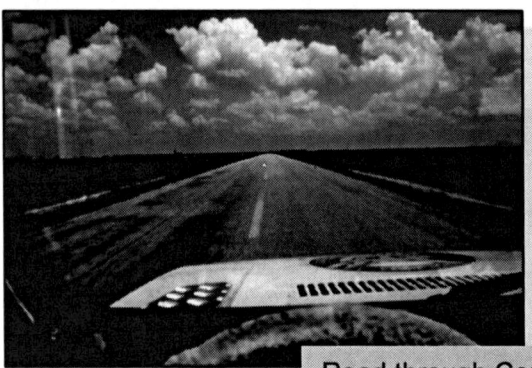
Road through Central Anatolia

Also road construction sites, which are sometimes miles long, turn out to be excellent road obstructions. First, molten tar is sprayed on the old road surface for some miles, with the traffic going on as usual. If your car needs a new underbody coating, you should step on the gas properly here. But be careful, this is slippery stuff. Afterwards, gravel is distributed over it and rolled in only slightly, expecting the wheels of the cars to finish the job of compressing. On such parts of the road the motto is: keep your distance, and drive slowly. On one occasion a heavy truck managed to shoot a hole the size of an egg into our minibus, right below the windscreen.

As mentioned before, motor traffic has increased rapidly during the past few years. This makes itself felt particularly in bigger towns. But when driving long distances, you sometimes seem to be all on your own on the road. The exorbitant fuel prices, which are even higher than those in Western Europe, are the reason for this. If you consider the average income of Turkish people, which is much lower, these prices are practically unaffordable to the normal consumer, so that he mostly will refrain from long distance trips.

The quality of fuel is excellent, but it is nevertheless still advisable to buy fuel only at bigger filling stations. Owners of small gas stations sometimes tend to dilute their fuel. By the way, "Diesel" is called "Motorin" in Turkey.

Just a word about the American tyre pressure machines. They use "psi" as a working unit, 14.5 psi corresponding to 1 bar. You choose the desired pressure and put the hose on the tyre valve, and immediately the machine starts working until the requested pressure has been reached.

If you are involved in a car accident with either damage of persons or of property, always call the police and make them take it down on record. Otherwise it could happen that your insurance company will refuse to accept your claim. Moreover, damaged tourist vehicles always arouse the interest of the police, and then it is very useful to be able to show the police report.

If a total loss or even something worse has happened, it is very advantageous to be an AAA or ARC member and to have international travel cover. This saves you a lot of trouble with the customs authorities if your car has to be scrapped. The international travel cover also includes the return transport of your car and the possible return transport of injured persons – a thing that, most hopefully, will never happen.

As for the problem of car theft, we can assure you that you can leave your car behind at any time without worrying. Just always make sure that it is locked! Firstly, doors left open invite thieves and secondly, children are very fond of playing car-driving. On one occasion we forgot to lock our car, too, and our windscreen blotched with spit on the inside bore witness of an exciting imaginary car ride afterwards. But not a single thing had been stolen.

Traffic signs and their colours:

Green:	signs on public motorways
Blue:	long distance signs
White (outside built-up areas):	signs for small villages
White (inside built-up areas):	town quarters or important institutions
Brown:	tourist sights
Orange:	road maintenance authority signs

American Automobil Association - AAA: www.aaa.com
Europe Automobil Association   - ARC: www.arceurope.com

By Motorcycle

To motorcyclists, we advise the greatest possible caution. Turkish traffic has a very hierarchical structure. Way up on the top there are the long-distance coaches and trucks, and in this order cycles come directly behind donkey carts. Almost no Turk would ride a motorbike if he was able to afford a car. Therefore, motorcyclists are an inferior social class that is looked down upon. Additionally, again and again there are objects lying on the roads: rocks, branches of trees, relics of road construction sites or only just parts of cars that have been lost. Turkey provides lots of dream routes for motorcyclists with serpentine roads and continuous ups and downs, but – PLEASE DO be careful!

You should never leave your motorcycle unobserved, either. Not because it might be stolen - but children always have a lot of fun climbing into the seat, putting everything in disorder, and rubber lashing straps can make excellent slingshots. At night, too, when you are putting up at an accommodation, you should take all objects with you that can be removed without using tools.

By Rented Vehicles

In Göreme and in Ürgüp there are numerous rental agencies which provide various kinds of vehicles. The most common type is the miniscooter, which however is already rather overloaded with two passengers on certain hills. Those scooters can be rented by the hour, but also by the day. The longer the rental period is, the more the price can be negotiated. Prices vary considerably, especially in the off-peak season.

The technical reliability of the vehicles is not very good, however, and you should check the vehicle carefully before starting. You should rather keep your hands off the Chinese models, which are cheaper as a rule, as they are unreliable and are real gas-guzzlers. Inexperienced moped riders should proceed very carefully and slowly at the beginning, as the road condition, which is sufficient for car drivers, demands considerable attention of the miniscooterist. Bumps in the road and potholes, which flourish especially at the edges of the road, are not altogether unperilous for the overloaded vehicles and for their passengers. The rental fee is mostly due on signing the hiring contract, plus 50 TL of bail money, and a passport must be handed in. A driver's licence is not required.

For aficionados of German 'Eastalgia', there are sometimes 'MZ' motorcycles of Turkish production on offer. In 1993 a Turkish businessman bought the brand name together with the complete production equipment and restarted production very successfully in Istanbul. In contrast to the miniscooters, there must exist a licence for motorcycles for these. If you rent a car from one of the small rental firms, you should also check the appropriate technical condition of the vehicle. Of course one should refrain from being too pernickety here. The cars are in running condition, the brakes and the steering are in working order, that must do. Even if AAA safety fanatics strike up a howl of protest now, we are in Turkey and so we will just drive a bit slower and more carefully than usually. People who have problems with that, for them there are the big European car rental companies, "AVIS" and "Eurocar", at Ürgüp, but rental prices are significantly higher there. However, you can also book the car from your home country already.

"Görtour" near the bus terminal in Göreme offers a special treat: years ago the owner had his 1973 Ford M 20 altered into a convertible and also offers it for hire. Members of the Technical Control Board should not hire it, but apart from that it is great fun, isn't it?

By Long-distance Coaches

Turkey has a giant closely-meshed bus network that covers the whole nation. It makes travelling from one corner of the country to the other possible without any problems. Atatürk, the founding father of the Republic of Turkey, regarded improving the infrastructure of the country as fundamentally important and thus attached absolute priority to building roads. The railway network was largely financed by the German Empire, and the young Republic could not afford any further enlargement. Thus, huge numbers of tracks and roads were pushed every which way all across Asia Minor. This gave some clever entrepreneurs the idea of starting private bus lines which connected the big cities with each other.Thus it happened that all long-distance bus lines have been privately owned up to the present day. Today their number is almost uncountable. Just a visit to the central bus terminals of Ankara or Istanbul gives you an impression of the abundance of offers. The ticket office stalls spread along the huge halls in an endless row, with the smaller bus lines even sharing stalls with each other. From the enormous size of those bus terminals it can be seen how important the bus is as a means of transport. No airport terminal in Turkey is so huge. Thus, the bus terminals are designed like airport terminals: the departure gates are upstairs, below them are the arrivals, and at the very bottom there is the service and repair sector. The coach terminals of the smaller Cappadocian towns are a lot more unobtrusive, though.

The coaches are mostly almost new vehicles, which are serviced with meticulous care. Because of the fierce competition the companies cannot afford any inconveniences to the passengers or even any accidents. Nevertheless reports of bad accidents with Turkish long-distance coaches are frequent in the European media. In this case you must imagine that hundreds of these vehicles are on their way through this huge country day and night, 365 days a year. Additionally there is the fact that buses have no special lanes or paths like railways, and thus frequently come into conflict with other road users. With about 10,000 tours per year, some of them will end in serious accidents, which are seized upon eagerly by the media. In any case it cannot be said that bus driving in Turkey is highly dangerous.

Travelling by bus is also so popular because the price-performance ratio is second to none. Bus lines are punctual, connections are fast and quick, and the prices are affordable to Turkish people. Competition simply enlivens the market. A trip of 800 km from Istanbul to Cappadocia thus costs only about $40.

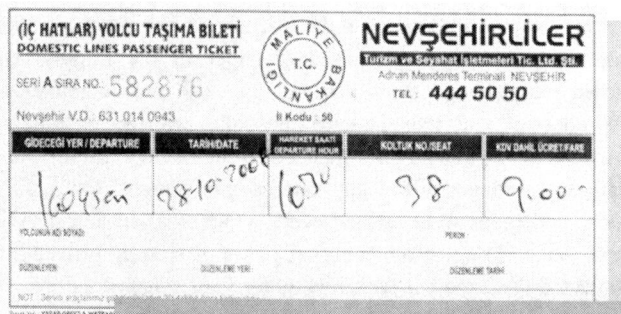

Bus ticket with information about: destination / date / time of departure / seat number and price

Travel Informations 109

How do you get to Cappadocia, now? At the bus terminal of any larger town of some size you go to the office of one of the Cappadocian bus companies, NEVŞEHIR-SEYAHAT, NEVŞEHIR-METRO or KENT. Having bought a ticket there, you then go to the platforms and select the platform (Peron) that is printed on the ticket. The coaches of the selected line mosty arrive there at hourly intervals. Your seat number is on the ticket, too.

The reason why you should not in any circumstances book a ticket with a different bus line is that you will be getting on the bus in the afternoon or in the early evening and you will reach Cappadocia in the middle of the night. Other bus lines will drop you off just somewhere in the pitch dark countryside. Not so with the recommended bus companies. Perhaps you will have to change to a minibus in Nevşehir, but it will take you to your destination, and that is included in the fare. Furthermore, the bus terminal of your destination will be open all night, there are taxicabs on site and you will always find people who can help you to find accomodation.

The trip from Ankara to the provincial capital of Nevşehir takes about 4 hours, from Antalya, 10 hours, and from Istanbul it is about 12 hours. In Nevsehir all passengers are put on various minibuses, which take about half an hour. Contact the bus personnel and say distinctly to which place you want to be taken, as the big bus also goes to various other places. These are mostly Uçhisar, Göreme, Çavuşin and Avanos.

Just a word of advice: women should always get a seat by the window, protected from the curious eyes of the male passengers, or always in the front rows and together with another woman. If you happen to fall asleep on the trip and sink into the arms of a stranger, that would be rather embarrassing – for both of you.

Websites of the Cappadocian long-distance bus lines:

NEVŞEHIR-SEYAHAT: www.nevsehirseyahat.com.tr
KENT: www.kentturizm.com.tr
NEVŞEHIR-METRO: www.metroturizm.com.tr

Survey map of bus lines inside Cappadocia

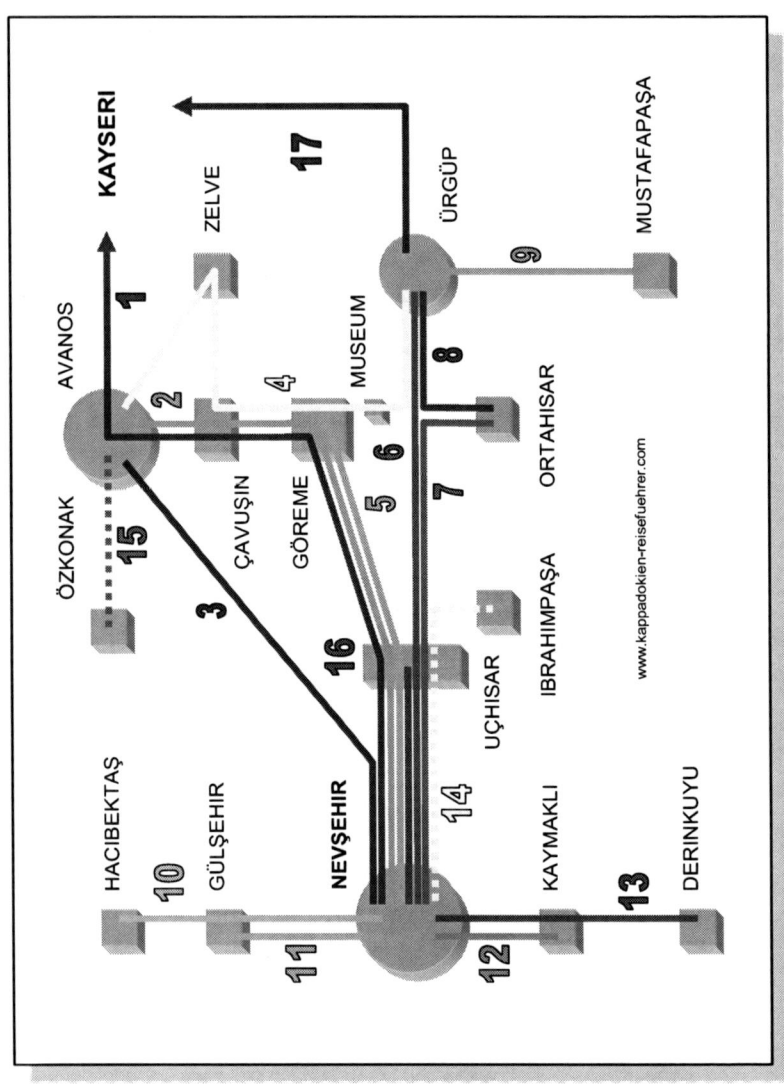

Travel Informations 111

	Connection from - to	Interval	Departure from	Terminals
1	**Nevşehir** – Kayseri*	60 Min.	00	00
2	**Avanos** – Çavuşin - Göreme – Uçhisar - Nevşehir	60 Min.	00	00
3	**Avanos** - Nevşehir	60 Min.	30	30
4	**Avanos** – Zelve – Çavuşin – Göreme**- Ürgüp	120 Min.	00 every uneven hour	00 every even hour
5	**Göreme** - Nevşehir	30 Min.	30 / 00	30 / 00
6	Ürgüp - Nevşehir	15 Min.		
7	**Ortahisar** - Nevşehir	60 Min.	00	00
8	**Ortahisar** - Ürgüp	30 Min.	30 / 00	30 / 00
9	**Mustafapaşa** - Ürgüp	60 Min.	45	15
10	Hacıbektaş - Gülşehir- Nevşehir	60 Min.	00	00
11	**Gülşehir** - Nevşehir	30 Min.	30 / 00	30 / 00
12	**Kaymakli** - Nevşehir	15 Min.		
13	**Derinkuyu** – Kaymakli - Nevşehir	60 Min.	30	00
14	Ibrahimpaşa – Nevş.	irregular	3 times	per day
15	**Özkonak** - Avanos	60 Min.	00	30
16	**Uçhisar***** - Nevşehir	30 Min.	30 / 00	30 / 00
17	**Ürgüp** - Kayseri	60 Min.	00	00

*) also stops at Uçhisar, Göreme, Çavuşin and Avanos
**) only stops at the crossroads at the museum, no stop at bus terminal
***) only bus which stops in the town centre, all other stop at the ring road

Place names **in bold print**: municipality is owner of the bus line

By Lokal Buslines

If you change from a long-distance coach to a Cappadocian local bus, you will time travel back into the 1980s. Away with onboard service and air conditioning; instead, we have loud noise, lots of draught and unfailing contact with potholes. Uniform colour or serial bus numbers will not be found, and the destination is mostly written on a small sign fixed behind the windscreen. The enormous difference in technical standards can be explained by the fact that these bus lines are operated by the individual communes or towns, whose treasury is often a bit hard up. Therefore the vehicles are used until they fall to pieces, trying to invest as little money as possible for them.

And thus almost every municipality in Cappadocia has its own buses which connect the township with the provincial capital of Nevsehir. People who want to go to Ürgüp, for example, should watch out for the bus with the legend "Ürgüp Belediye" (municipal administration of Ürgüp) on its side panel.

All bus lines end in Nevsehir at the crossroads to Lale Caddesi in the town centre (see city map of Nevsehir, page 237). Some smaller bus companies have their offices and waiting rooms there. The local lines do not stop at the bus terminal directly. If you are coming from Ürgüp; Göreme or Avanos and want to continue travelling by long-distance coach, you get off after the big crossroads in front of the 'Tansaş' supermarket or the 'Total' filling station and go down the hill towards the ring road for about 100 m to the bus terminal.

The public local bus system is not so inflexible, however, as we know it from Europe. The buses represent a good mixture of a scheduled bus system with fixed departure times and ramshackle bus shelters, but nevertheless you can thumb down a bus en route like a dolmus. Your luggage is stowed away under the floor in the luggage department as in the long-distance coaches, and there is always someone who helps you with it. Tickets are bought from the conductor during the journey, who makes his tour through the bus just like in the old days. It can take him a while to get through to you, especially at peak time. And please, have the necessary change at the ready, as you will cause embarrassment to him with larger banknotes. There is often no conductor on smaller buses. There you pay the driver on getting off the vehicle.

Travel Informations 113

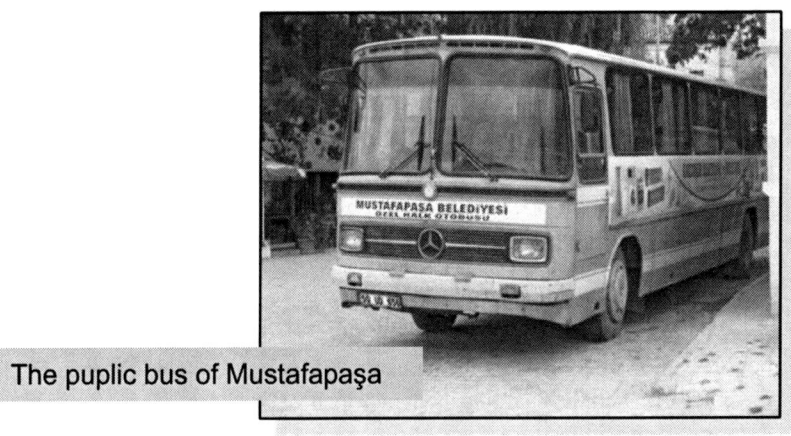

The puplic bus of Mustafapaşa

The departure times given here by us in this chapter are valid from 8.00 a.m. to 6.00 p.m daily from Monday to Friday. You should ask for information about later departures and winter or Sunday schedules well in advance. Especially during the last tour of the day, the times and the route are handled rather liberally by the driver. And during the fasting month of Ramasan there is no stopping him at all any more when, in the evening, the end of fasting is drawing near.

Bus Schedule (line 2 and 4) from :

Avanos	to	Nevşehir	Avanos	to	Ürgüp
No. 2 Every 60 min	direction Nevşehir	direction Avanos	No. 4 every 2 hours	direction Ürgüp	direction Avanos
Avanos	.00	.30	Avanos	.00	.40
Çavuşin	.15	.20	Zelve	.10	.30
Göreme	.20	.15	Göreme	.20	.20
Uçhisar	.25	.10	Museum	.25	.15
Nevşehir	.35	.00	Ürgüp	.40	.00

Accommodations

It is easy to find accommodation in Cappadocia. When the first tourists invaded Cappadocia in large numbers in the mid-eighties, numerous boardinghouses were opened. After some years they were followed by the first hotels. Today there are so many tourist beds that you can always find a room even in the peak season; perhaps not in the chosen lodging house, but there will always be similar accommodation only a few hundred yards away from it. The supply is manifold, from five star hotels to simple boarding houses with shared toilets on the landings. Prices are also wide-ranging. First there are the simple boarding houses which offer a bed in a community dormitory from $7 per night, and at the top end there is a hotel which offers its best suite for $1220 per night. The distinction between a hotel and a boarding house is not always clear in Cappadocia, as there are no definite limits between both, especially since so-called 'boutique hotels' have become increasingly popular in Turkey. They combine the characteristics of a small boarding house with the service of a big hotel, but without being categorized with stars. Their room rates are only somewhat higher than those of the boardinghouses. As most of these hotels were built within the past ten years, they were forced to adapt to the stricter town planning preservation rules and therefore had to adopt the local architectural style. Because of this, now and again little enchanted complexes, as if from 'The Arabian Nights', were built, composed of historic rows of houses with caves in them or even with real cave rooms for the guests. But it must be said that generally boardinghouses are cheaper. And, let us be honest, who is a greater help in the case of problems or questions, a benevolent hostel owner or a stressed and underpaid hotel receptionist?

In this travel guide we have avoided mentioning those hotels in which travel groups from the seaside are accommodated, because there is nothing worse than being awakened at eight in the morning by a noisy group of sun-seeking tourists on their way to the breakfast room or than being forced to inhale the diesel soot of warming up tourist coaches. Similarly, we could not list all hostels in Cappadocia which offer rooms. This book would have become a lot more voluminous then, as there are said to be more than 200 hotels and boardinghouses in the area. In any case you should ask to be shown the room before checking in, even though the times have gone by when the bedclothes were turned inside out instead of washing them. Ask about vaulted rooms or even a cave room. Such rooms convey a good impression of the old Cappadocian style of living without having to do without the conveniences of our modern century.

In the third part of this travel guide - called " Sights and Places" - you will find a list of places of accommodation with each town or village, and under the description of each there is a bar with figures and abbreviations.

And here is an explanation of this codification:

The first number is for finding the accommodation on the town map. After that there is the price per night for a double room for 2 persons in TL, including breakfast. The third specification refers to the size of the place and lists the number of double rooms available. The signs 🍽 and 🍸 stand for a restaurant or a small bar in the house. E – F – D or other letters stand for the foreign languages spoken by the personnel. The number code in the last column refers to various details and amenities (see below).

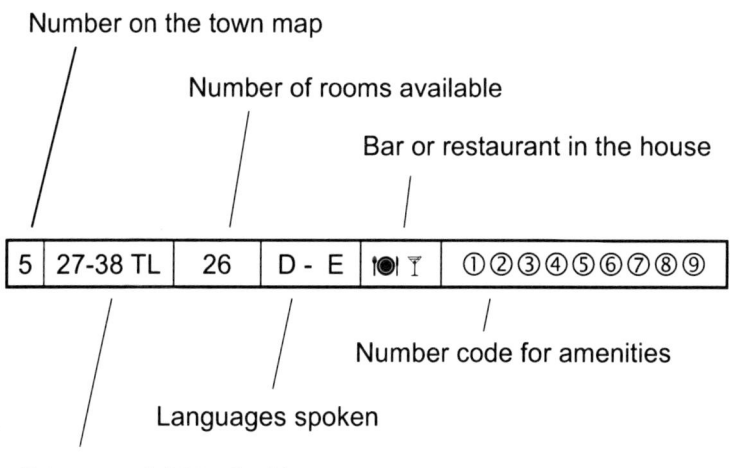

116 Travel Infomations

Letter code for languages spoken:

E	English		NL	Dutch
F	French		I	Italian
D	German		TR	Turkish only

The equipment details are represented by a number code:

① - open all year
② - historic building
③ - partly with cave rooms
④ - with swimming pool
⑤ - with central heating
⑥ - international TV available
⑦ - access to internet
⑧ - with washing machine or laundry services
⑨ - not all rooms with shower or WC

Camping

Turkish people are far from connecting this term with a philosophy of life, as some other people do. They would never crawl under a flapping cloth cover to stay there for a night and then proudly tell themselves what great nature enthusiasts they are. You only go to a camping site if you cannot afford to stay in a hotel or guest house. And even there you rent something in a house. Thus many camping grounds consist instead of a conglomeration of plain little houses. Often such sites are also frequented by day trippers. What the Turks love above all other things is a picnic out in the open and thus some camping grounds have hardly any room for tents any more because of all the barbecue sites. Turkish people travelling by caravan or campervan hardly exist. Accordingly, the choice of camping sites is very small. Cappadocia is an exception, as there are no less than 8 camping grounds within a radius of 10 km here.

Before we introduce the individual camping sites, a word on 'wild' camping. Basically this is possible wherever it is not prohibited by special signs. There are many farm tracks or field cart roads at whose side you can put up your tent, or in other dusty open spaces. Owners of campervans should always remember not to obstruct the way, otherwise the night could be very short, as there will always be a tractor passing by at five o'clock in the morning. You should also be prepared for a short visit of curiosity in the evenings. Be nice to the people in spite of the disturbance, as the owner of the piece of land could be among them.

A word about the camping gas supply: the Turkish gas cylinder system is not compatible with the European system. Owners of campervans should make sure that their gas cylinders are full before starting on a journey.

Now, some details about the camping grounds, with all prices being in Turkish Lira and the fees for one campervan plus two persons:

➢ PANORAMA-CAMPING (Göreme)

Little terraced site above the road from Göreme to Uchisar. As the name says, you have a marvellous view over Göreme from here and there is even a small pool. The trees, too, have grown a little during the past 15 years, so that there are some shady places. The way to the village is only short, but steep. The position closely above the public road which has some traffic even at night is a disadvantage, and unfortunately the site has been around for quite some time. Price: 20 TL.

Phone: 0090 384 271 2352
Fax :   0090 384 271 2632
E-mail: panoramacamping@hotmail.com

➢ BERLIN-CAMPING (Göreme)

This site is at the northern end of Göreme. It provides some shade, and there is enough room for camping vehicles. The site is ideal for nightbirds, who want to enjoy Göreme's party scene. You are only 5 minutes walking distance from the town centre, where the bars and discos are. The shopping distance is also short enough for campers without vehicles. Price: 24 TL.

Phone: 0090 384 271 2249

➤ KAYA-CAMPING (Göreme – Ortahisar)

By far the best local camping site. Unfortuately, it is quite remote from all towns or villages. But therefore perhaps the best site for lovers of nature and quietness. There is almost no traffic on the narrow road to it at nighttime. As the place is situated very high, there is an excellent view over the surrounding hills and valleys from it, which turn deep red in the setting sun. The site has modern and clean sanitary facilities and a restaurant and a small shop are connected. Everywhere there are large shady trees, and there is also a swimmingpool. Coming from Göreme, you follow the signs for the museum, drive past it and then up the mountain on the extremely steep serpentine road. It is about 2.5 km from Göreme to the camping site. Drivers of car-trailer combinations are recommended to approach the site from the opposite direction. This means that coming from the Ürgüp – Nevsehir road, near Ortahisar you follow the roadsigns towards Göreme. Price: 30 TL.

Phone: 0090 384 343 3100 or 3983
Fax: 0090 384 343 3984
E-mail: kayacamping@www.com

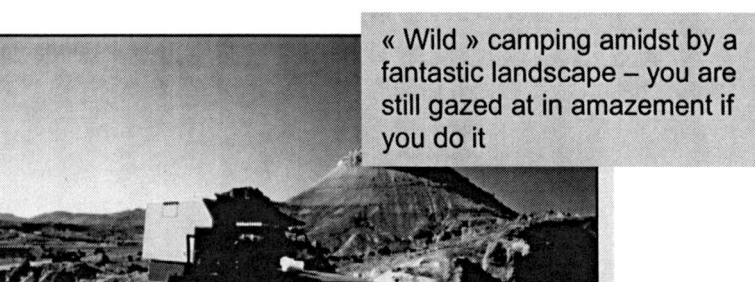

« Wild » camping amidst by a fantastic landscape – you are still gazed at in amazement if you do it

➢ ADA-CAMPING (Avanos)

A somewhat larger site near Avanos, separated from the river by only a narrow reed belt and secluded from any through traffic. The site has some shady trees but a highlight is the large pool, which is 25 meters long. Once a week the water is exchanged by means of a nearby well. This site is ideal for a couple of lazy days by the water and for sunbathing. It can get somewhat noisier during the day, as the pool is also used by non-campers who pay an entrance fee. But the fee is so high that only well-off Cappadocians can afford this luxury. There is also a small restaurant which belongs to it. As the site is somewhat out of the way, you need about 10 to 15 minutes of walking to get to the village. Fans of fishing are in good hands here, as the adjacent river is full of fish and a fishing permit is not necessary.

The owner takes 20 TL per night and keeps his site open from April to October.

Phone: 0090 384 511 2429
E-mail: info@adacampingavanos.com
Web : www.adacampingavanos.com

➢ GREEN HOTEL (Cavusin)

This camping site belongs to a motel. Unfortunately, despite the name, there is very little green there and shade is a rarity, but the price of 6 TL per person cannot be beaten in all of Cappadocia. If you need electricity for your camping van, you pay another 5 TL for it. Without electricity, tents and all kinds of vehicles can be put up for free.

Phone: 0090 384 532 7050
Fax: 0090 384 532 7032
E-mail: info@motelgreen.com
Web : www.motelgreen.com

120 Travel Infomations

> **SEVIN ROCK HOUSE (Göreme)**

As with the Green Motel, here also the owner of the guest house offers the possibility of camping in his spacious garden area. The advantage is that here you are right in the centre of Göreme with your camping van and all distances are very short because of that. A small swimmingpool belongs to the garden and the fee breaks all records: 5TL per person with electricity included.

Phone: 0090 384 271 2462
E-mail: sevinrock@hotmail.com

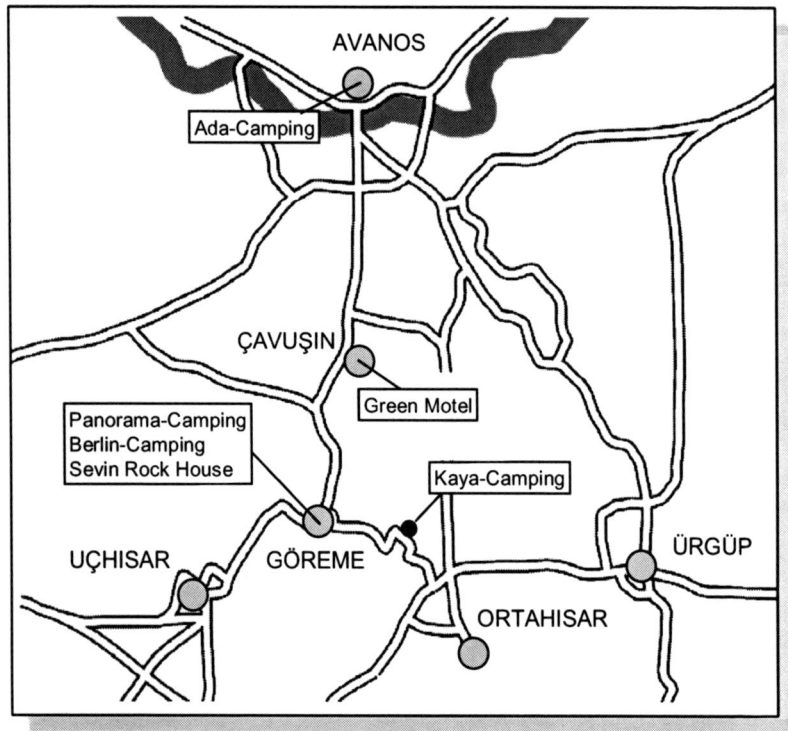

Monetary Questions

In the year 2005, the number of millionnaires in Turkey decreased rapidly. In that year the government deleted the unnecessary zeroes on the banknotes. Turkey had possessed the highest banknote in the world, as far as the number of zeroes is concerned. But this 20,000,000 Lira note was finally worth only $12,50. Inflation had been soaring for decades in the country. On our first journey in 1986 we got 300 TL in exchange for one Deutschmark; 16 years later, shortly before the Euro was introduced, we were paid 750,000 Lira for one Mark. After the AK Party took over government in the year 2003, the fall in value of the Lira has slowed down considerably and thus the government decided to delete 6 zeroes. From now on the currency was called "New Turkish Lira". At the beginning of 2009, new banknotes were introduced again and the addition "New" was again deleted. Thus, now the official Turkish currency is called "Turkish Lira" (TL) again as before.

The following coins and banknotes are in circulation at the moment:

      Coins: 1 / 5 / 10 / 25 / 50 Kurus and 1 TL
      Banknotes: 5 / 10 / 20 / 50 / 100 / 200   TL

At the beginning of 2009, 1 US $ was equivalent to 1,64 TL

(TL = türk lirasi = Turkish Lira)

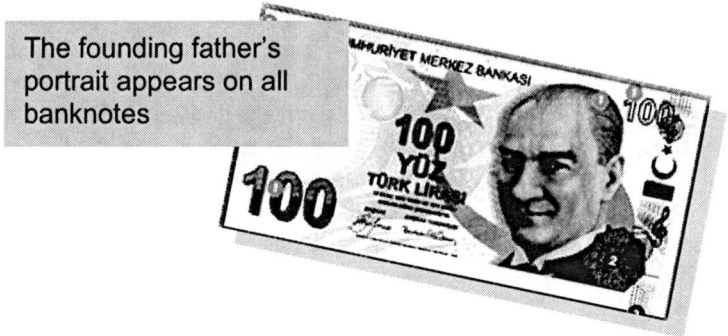

The founding father's portrait appears on all banknotes

In order to get Turkish Lira, there are several possibilities. First, in every town there are several banks which accept credit cards and which of course also exchange money. If you intend to stay in Cappadocia for a longer period of time and are dependent on money transfer from your home country, you can open an account at the bank. It will not bring any profit from interest, but as it is run in Euro, there is no danger of inflation. Banks are open on all five working days, but you should avoid exchanging money on Mondays or on Fridays, as on those days the onrush of customers is very great and there are extremely long waits.

Meanwhile all important banks have installed cash machines which are accessible 24 hours per day. Unfortunately this method is quite expensive, as there is a fee of at least $5,50 for each withdrawal of money. Service in English is possible on demand, and the procedure is almost the same as in all other countries:

1. insert your card
2. choose language
3. enter PIN code
4. choose 'withdrawal'
5. choose amount
6. don't forget to collect your card and money after finishing !!!

Finally, one last tip about using your bank card (credit card). Credit card fraud is increasing more and more all over the world, and unfortunately, Turkey is no exception. Please use your bank card only to withdraw money from ATMs. Never let yourself be misled into paying with your card in a shop or restaurant, as all data on your card can be read and copied by means of a simple card-reader within a split second. If then you are also watched when entering your pin-code number, the crooks will have gathered all the information they need for creating a so-called duplicate. Now it can happen to you that – perhaps months later – your bank account will be cleared, including the total amount of your overdraft facility. In contrast to European cash machines, the Turkish ones do not check the authenticity of cards. On the whole the tourist should treat his bank card like a packet of $500 bills, not only In Turkey or Cappadocia, but everywhere and at all times.

Exchange is still most uncomplicated in cash. Besides banks there often are also private exchange offices, whose exchange rates can however be considerably worse than those of the banks. Gold and jewellery shops are another alternative. Their exchange rates are only a little lower than the official ones, and they are also open on weekends. The gold shop is the fastest and easiest way of getting Turkish Lira. Many travellers, however, are afraid of carrying large sums of money with them. In this case, we strongly recommend reading the chapter on "Security" p.125. We ourselves have always used a money belt. Its secret is not visible from outside, as it is worn like any normal belt. It is double-lined and there is a zipper inside. You only have to fold the bank notes twice, and then you have an ideal hiding place for large notes. There is only one thing you should not do under all circumstances: that is, take the belt off on a busy street in front of a souvenir shop for paying with a large bank note. That your pants might slip down will probably only be your smallest problem then.

Bank opening hours:

Monday to Friday from 9.00 a.m. to 12.00 a.m.
and from 1.00 p.m. to 5.30 p.m.
Banks are closed on Saturdays, Sundays and on public holidays.

Medical and Health Care

Cappadocians say that there are only two categories of people who would run hectically through the town: The first are thieves on the run and the other are tourists in search of a toilet. It is a fact that diarrhoea is the disease travellers mostly suffer from. Various aspects are responsible for this. First, the abrupt change of climate is a stress factor to many people. If you have left the dirty weather in Europe or elsewhere just a few hours ago and now have landed in the dry heat of Anatolia, you are exposed to intense physical strain. If now you decide to drink from the nearest water faucet, to go to the nearest köfte (meatball) stall and to round up your meal with ice cream and fresh fruit, you have laid a perfect foundation for successful diarrhoea. There are people who go through with this the hard way and who cannot be harmed by anything after two days of suffering, but this only works for very tough guys. Taking things a bit easier is much better. First, you should be careful with water.

Water from the water faucet or from a well is not spoiled, but it contains substances our digestive system is not accustomed to and which it regards as a reason for becoming mutinous. Therefore, care must also be taken with loose ice cream or ice cubes, because all this is also made of water. Only drink water bought in a shop in plastic bottles during the first days. Fresh fruit is also an excellent catalyst, especially if it has not been washed carefully before. Turkish people are merciless in the usage of pesticides. Finally, the visitor must be warned against Köfte, that is, meatballs. Admittedly, this specialty consists of beef, but lying around in a showcase exposed to the sunshine for hours does not make them any healthier. All these tasty things should be avoided at the beginning. Later on, when your body has got accustomed to the environmental conditions, you can turn towards this food, too. But there is no guarantee that you will not get caught still.

Travellers to Cappadocia do not need to have themselves vaccinated. Diseases like malaria or the yellow fever belong on another continent. There is only one unpleasant disease that is common in Turkey; jaundice. Turkish people work off this illness as we do the flu. Contrary to European regulations it is not covered by the Infection Protection Act here. As a visit to the doctor and expensive medicine would cause a large hole in the Turkish family budget, the people just try to ignore the disease. Many people try to calm down their stomachs with large amounts of Raki, which their livers do not think to be funny at all. So, avoid drinking from one glass or eating from the same bowl with other peole, as the symptoms of the disease are not always recognizable. If your counterpart has bright yellow eyes and complains of stomach ache, the situation is obvious, however. One morning we passed by a small building site where the workmen were just having their first tea. They waved us nearer and put the only two tea glasses they possessed in our hands. We thanked them and carelessly drank our tea. When we returned the glasses, we looked into the goldish yellow eyes of the workers who smiled at us in a friendly manner. We spent the rest of the day worrying about quarantine facilities, an exploding liver and twelve months of diet food – but, for once, fortune favoured fools; nothing happened.

Medical care in Cappadocia cannot be called really excellent, but it is sufficient for the little ailments of everyday life. Numerous doctors from various medical fields are to be found. Avanos, Ürgüp and Göreme have small hospitals, Nevsehir has one state-owned and several private clinics, and there is even a large university hospital in Kayseri. This is the one you should absolutely go to if there are really serious problems. Antibiotics seem to be a panacea to most doctors, and they administer them immediately and without any hesitation. Once I suffered from a terrible and inexplicable headache and went to see a doctor. The only word I understood was 'antibiotic', whereupon I left the practice in a hurry. An acquaintance advised me to see a dentist. And lo and behold, a very bad tooth had to be pulled and the headache was gone immediately. The whole procedure took 20 minutes and cost about $15, anesthesia included. Generally, prices for doctors and medication are very low. If you need a medicine that is very expensive in your country, try and ask for it in a Turkish pharmacy. But you should not buy it in large quantities, as the European customs (among others) will have objections to that.

Costs of treatment and medicine have to be paid by you directly on the spot. Therefore it is important to inform your health insurance company of your travel destination in advance and to ask for a special health insurance certificate. After your return you must submit the receipts to your insurance provider, and in general the costs will be reimbursed.

For very serious cases having a certificate of international travel cover is useful, as transport back home is included in it. However, the local doctor's consent is necessary for this.

Unfortunately, the language difficulties are an irksome problem. It is true that medical students are expected to have learned a foreign language at university, but this seems to be only an unpleasant and unwelcome obligatory they are subjected to. Thus very few doctors in the country have any knowledge of a foreign language. If seeing a doctor is absolutely necessary, you had better find a companion who can translate for you.

Security

We know horror stories about vanished or even murdered tourists from Turkey, too. But similar news could also be heard from the USA, Italy, or from the municipal park of any big city in Germany. A trip through Cappadocia is no more dangerous than staying in a small town somewhere in Europe. On all our journeys through Turkey we have never got into a situation which seemed threatening to us in any way. Our belongings were never stolen, although often enough we forgot to lock our car. A loss of property was always related to our own scattiness. Once we even left our belt bag with all our personal documents including our passports in the restroom of the Istanbul airport. We were informed by the cleaning woman, who came running after us, breathing heavily, to hand over the bag. Only once a lashing strap was stolen from the luggage rack of our car in a little village at night. But we are sure that somebody desperately needed it and just did not manage to bring it back before we left next morning.

Of course there are black sheep, as everywhere else in the world. Especially in those corners of the globe where the income differentials between locals and foreign visitors are especially great, this tends to wet the appetites. Therefore the proverb 'opportunity makes the thief' is still true today. You yourself can contribute most to your safety. Leave your crown jewels at home. You will hardly find an occasion for wearing expensive jewelry in Cappadocia. And never pull wads of banknotes from your pocket, but carry only as much money with you as you are actually going to need. An expensive camera should always disappear in your bag whenever it is not used, and other electronic equipment should not be shown in a provoking manner, either. We are sure that if you do **not** take heed of all this, none of your things will get lost anyway.

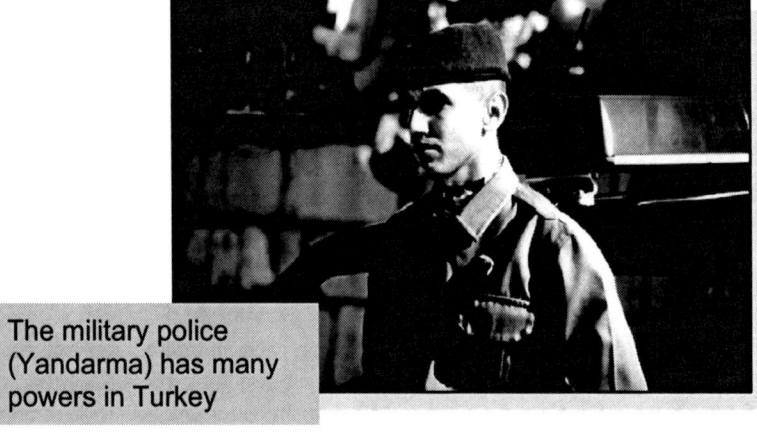

The military police (Yandarma) has many powers in Turkey

Where to put cash and personal documents? If you are staying at a big hotel, you can deposit them in the hotel safe. A belt bag or a neck pouch worn under your T-shirt is a good alternative. Also a pouch that is worn

permanently on the body makes sense. But it has one disadvantage: it has to be taken off
in the restroom. There many tourists do not know where to put them. Especially in public lavatories with primitive toilets and problems of hygiene (see the chapter 'toilets' p.183) a peg on the inside of the door invites you to hang it there. This is a fatal mistake. Now anybody can reach over the door with his hand and grab it, and suddenly all your documents and the money are gone. When your pants are up again, the thief will be miles away. But such stories can be heard from all over the world and they have nothing to do with Cappadocia in particular. One rule applies all over the world: never leave your car unlocked, and always keep an eye on your luggage. If you follow those rules, you will always be on the safe side.

If in spite of all this you should get into some kind of trouble, ask somebody to call the police or dial **155** yourself. Look if there is somebody around who can help you, or try to find someone who can explain your problem to the police when they have arrived. Unfortunately most policemen do not have any knowledge of foreign languages. Within the boundaries of Göreme National Park the Yandarma, the military police, is in charge of public security.

Travelling women

Turkish Women travel alone also, to their relatives or to a distant hospital, and students explore their own country. But there is always the principle that women have to stick with other women, and men with men. So, always sit next to other women, whether on the bus, in a cafe or on a park bench. If there is a choice, talk to women, ask women for the way.

In Islam (which also means in Turkey) there is a living solidarity of women, perhaps a virtue caused by the pressures of patriarchy. Women care for each other and help each other. In the Turkish bath, the hamam, they even wash each other. Women in the company of other women deal with one another more confidentially and more lovingly than we Western women are accustomed to.

And while shopping, women help you so that the shopkeepers do not rip you off. Turkish women are often confused by us, the Western women, because of the great efforts we make to understand our husbands or partners and even to lead a life based on partnership and equality with them. Such an absurd idea would never occur to them.

If you have been invited by a traditional family, the men will do all the talking there. Try to establish contact with the women, sit next to them, admire their cooking, their needlework and the well-behaved children. Invite them for a walk in company. The interior decoration of the home is strictly functional in traditional living, and remarks on the beautiful house, as they are customary in our countries do not find any sympathy and could even appear insulting, as it is not the most wealthy people who mostly live in the traditional houses.

When visiting a traditional family, give the men the cold shoulder and show the women your sympathy. And often there also will be more fun in the women's corner than in the patriarch's corner. On taking leave, the new friendship will finally be sealed with some tender kisses on the cheek. But never kiss a man on the cheek. If the patriarch indicates this gesture of friendship, react with friendly reserve: a short smile, a nod and words of thanks for the hospitality are sufficient.

Women in Turkey deal with each other on a very emotional level: show your affection, show your feelings, smile, and immediately a warm feeling of familiarity will pervade you without your necessarily having to understand the language.

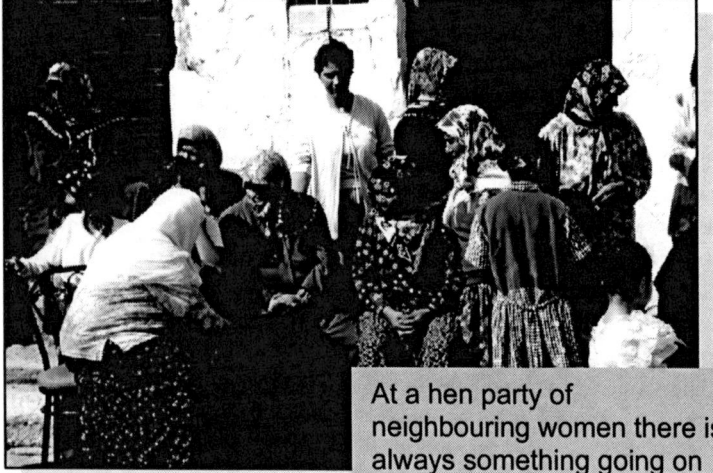

At a hen party of neighbouring women there is always something going on

Exactly the opposite rules of behaviour apply towards men. Only women with obviously indecent intentions would like to be in the world of men, that means on the streets, which we tourists on the other hand are forced to do. But even decent Turkish women are sometimes forced to leave the house. They would never think of smiling at men in public or of talking to them more than required by politeness. A decent man treats a woman with respect by bowing slightly from a certain distance, greeting the lady without staring at her and asking about her wellbeing in a serious tone. The woman can express all her wishes directly and seriously in public. It is the gentleman's job to fulfill all her wishes at once without any great ado. A short word of thank you is enough for his efforts.

Thus, do not show too many emotions towards men in public. Compliments or even physical contact with strangers have to be regarded as impudent and indecent and have to be rejected loudly by women, also in order to show the impudence to the passers-by. Strangers who laugh in a women's face in the street show this woman what they think about her, that is, nothing at all. Defend yourself, show your outrage by scolding noisily and treat those ruffians like vermin or chase them away: only then will you have saved your honour and your respectability and there will be nothing that prevents a friendship with men who have serious intentions towards you. You do not have to wear a headscarf for this, just your behaviour gives enough information about your status as a woman. But this should not be totally unknown to us in our Western culture. This is only true for behaviour towards strangers. If a friendship already exists, the behaviour of men and women is in no way different from our own conventions: you hug each other, kiss each other on the cheek, and you also make the occasional crude joke. There is always a lot of fun among friends in Turkey.

Women and Islam

- a Different View

by Susanne Oberheu

The roles of men and women are strictly separated and subject to the constraints of everyday life in most societies of the world: the men provide for the family, and the women have children. There is hardly any room for experiments.
Only the well-educated women of the Western world, where physical strength plays an increasingly unimportant role, can economically afford to go without men. Their relation to men is therefore completely different from the rest of the world. Their relation to men is primarily influenced by affection and by emotions. In other societies, where women do not have the opportunities of good training and a good professional career, the men are still what they always used to be in the patriarchy: maintainers, providers of economic security, often no more than that. Love and affection for men play a minor role there. Western women now could feel sorry for those poor creatures, but perhaps our sisters in Islam do have something ahead of us. As an example, I would like to report two of my key experiences in Cappadocia: Once Michael and I had been invited to their house by a family. But we had had a terrible argument before, so finally I decided to go there alone, which made me feel quite embarrassed. The landlady saw my tear-stained face and, startled, asked for the reason of my sadness. When I told her that my husband did not understand me, she shook her head in amusement and exclaimed: "Why are you crying? He is only your husband!"
On another occasion I was invited – alone this time – by a woman to her house. Many women, friends and female neighbours were already sitting on the floor on soft carpets and cushions and there was a relaxed mood: Steaming tea and lots of cookies were passed around and after a while, the Raki bottle was taken out from under the bed with a lot of laughing and cheering; in addition, there were cigarettes. Apart from talking, we were all busy preparing a meal for ourselves. The scars of pregnancies and Caesarean sections were proudly presented, pieces of crochet work were exchanged. The mood could not have been better, there was much laughing. And then the inconceivable thing happened: the landlord came home, totally unexpectedly;

he was hungry. With consternation, he saw his Raki bottle, but said nothing. The good mood was gone immediately. The sour looks of the women clearly showed their disrespect and the lady of the house became even more explicit in just throwing her husband out. As a Western woman, I was speechless how impotent the so-called patriarchs are in their own four walls.

It was obvious that this married couple was not exactly dearly in love with each other, but this was not necessary for the self-image of the women. In any case, they did not appear to be weak and subdued dumb females to me. If the husband had brought any visitors with him, they would have got a totally different impression: the wife, who devotely serves the tea and keeps her mouth shut; the husband, who would seize every opportunity to show the guests that he is the man in the house, including little acts of revenge.

In public, the deceptive image of a perfect world with a strong patriarch and an obedient family is gladly presented again and again by the husband, and unfortunately, quite successfully, too. By tradition, men and women in Turkey live in totally separate spheres. Everyday life separates them, but their common attempts to cope with it also unite them, as I was able to watch many times, too: tender respectfulness can be seen even in marriages that have been arranged by the parents.

Endearments between husband and wife are taboo in public. In contrast, you see men walking through the streets hand in hand; if you called them homosexuals, you would have a problem right away.

Public life belongs to the men, as the private home does to the women. This is why we tourists often see only men hanging out in the streets or in the cafès and the teahouses. The men do not even come home for the daytime meals; for those, there are Lokantas everywhere – canteens which provide the men with cheap meals. Besides, the men have to worry about earning money. With this, the women have no mercy either. If the husband returns home in the evening without the money which is needed for oil, gas bottles and the housewife's next trip to the market, there will be a noisy argument. A husband who is not able to support his family is worthless – at least in the women's eyes – and things will get quite uncomfortable in front of the family tv set in this case.

Thus, friendships between men, like those between women, are much closer than in the Western world. Despite their economic independence, Western women's focus is still directed solely on the man of their love. Friendships among women have become less important, if not, with all the daily competition – for men, too – altogether impossible. What distinguishes us

Western women from the women in Islam is not the submissiveness prescribed by the patriarchal law, which incidentally is required in the same way in the Bible and by the church: women in Islam are not permanently concentrated on the male world. Whenever women in Islam achieve economic independence, they have the advantage of emotional independence from men compared with us Western women. This is perhaps the reason why in the Islamic world there are so many more women in political positions than in the Christian Occident – up till now, that is. Education and assets provided, they have no bad conscience towards men. To women in Islam, the behaviour of Western women towards men appears like currying favour. The Islamic woman is rather cool and unapproachable in public. Men are kept at a distance, not because they fear them, as is often supposed in the West, but because men are simply not so important. Islamic women's lives take place among other women, and thus the woman from next door can achieve greater significance than one's own husband. The Islamic husband would see this in a totally different way, of course. And as we Westerners are so much focused on men, we listen only to them. And that is the crux of the matter.

Also, women from the West regard themselves as sexually more liberal, as they equate the veiling of Islamic women with prudery. The contrary is true: especially in Islam, sex is a real women's issue that is discussed in great detail between cooking, recipes and family gossip. Here, too, the spouse is not spared. If things do not work in the marital bed, the wife will discuss this topic quite openly at the next afternoon tea party. Thus it is no wonder that the husbands like to escape from the domestic hearth.

Wearing a headscarf is not a point of interest in Cappadocia, nor a sign of special religiousness. Older women wear headscarfs, the younger ones don't. At home in company, the lovingly embroidered scarfs are put casually over one's shoulders. In rural areas, scarfs protect the hair from dust and dirt, as there are no bathrooms in many houses and as the only water tap is outside in the yard – also in winter and always with cold water. A weekly visit to the hamam must be enough for the care of the dense head of hair. But headscarves are a matter of tradition and if the women have got used to them from their childhood, they do not feel properly dressed without them. No modern daughter with dyed blonde hair would expect this of her mother. Going outside bareheaded would not only cost you quite an effort, but would also require a visit to a hairdresser, who are increasingly found in the villages, too - another sign of change. Headscarfs are worn in a special style in Cappadocia, by the way, which is quite unique to this region. A traditionally dressed Turkish woman wears a headscarf, comfortable Turkish harem trousers (şalvar) or a long cotton skirt with long underpants under it, a pullover and, if necessary, a knitted waistcoat over it, and slippers. Not exactly the latest craze in the fashion world, but comfortable, and who cares? As we know, it does not matter what the men think about this. Never have I regarded these women as less strong, less courageous or less fun-loving. Quite the contrary, their hard daily work, their coping with the hardships of family life without any social and health insurance has always compelled the greatest respect from me. Those women still bear the full responsibility for their actions, with all the tragic consequences and without any help from outside. One can easily imagine that many a grandmother turns into an old gorgon and many younger women break down under this burden.

The better education of women in Turkey actually has very different consequences than expected by the West: Educated young women wear the headscarf again. The veiling of women was not common at the time of Mohammed and is not mentioned in any line of the Koran. Sometime it became elegant in the East to wear a headscarf. Only during the decline of Islam in recent centuries has disguising been prescribed by fanatic believers of different religious groups as a sign of oppression of women.

In Turkey, at any rate, the hard daily life of the women is not Islam's fault but the fault of the social circumstances, their dependency cannot be blamed on the men, but on their lack of education. But the next generation of women will do everything differently, supported by their mothers in their headscarfs. Unfortunately, higher education in Turkey still has to be paid for, and thus it is often unaffordable for those who are poorer.

Today, the modern emancipated Turkish woman wears a headscarf as a sign of protest and because it is chic again. She wants to distance herself against the Western woman's role and to give Islamic culture a fresh impetus. These women are professionally, politically and socially active and feel equal to their husbands. They also differ outwardly from their Şalvar-wearing grandmothers: under the headscarf the hair is tied up in a bun, giving the head a very elongated shape. In addition, a slight, almost floor-length coat is worn. All this is made from the finest cloth and elegantly cut, and according to the latest fashion. Thus at family celebrations, all styles are present: the grandmother wearing the traditional crocheted Anatolian headscarf, the mother with her hair dyed and permed in Western style, and the daughter with pinned-up hair and dressed in finest silk.

Food and Drink

The gourmet speaks of three great cuisines in the world with an excellent reputation. These are the Chinese or Asian cuisine, the French cuisine and finally also the Turkish-Ottoman way of preparing food. As you see, they are all countries where monarchical pomp and decadence brought forth its strange blossoms for centuries. And, as scholar Ibn Haldun has written: "In due course, the population will assume the religion of the ruler", this also happened to the Turkish cuisine. If you add the rich flora and fauna of Turkey and its regional differences, you will have got everything that makes a world-class cuisine. In addition to the great creativity which the cooks at the Padisha's court developed in paying homage to his spoilt palate, they were also very inventive when naming their products. Stuffed Aubergines are called "The Imam was sick" or "The Imam fainted". Other dishes are called "Women's Thighs", or sweets are called "Nightingale's Nest" or "Wound Turban" or even "Woman's Navel".

Of course the elaborate cuisine from the Topkapi Palace in Istanbul did not pass on to the bowl of the Anatolian farmer completely unchanged. The menu here in Cappadocia depends on the seasonal and the geographic peculiarities. On a winter's day you will look in vain for strawberries flown in from South Africa. Instead of that, things that are low in price and available in large amounts on the weekly market are put on the table. Especially in winter, the diet is dominated by preserved food or food prepared in autumn.

The Turkish cuisine is regarded as very balanced. Traditionally you will not find large heaps of meat on your plate here. The doner kebab, which is regarded as the standard Turkish food by some people, is only found in big cities or in areas with tourism. 25 years ago the giant spits rotating in the shop windows were a rarity here in Cappadocia. Vegetables, rice and potatoes still constitute the majority üon Anatolian plates. A family of five consumes at least 10 kilograms (22 lbs) of potatoes per week, and the omnipresent white bread serves as a 'filling side dish'. It belongs on the table in any restaurant, inextricably linked with a bottle of water. Neither should appear on the bill, however.

The 'Lokanta' is the simplest form of public feeding. Here, the local dishes are on display directly at the entrance in a heatable counter. You choose your meal there before taking a seat. Afterwards the waiter will bring your chosen meal to your table. Often we Europeans are a little disappointed because the servings are not very large here, but for filling there are mountains of slices of bread lying ready for use. Moreover, the food is not as hot as in our country, but just warm. You do not pay at the table by the way, but at the checkout, which is next to the entrance door and where, beneath a protrait of Atatürk, the master of the house himself collects the money.

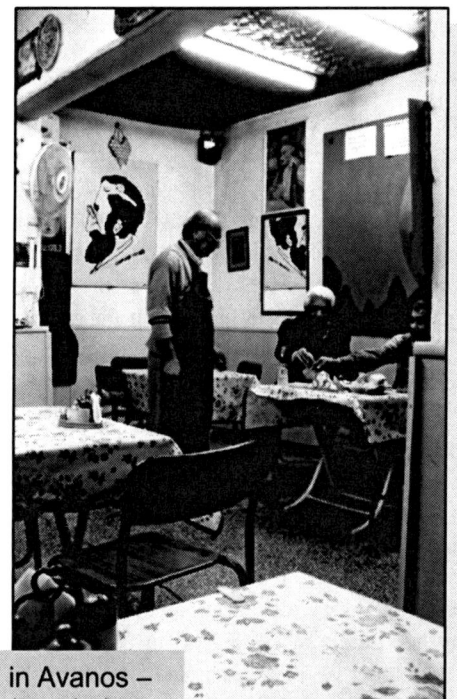

At ‚Ibrahims Place' in Avanos – here you get fresh draught beer

"Soup drinking" in the morning is a Turkish specialty. Lentil soup (mercimek) as part of it is something that still comes closest to our middle or west European eating habits. The "paça", a sheep's head soup whose meat components you should not examine too closely, or even the "işkembe", a tripe soup, are not for everyone. The Turks, however, have absolute

confidence in them. Especially after a night spent drinking, these soups will replace any coffee or headache pills.
If you want to know if the Lokanta has a clean kitchen, just look at the number of local guests. You can unhesitatingly visit a location that is well-frequented in the mornings and at lunchtime. In the evening it is more advisable to go to a restaurant, however, as in a Lokanta the choice is not so large any more and the food often has been overcooked by then. You also should be a bit careful with the dishes you choose there in the first few days. In the chapters on "Medical Care" and "Toilets" you will learn more about the reasons.

In a restaurant things are a little bit more tasteful. Here, too, you should have a look at whether it is frequented by Turkish people. The Turks are very critical regarding the quality and freshness of food, and any shortcomings of a restaurant get around among them fast. In a restaurant there is also a menu again, and it is no problem to have a short look into the kitchen if you have difficulties with the language. Here the menu will look a bit different than in a Lokanta. More meat dishes appear on the menu. You will find the well-known "Sis Kebab" in several variations, but also specialties like the "Saçtava" a mixture of meat and vegetables that is cooked and served on a vaulted platter. You will find the local specialty, "Güveç", a stew that is boiled in special earthenware pots from Avanos for hours on end, as well as the widely known "Döner" spit. The "Testi Kebab" is a special attraction. For it, meat, potatoes, garlic, onions and tomatoes are seasoned with salt and pepper and boiled in the oven for two hours. The clou is that the whole thing is inside an earthenware jug whose mouth is closed by bread dough. The jug is opened theatrically with a swinging blow at the table and in the presence of the astonished guests by cutting off the top part with a knife, the delicious content landing on the plate, steaming. The streets in front of the restaurants are lined with those headless jars, which are all produced by hand and exclusively in Avanos.

After the meal the waiter will mostly ask you if you want a dessert. Fresh fruit, sugary Baklava (puff pastry soaked in honey with nuts and pistachios) or Sütlaç (rice pudding baked in the oven). If you are with several persons and want a dessert you should order the fruit platter as the final culmination.
Apart from the restaurant, there is also the "Pide-Salonu". Here the Turkish variety of the pizza is awaiting you. It is oval and is served with cheese,

minced meat or fried eggs. Hot and cut up into handy portions, it will finally reach the guest's table.

For people with a sweet tooth the Turks have invented the "Pastahane". Confectionary is available here and friends of coffee and cake will get everything they want. Besides the "Baclava" mentioned before, there are also tarts, cookies and similar treats on display. But be careful: Turkish pastries are almost always very sweet. The local cake rather reminds one of the good old butter-cream cake with its exorbitant calorie value.

Besides this we can recommend a visit to the mobile "Köfteci". Here the little meatballs – the Köfte – are fried over charcoal on a little pushcart directly by the side of the street. Afterwards they are put into a sliced half of a pita bread together with onions, paprika and tomatoes, then wrapped into a piece of newspaper and handed to the customer for eating. The bread with Köfte is an inexpensive and very tasty alternative to a visit at a restaurant.

But now we will come to the drinks. You will not get any alcoholic beverages at the Lokanta – a fact which does not make an evening meal in a Lokanta more attractive. Coffee, tea, fruit juices or the usual international lemonade drinks are available there. The "Ayran", a drink made of diluted yogurt, can be strongly recommended. If it is served chilled, there is no better thirst quencher far and wide.

In a restaurant, however, the whole range of alcoholic beverages is available. Besides local wines and the tasty Efes Lager, of course the Turkish lion's milk, the Rakı, is on the menu. 'Lion's milk' because this high percentage anise schnaps is mixed with water, thus assumes a milky colour and is believed to give you the strength of a lion. The Rakı has 40% of alcoholic content, or sometimes even more, and there cannot be enough warnings against excessive consumption. The vigours that you developed in drinking the previous night will surely be lacking you next day. But there are very high taxes on alcoholic beverages, so that the obligatory glass of Rakı in the evening is not affordable any more to many locals; consequently, an invitation will mean a great treat to many Turkish people.

With its average altitude of 1000 m above sea level, with its hot sun and its porous soils, Cappadocia is the ideal wine-growing region. Vines cover the hillsides and are growing on the walls of almost every house. The grapes are sweet and juicy and a real treat. Many a household had its own winery in former times. Cappadocia's great wineries sold their products all over the country. Thus Cappadocia should be an eldorado for real connoisseurs – but unfortunately, this is not so.

What the wineries do with the sweet grapes is a complete mystery to us. Some of the cheap Spanish carton wines are better than the wines that are sold here in the shops for 20 TL a bottle. You have to pay quite a lot for a good wine in Cappadocia, and then this wine is often from another region of Turkey. (For more information on viticulture in Cappadocia, see the text in the previous chapter, page 140).

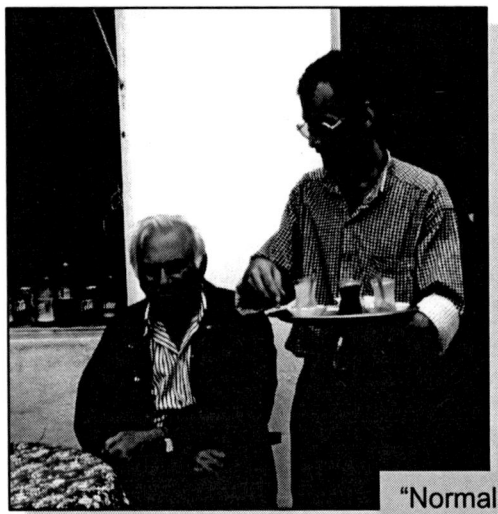

"Normal Çay or Elma-Çay ?" - The Çaycı at work

So, you should rather eat the fresh grapes and have a nice glass of tea (çay) with them. It is the national drink of the Turkish people and it is cultivated in the tropical humid climate at the Black Sea coast. It has not always been like that. Actually the Turkish mocha (kahve), which was consumed en masse up to the end of the Ottoman Empire, is much more well-known. But Atatürk, the founder of the Republic of Turkey, very soon noticed that the import of coffee was much too expensive. So he ordered tea to be planted in the northern parts of the country as an inexpensive alternative for the people. The success of this plan was immense, and within a few years the Turks became a nation of tea-drinkers. Of course you are still served the famous black and strong Turkish coffee. People with a high blood pressure should be very careful however, as the black venom is not harmless altogether.

Finally, we have a recipe for Güveç for you. You can buy almost all the ingredients in a good supermarket. The only thing you should have bought before is the necessary traditional Güvec pot, as a souvenir from Avanos.

Güvec – for 2

By Ayşe Neumüller from Avanos

Use an origional Güveç pot of about 16 cm (6.5 inches) in diameter and a content of about 1,5 l (0.9) pints.

Ingredients:

3 potatoes (medium size), 2 onions, 1 aubergine, 3 tomatoes, ½ garlic, 4 green thin bell pepper pods (not hot), one tablespoon Turkish tomato paste (salca – perhaps from a Turkish shop), spice and herbs: marjoram, thyme, parsley, salt and kırmızı-biber (from the weekly market in Cappadocia), ca. 300g (½ pound) of lamb.

Preparation:

Put potatoes and peeled eggplants in cold salt water for some time. Then cut into small pieces and put into the pot. Cut the lamb into rough pieces and put on top of the potatoes. Mix tomato paste, herbs and salt with ca. ½ pint of water and pour over it. Allow to simmer for about 1 hour, add some water if necessary.

The pot can be put on the hot plate of the stove without worrying. Otherwise it can be shoved in the oven like a chicken brick. If you want to try out the recipe in your holidays, get the mixture from the nearest "Pide-Salonu" and put it in your oven.

Cappadocian Wine

- the Rediscovering

by Ines Rebentrost

Asia Minor is the cradle of winemaking. Grapes have been cultivated in the Euphrates and Tigris region for thousands of years. From here they made their breakthrough into Europe and the whole world, first because of the Greeks and later the Romans. Because of this, Anatolia, and more especially Cappadocia, became a winegrowing region at a very early time.

Despite religious restrictions with the advent of Islam as a state religion in the 12th century, viticulture was able to be continued in Turkey. However, the focus was now on the production of table grapes and raisins, and the ancient know-how of wine production was lost. A wine culture in the proper sense of the word has only been able to redevelop in the past 70 years, since Atatürk's attempt at secularization.

But the cultivation of grapes for wine production is still of very little importance in relation to the total area of vineyards in Turkey. Thus Turkey is still number 4 in the world's production of grapes, but as a wine producer, Turkey is mostly not even mentioned in the statistics and, if it is at all, then it is among the 'also-rans'. At the moment, the production of wine is just 3% of the vineyard cultivation in the country, however with a strong upward trend. Wine enjoys an ever-increasing popularity among members of the newly emerging and well-paid urban middle class.

Although wine production has a great tradition in Cappadocia, however today's younger generation does not see many opportunities in agriculture. They would rather turn to tourism or migrate to the cities. No wonder! A farmer who sells his grapes to a Raki factory or a wine press cannot even cover his basic costs any more by doing this. That is why many of the ancient vineyards are overgrown today. Up to the 1960s there was a wine press in every bigger community; today you can count them on the fingers of your hand.

This is extremely unfortunate, as, being wine experts, we are sure that the geological and climatic conditions in Cappadocia are especially suitable for the production of top qualtity wines: at an altitude of between 800 and 1200 m above sea level, during the growing period cool nights alternate with hot and dry days. These day-night fluctuations promote aroma development in the grapes during the ripening period in an ideal way, and they minimize the reduction of acids, as is the case at the Turkish Aegean Coast, for example.There, the results are more or less dull and uninteresting dessert wines.

The soils of Cappadocia are of volcanic origin. Thick tufa layers formed by volcanic ash rain cover the original sedimentary rocks. Those soils are deep and easily penetrable for roots. In addition, their porosity enables them to store humidity, which thus can be used by the deep-rooted vines also in the dry summer season. Thus irrigation, which would be ecologically senseless because of salination and the general scarcity of water, can be omitted. It would only result in "laziness" of the vines, so that they would become shallow-rooted. Good, concentrated wines are produced by those vines that grow on rather barren soil – by positive stress, as it were.

The great rains in Cappadocia are limited to the winter and the spring. The soil is refilled then in a way.

The dry summers also minimize the problem of fungal infestation, which, quite naturally, pleases the winemakers.

So why are the wines from Turkey and from Cappadocia lagging so far behind the wines of the rest of the world? And why are they so expensive, so that there is an extremely poor price-performance ratio? Many tourists interested in wine bravely taste various Turkish products before they disappointedly change to beer or Rakı very quickly.

The exorbitant prices are not the winemakers' fault, they are a result of the present Islamic government party's policies, which put an extremely high luxury tax on alcoholic beverages, in addition to 20% of value added tax.

But the poor quality can be blamed on the winemakers. In recent years a positive development has become visible: work in the wine cellars has become cleaner and there has been a quantum leap in technology. Larger firms often employ foreign oenologists as advisors, as for example family-run firms like "Turasan" in Ürgüp and "Kocabag" at Uchisar. The "Kavaklidere" group from Ankara has recently been investing money in Cappadocia. Those corporations, of course, have the necessary means for investing money in new technologies and foreign know-how. But also many smaller firms, like those in Ürgüp and in Mustafapaşa take great pains to improve the quality of their products. In Mustafapaşa for example, there has even been a technical college for winemaking for some years. The reason for this of course is the fact that no other region of Turkey can hold a candle to Cappadocia's qualities in the field of viticulture.

All the same: we have not yet found a Cappadocian wine which is really fun, which is many-sided and exciting, and which even increases in its facets on drinking and which has been produced straight and pure. It can be said that winemaking in Turkey lags behind Europe and the New World by some years. For example, 15 years ago, average German wines were regarded as sour in comparison with products from the famous wine nations, France or Italy. Increasing competition and a change in consumer behaviour – drinking less, only on special occasions, but with products of better quality – finally led to a quality improvement of German wines. We must allow Turkey this learning process, too, as the country has not been able to develop a continuous wine tradition due to the Ottoman rule.

In any case it would be extremely unfortunate and a huge waste of potential if a perfect winemaking region like Cappadocia did not produce any top quality wines – wines which would enjoy a high international reputation but which would above all bring us, the Turkish and foreign wine lovers, much joy.

Ines Rebentrost, the German oenologist, has lived in the region for many years. Presently she commutes between Switzerland and Cappadocia with her Swiss partner, Philipp Gfeller, in order to build up a new winery near Ortahisar. From there, an excellent Cappadocian wine is to be expected in the next few years. Everything on the state of development can be found on the Internet under:

www.ortahisarwine.com

Shopping

The topic of "shopping" is primarily meant for self supporters. As for buying souvenirs, there is a corresponding chapter later in the book.

Those who want to buy fresh vegetables should wait for the weekly market day in the various places. The weekly market is unbeatable as far as freshness and low prices are concerned. This is proved by the onrush of the local people on those days, so that you can hadly put your foot on the ground there. Cappadocians often buy their whole week's supply of fresh fruit or vegetables at the market.
Do not have any scruples about testing the fruits on offer extensively with your fingers. If there is a big rush at a stall, ask for a plastic bag and select the best fruits without any hurry. Experience shows that older sellers often try to cheat tourists by showing them perfect products but then puttting faulty products from another crate into the bag. We recommend taking a large shopping bag with you, as you will be given at least one or two plastic bags at each stall and handling them will become increasingly difficult if you have several of them.
Also your year's supply of spices can be excellently bought here on the market, as there is a huge choice and the prices are many times lower than at the supermarkets in your home country. Apart from that, the weekly market offers also housewares, textiles, shoes and tools. Actually, you can buy anything you forgot to pack in at home here, from a simple sewing kit up to a 10 kilogram sledgehammer. The only thing that you will not get at the market is meat.

Market days in Cappadocia:

Monday   - Nevşehir
Tuesday   - Uçhisar
Wednesday - Göreme
Thursday   - Gülşehir
Friday   - Avanos
Saturday   - Ürgüp

Those who have no possibility of going to a weekly market need not go hungry either. In the villages there are shops where small quantities of fruit and vegetables are on sale during the whole week. Additionally some mini-markets have established themselves where you can also do your daily shopping and where everything your heart could desire is available. Those shops are open seven days a week, at least from eight o'clock in the morning till eight at night. You can also get freshly baked bread here almost the whole day long, as there are no baker's shops in the usual sense. Some of those shops also sell fresh meat, but it is shrink-wrapped and sometimes not really fresh any more or has even been defrosted from the deep freezer. You are safer at your butcher's there, so long as the last butchering day was less than a whole week ago. The meat is mostly cut up into small pieces in Turkey. So, if you are hungry for a big steak, you will have to hold back the butcher from doing this.

Beer and wine are also available at some mini-markets, but in general they are sold in special shops for alcoholic drinks. They can be identified by the supersize advertising signs for the tasty "Efes" beer, but they also sell harder stuff like Rakı or awfully sweet cordials. Real wine experts will be disappointed in Cappadocia, because the wine is expensive and mediocre. This is really an impossibility, considering that you are in an avowed wine producing region.

And, please do not get frightened if you hear a salesman talk about millions or thousands when talking about the price. This comes from before the monetary reform in 2005, when the banknotes had six zeros more than they have today.

Here is the English translation of some important shop names:

kasab	-	butcher
eczane	-	chemist, pharmacy
bakal	-	large kiosk with huge assortment of goods
pastahane	-	pastry shop (no bakery)

Exotic Services

The Berber (hairdresser)

The word 'berber' is derived from the French 'barbier'. As people did not shave their beards for religious reasons in former times, this profession is not yet very old. Only after the foundation of the Republic and the related reforms did the profession of the barber become popular. Today it is courteous behaviour to have a regular shave. Razors are rarely found in Turkish households, even those for wet shaving. And as one cannot afford going to the barber every day, many Turks have a stubbly beard on their faces, which is several days old.

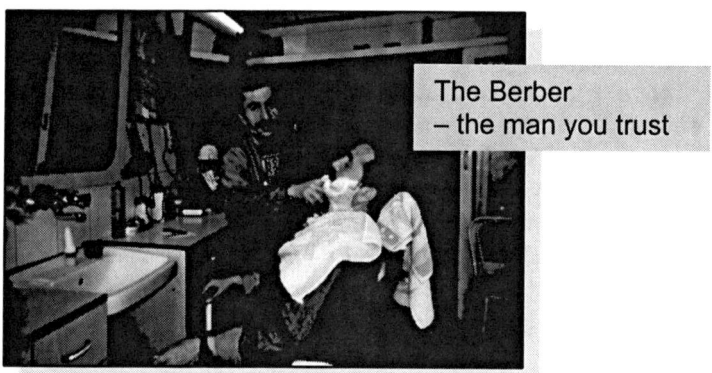

The Berber – the man you trust

For tourists, a visit to the hairdresser's shop is a must. You feel like being in the Wild West there. The shaving is done with the old familiar razor blade, which is occasionally sharpened on a leather strap. Covered with lather and attired in an apron, you are sitting in a chair, the knife at your throat and totally at the mercy of the master's steady hand. The shaving is thorough and almost never bloody. Afterwards, the remaining fluff is burned off by means of cotton sticks drenched in alcohol and set on fire. Finally, the tortured skin is drenched in aftershave and powdered slightly, and immediately you feel like a different person. If a massage is offered, you should be careful, as temporarily dislocated cervicals are not for everyone.

Recently, the berber has developed into a "Show-coiffeur" for the male youth, where you meet your friends in the evenings. You can see the young men sitting there until late at night, debating, cracking jokes and trying out all kinds of creams and cosmetic care products. Do not be surprised when you see those youngsters' faces through the windows of such a hairdresser's shop, covered with sliced cucumbers.

The Ayakkabi Boyacisi (shoe polisher)

This profession is totally unknown in Central Europe and thus seems suspicious to most travellers. But mostly this is only because of the seemingly submissive working posture. If you feel embarrassed by this but want shiny shoes all the same, you can make the shoeshine boy give you a pair of flip-flops. Then you can take a seat a little off in the shade and the shoe polisher will take your shoes in his hands. Another advantage of this method is that your socks will remain unstained. This should be done especially with children, who often work as shoeshine-boys in the summer holidays. They like to transgress the dividing line between the black shoes and the white socks, a popular combination among Turks. You should not have any scruples about letting young children do this job, as they are often from poor families and help to increase the family budget this way. But this only applies to the three months of summer holidays. At other times, lessons are compulsory, and this should not be avoided.

The Çaycı (tea seller)

Would you like a glass of tea without having to sit down at a teahouse or tea garden? Then you should see a cayci. Finding one is very easy. Look for the intercom system at the entrance of any shop, and follow the cable. More and more cables will come together and will finally lead you to some dark entrance door. This is where he works, often in a tiny room together with his delivery boy. The fastest way of getting a glass of tea is here. But normally he supplies the businessmen of a certain area with tea, and this is what the many intercoms are for. The shop owners or their assistants announce themselves by a slight knock on the microfone and then transmit their orders. Customers who have been in a shop for a longer period are always offered a glass of tea, and this of course also applies to tourists. If there are several rounds of tea, try to order and pay for one yourself. You will not be given the chance, but it is the good will that counts.

Travelling Dogs

Principally you must ask yourself if you wish to expect such a journey from your favourite. People who are travelling in their own camper van will have the least worries. Those who travel by plane should consider leaving their dog at home with friends or relatives. Dogs are only admitted to the passenger section up to a weight of 6 kg and in a special handbag as carry-on baggage. For all bigger dogs a special box in the luggage room has to be organized. Make sure in advance how many animals will be on board besides yours, as Turkish airlines do not transport more than three dogs at a time. If there happens to be a cat on board, no dogs at all will be transported. But your dog's odyssey will not be over with this. In public transportation, dogs are not allowed in the passenger section either, and will wind up in the luggage compartment with their boxes. This means in the baggage van on trains and in the underfloor stowage room on buses. Taxi drivers are not too happy about transporting a dog, either.
Information about the importation of pets can be obtained in the chapter on "Entry requirements" earlier in this book.
The dog is an impure animal in Islam and therefore has a low status in Turkish life. Just the idea of touching a dog makes many Turkish people cringe. Women and children often have terrible fear of dogs, however small and cute they are. So please do not take your dog with you to a Turkish household without having been asked to do so.
Finding an accomodation will not be any easier with a dog, either. Many lodging house owners will shake with disgust at the imagination that a dog will live in their rooms or will even sleep in the beds. If Turkish tourists were staying there, they would cancel their rooms at once. You should also definitely forget the idea of taking your dog with you to a Locanta or to a restaurant. Only restaurants with tables outside on the street are possible for you.
Only take your dog with you if it is well-mannered. Dogs which always jump at strangers or begin to roam when off the leash will cause nothing but trouble to you. On the other hand, you can gain prestige with an intelligent and obedient dog. There was always great amazement among the locals when we were leading our dog through the chaos of Turkish traffic without any leash. We told him to wait outside the shops, whereupon he sat down dutifully and patiently waited for us to return. No sugarcubes or other

enticements offered by passers-by were able to distract him. Turkish people are not used to such an amount of learning in a dog, which, however, is certainly not the local dogs' fault.-
Feeding your dog is another problem. Canned dog food or dry food is very rare and only available in the supermarkets of some big cities. The only possibility of scraping up dog food is the butcher (kasab). There you can ask for bones (kemik) or intestines like lung (akciğer). Both are slaughter waste, which does not play any role in the Turkish kitchen, and are therefore often available for free. The bones do not need to be boiled, as they are not from pigs. It is a bad habit of Turkish people to feed tourist dogs with the surplus sugarcubes from their tea. Try to explain to the people that this feeding method is not good for the dog and undesired by yourself. And keep your dog away from raw meatballs (köfte), for nothing is worse than a dog with diarrhoea, above all in your own car. We could tell you a story about that, too; but we prefer not to write it down here.

Holidays and Festivals

Banks and administration offices are closed on public holidays. The same with shops that do not sell products of daily life, like fashion boutiques and household supply stores. On those days also more Turkish visitors are to be expected, so that all tourist facilities will be hopelessly overcrowded. People even come from faraway Istanbul to pass an extended weekend in Cappadocia. Ürgüp is especially overcrowded by them on such occasions, as the site and the scenery of a popular Turkish TV serial are located there.
National festival days on special dates have to be distinguished from religious holidays, which follow the moon calendar and take place 11 days earlier each year. The feast of sacrifice (Kurban Bayrami) and the sugar festival (seker-bayrami) at the end of the fasting month of Ramasan are the two most important religious holidays. For more information, see the chapter on "Islam" in the first part of this book.
Some places in Cappadocia organize regular festivals. Thus, every year on the first weekend in August there is the Pottery and Tourist Festival in Avanos. In Hacibektas a great feast with many cultural events is celebrated from August 16th to August 18th on behalf of the holy Haci Bektas Veli. And

in Ürgüp there is a great wine festival in every autumn. Almost every place in Cappadocia has its own festival. For more information and for the exact dates, ask at the tourist information of the particular place.

National Holidays:

1. Jan.	New Year's Day
23. April	Independence Day after the opening of the National Assembly in 1923
19. May	Atatürk Remembrance Day. Youth and Sports Day
30. Aug.	Victory Day after the victory over the Greek invasion army in 1922
29. Oct.	Anniversary of the foundation of the Republic

Religious Holidays:

	2010	2011	2012
Beginning of Ramasan	11. Aug.	1. Aug.	19. July
Sugar festival, end of Ramasan	10. Sept.	30. Aug.	20. Aug.
Feast of Sacrifice	17. Nov.	7. Nov.	25. Sept.

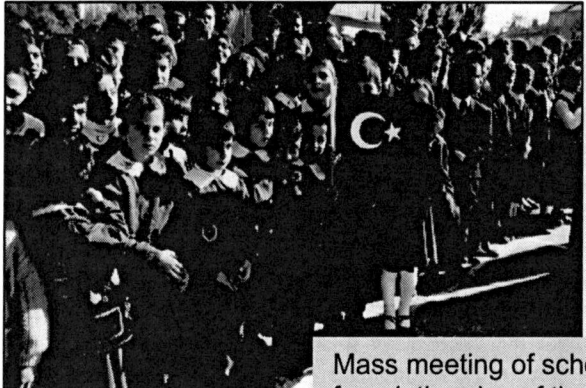

Mass meeting of school classes on foundation day of the Republic

Language and Communication

If you remain within the area of the tourist infrastructure in Cappadocia, you will not have any communication problems. Foreign languages are spoken in restaurants, hotels and in all other tourist places. Above all, English and French are spoken, and also some German. The whole tourism industry has set itself up for Western visitors, as they want to earn money from them.

Things are somewhat different with the normal population. There is almost no knowledge of foreign languages among them. In fact, English has been taught at school from the sixth year onwards for years already, but the language teaching methods can only be called disastrous. The teachers working there have hardly any command of the language themselves. Learning a foreign language is generally not very popular in Turkey. University language courses are an annoying compulsion even for future academics, and the few things you have learned are soon forgotten again. One important reason for this is the fact that Turkey is very much internally oriented in spheres like culture, economy and politics. Only very few young students are toying with the idea of going abroad later on. Most prefer setting themselves up in their own country with their own practice or office or working for one of the big companies in Istanbul. Also an executive position in the state administration is very popular. What are foreign languages needed for there? Even people who take up teacher training hope that they will never have to teach a foreign language. If this does happen, you just try to muddle through, to the detriment of the students. This is why communication with doctors, lawyers and officials, for tourists who are in trouble, is only possible with the help of a translator. We ourselves once had to extend our visa with the aliens branch of the police at Nevşehir. We had to traipse around more than ten different officials and counters during this procedure. Not a single person spoke a foreign language, neither the policemen who took down our particulars, nor the vice governor who signed our application.

Also policemen only very seldom speak any foreign languages. You are often more successful with plain soldiers or the Yandarma, as many Turkish emigrants from all over the world have to do their military service here. Basically we want to warmly recommend learning the most important Turkish phrases by heart. As the Turks have and employ numerous kinds of polite expressions of welcome, it makes a big impression if you, as a tourist, have a suitable answer in readiness. You will find a little language guide with the most common greetings and other useful everyday phrases at the back of this book. It probably does not need to be specifically mentioned that you should know the cardinal numbers, as nobody wants to be taken in when shopping.

Blunders

There is a wide range of these for visitors who are travelling to an oriental country for the first time. In spite of the risk of repeating things mentioned in previous chapters, we want to present the most important tips for avoiding inappropriate behaviour again here.

1. Please always wear appropriate clothing. Shorts and tank tops resemble underwear in the locals' eyes and are not apt to improve your social status.
2. For a visit in a mosque, clothing that covers your arms and legs is required; women should cover their head with a scarf. Shoes are taken off at the entrance of course. Before entering, make sure that it is not prayer time.
3. If you have been invited to a private household, a little welcome present for the wife (cosmetics, a box of chocolates, cake) and for the head of the family (cigarettes from abroad, some hard liquor) are gratefully received. Here, too, shoes must be taken off on entering the room. The presents, by the way, are only handed over. They are unwrapped only after the guest has left, in order not to appear greedy.
4. Do not eat or welcome somebody with your left hand, for it is used for cleaning your behind, and that is regarded as impure in Islam.
5. If you are sitting in the company of several persons, do not turn your back on somebody or show anybody the soles of your feet. Both things are understood as signs of personal aversion.
6. If you have been invited to a private household for a meal, go there with an empty stomach. Picking at one's food unenthusiastically could be misunderstood as a criticism of the housewife's cooking

skills. The obligatory praise after the meal will be of no use then, because nobody will believe you any more anyway.
7. Do not concentrate too much on the host of the opposite sex. This could be misunderstood. Flattering or even flirting with the wife or other female members of the family are signs of crude disrespect and contain huge potential for trouble.
8. Exchanging endearments with your partner in public is regarded as a taboo in small and remote villages. You will even rarely see couples holding hands there. This is however no problem in tourist places. Look at your environment for orientation, or restrict such things to the limits of your hotel room.
9. If you want to take photos of persons, ask for permission first. Devoutly religious persons have an adversity to being photographed, as Islam does not allow this.
10. Please refrain from swimming in the nude. Besides being contrary to good manners, this is also indictable, and you will never be alone in this huge country anyway.
11. If you have been invited for tea, do not try seriously to pay the bill. Apart from having no chance to do so, you would also insult your host.
12. If there problems should arise, try to keep calm. Be quiet, but determined in the matter. Shouting and name-calling only have the effect that the shutters go down and the matter is over for the other partner.
13. If you want to buy something or to make use of some service, please always ask for the price in advance. This is a completely normal procedure in the Orient. Only inexperienced tourists do not do this and are therefore still cheated too often.

On the whole we would like to suggest to you to confront people openly and in a friendly manner here in Cappadocia. Politeness towards others is a law of life in the Orient. If in addition you are able to use some Turkish words, then this might be able to smooth over the very few blunders which you will commit in spite of everything.

Like Dogs and Cats

Views of two Worlds

In Islam the social norms and standards originate from a totally different life situation than those of the Christian Occident. Islam is based on the necessities and demands of nomadism. In contrast to this, the demands of the Western civilization are on a totally different basis: the right of property, your own piece of soil as it were, that is, 'sedentariness' influences the ideas and the emotions of the Western world.

The Turks, too, were nomads, and the effects of that vagrant life still manifest themselves in the daily life of Turkish-Islamic culture, even today after 500 years. Then, the nomad tribes lived in large family clans; no state, neither executive nor judicial powers protected them when they were wandering across the open country with their herds of animals. There was no such thing as the superior authority of the state. Law and justice had to be defined within the tribe. This way of living was made even more complicated by the habit of all nomads to make raids on each other and plunder or kidnap the enemy's women in order to reduce in-breeding within their own tribes. Those raids sometimes destroyed entire families. How were they to be prevented by law and justice, and who was there to enforce their rights? As there existed no superordinated police, the tribes were forced to help themselves and thus, blood revenge was made a moral law: only the duty of the survivors to take revenge for a murdered or misused member of the family by bloodshed and murder could provide the security that prevented anybody from killing anybody else if he felt like it. This duty often was a difficult legacy for the following generations.

But other offenses, too, which were liable to endanger the fragile social norms, had to result in a strong moral obligation which nobody could evade even without any police authority, and they were meant to act as a deterrent. In the millennia of roaming about, of plundering and struggling for survival, the forced obligation for revenge has moulded people's character. Islam, which was founded in the 7th century by Mohammad, tried to soften this destructive power by superordinated and merciful laws and tried to unite the tribes. 1300 years have passed since then; tribal areas have turned into sovereign states; now there are police and law and order: the citizens do not need to defend themselves any more. But the former nomads cannot jump over their shadows.

And we settled people in the West, too, are subject to many constraints: this obsessive attachment to our own soil, this absurd hoarding of possessions and property, up to the present consumer terrorism, all this has already assumed neurotic traits. Appearance is reality - this is especially true in the Western industrial nations, under the motto: "you are what you have".

By contrast, in the Islamic world the people decorate themselves with perfect and honourable behaviour, which means total adaptation to or in the family. One can only really get ahead inside the clan, the approval by the family is at the zenith of all desires. The family has to be protected, individual liberties are not provided in this respect. Only 20 years ago, our travels in Turkey caused compassion and incomprehension among older Turkish women: Had our parents died in some kind of tragedy? Had we been cast out by our family? Nobody decides to live in a foreign land deliberately. We were given ample food then, as they assumed that we would hardly be able to survive on our own this way. The much-vaunted hospitality in Turkey and in the whole Islamic world is based on the wise experience that people in a foreign country need unlimited protection and support in their plight, as they would not survive being far away from their families. Unlimited hospitality, as one of the greatest and most honoured commandments, was even necessary towards enemies, even if this might have meant one's own destruction.

Vengeance versus Christian charity! Freedom of social or of material restrictions! Ruinous hospitality or cold-hearted striving for possession! As long as those two cultures do not understand each other, they will behave like cats and dogs: whenever the friendly dog wags its tail, the cat lauches an attack.

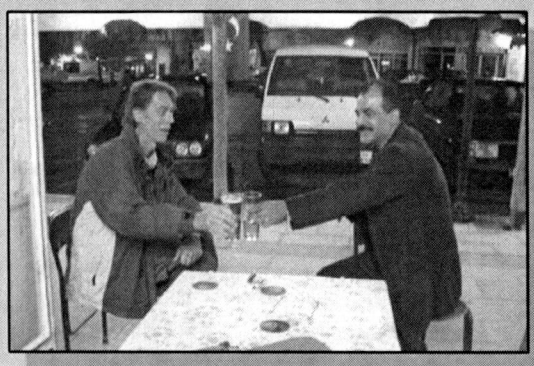

Begging

On the whole, begging is not an important issue in Cappadocia. The only thing is that the younger children have found out that adults sometimes have sweets with them. Unfortunately, we have frequently had the experience that tourists distributed large quantities of sweets among the crowd without any special reason, just because the little ones seemed so cute. We should like to ask our readers to refrain from doing such things. You cannot carry as many sweets with you as the children will take from you, as the children will not stop pestering you until after the last candy has been given away. Additionally, the throng of the little ones will get bigger and bigger so that it soon will grow very shady around you. Putting an end to this feeding of predators will always more and more resemble a hasty retreat. If you want to make a donation, always combine it with a little duty. Let older children go on an errand for you and give them the change afterwards, or ask them to stand sentinel over your vehicle, even though this is quite unnecessary. The indiscriminate distribution of gifts only puts stupid ideas in their heads and makes them pester the next group of tourists.

With elderly and infirm persons or sometimes also with unmarried women with children, things are different. Their sustenance is not always guaranteed in Turkey. Especially in cases where no other family members exist they will have to rely on other people's generosity. Begging at exposed sites, like the mosque or the market square, is related to this. The fact that these persons have to go begging does not have the same negative reputation as in our countries, but is regarded as a dire necessity by the population. One important reason for this is based on Islam, to whose five supporting pillars the giving of alms to the poor belongs. The begging person has a right to a small contribution guaranteed by the Koran in a way that he or she is not obliged to make a long speech of thanks to the giver. Also as a tourist one should make a small contribution in such cases, some small coins being perfectly alright. Please do not take out a large bank note because you would just shame the person with it, and do not expect a beggar to be able to change your banknote. It has happened to us that our contribution was refused with indignation because it was regarded as being too large.

Leisure Activities

Walking

The beach, sunbathing and the sea – these are words that dominate the tourist image of Turkey. Only very few people know how many possibilities for walking are available here. For example, in South West Turkey, there is the "Lycian Hiking Trail". Excellently marked with signs, with many resting or accomodation facilities, it meanwhile extends for hundreds of miles along the almost untouched coast. You will frequently find the remains of historical monuments on it.

Cappadocia, too, is a dream destination for walkers, but still not many people know this yet. No wonder, if you have booked the "Cappadocia in 2 days" program, there will not be enough time for walking. Besides, walking as tourism is not advertised or promoted intensely enough by the official authorities. Thus there are hardly any signs and the paths are not maintained regularly. Nevertheless, or just because of this, a walking tour through the serpentine valleys is a unique experience of nature. And signs are not necessary if you follow the valleys downhill. Like branches of a tree that join together to form the trunk, the many side valleys unite, forming a broad valley towards the end. You simply cannot lose your way in them. There are mostly even two paths: the first one goes through the gardens that cover all valleys. Sometimes you have to look carefully at where the path continues, as it is only a beaten path for the locals. The second path follows the dry bed of a creek and often goes through the rocks through which the water has drilled huge tunnel systems in thousands of years.- But there is one thing that must be clear to you: These are no official hiking trails, but paths that go through other people's gardens. But this will not cause any problems, provided you do not step on the vegetables. If you meet any local people in those gardens and greet them with a friendly 'merhaba', you will only have one problem: you will be showered with fruit and vegetables ad nauseam.

Walking up the valleys is more difficult, as many side valleys rise abruptly, putting an end to the path.Thus it can take you a very long time until you have found an exit, and then you will often be far away from any road or inhabited place.

There are said to be hikers who need twice as much time for such a walk. The caves on both sides of the valleys are a reason for that. Even here in this secluded place, far away from the hustle and bustle of tourism, ancient frescoed churches can be discovered.There is mostly an ancient decaying irrigation system running along the valley in the tufa rocks which sometimes can still be walked through. Thus it is not surprising if such a walk takes a whole day. If now there is additionally a hobby photographer in your group, then faster advancement will be totally out of the question. On both sides of the valleys, countless wild rock formations in all colour shades make the heart of the photographer beat faster. Every five minutes he will begin to put up his tripod and camera and will put his fellow travellers' nerves to a severe test. Photo fans should do those tours with their spouse only, provided that the spouse is willing to tolerate this kind of hobby.

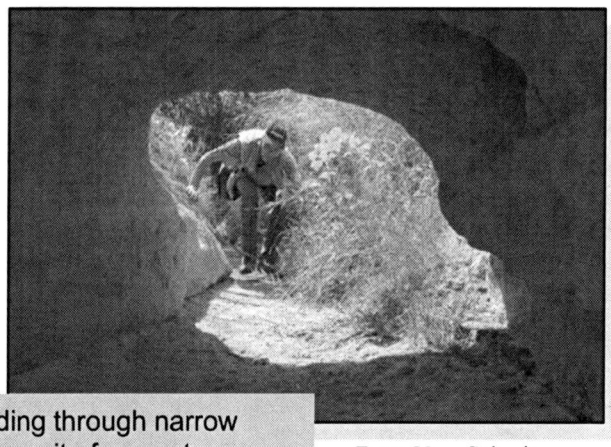

Paths leading through narrow tunnels are quite frequent

Foto: Uwe Schmitz

All big valleys finally end in an asphalt road that will take you back to civilization. Often the nearest inhabited place is not far away then.The longest walking trip takes 3 hours, that is, without any cave explorers and hobby photographers by your side.
If you do not dare to undertake such a tour on your own, you can book a guided walking tour. The advantage of this is the guides' familiarity with the area. They can show you things that escape the untrained eye. The guides know the secret and hidden entrances of many caves. Moreover, they are

willing to answer any questions or to explain the sense and the purpose of the various caves.

Being a good walker is the precondition for all routes. The upper entrance is often the most difficult part. You walk over steep and crumbly tufa there. The eroding rock crumbs form a slippery layer on top of the rock, like the little balls of a ball bearing. Only seldom have steps been hacked into the rock, and if they have been, they were worn down and eroded after a few years. There are also sections where you have to climb over ladders, or a steep wooden log path has been built so that you can only go on crawling on all fours. Therefore, durable trousers are as important as sturdy shoes. Apart from this you should wear as light and loose clothing as possible to allow your body to remain cool. A headcovering is absolutely necessary, too. There are in fact enough shady places on your way, but remember you are at an altitude of about 1000 m above sea level. Finally, the most important point: always take enough water with you, because we cannot advise you to drink from the occasional cisterns by the side of the trail. The consequences would become obvious the next morning at the latest.

If you want to explore the valleys of Cappadocia without using a guide, you will find some proposed routes with detailed descriptions, time information and a little map at the back of this travel guide. Unfortunately, there are no acceptable walking maps available yet.

Ballooning

It is still very early in the morning and the roosters in the nearby villages have only just started their early morning concert. The silent landscape lies in front of our eyes, spread out widely in the first light of dawn. We have spent the night in our motor home on a hill next to the museum in Göreme in order to witness a unique sight. Suddenly the morning mood is interrupted by the rattling noise of a propeller. Another one is fired up, and soon more and more small airplanes seem to be preparing to take off from the valleys around us. Shortly after, we hear the frightening hiss of a fire-spitting dragon. Will it attack the planes? The hissing replaces the propeller noise, until one after another they fall silent again. As every morning, the dragon has won the fight also today. Now its fiery tail can be seen clearly amidst the green of the valleys. There must be several monsters, as the fires begin to spread out around our hill. Suddenly huge mushrooms begin to rise from the ground, growing bigger with the increasing fire from the dragons. They tower before us in the light of dawn, bulging and illuminated by the fire inside them: the hot-air balloons.

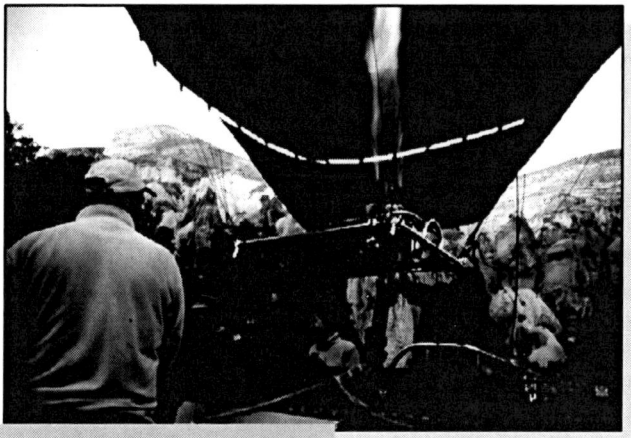

Takeoff is shortly before sunrise

Nothing has changed Cappadocia's morning landscape as deeply as they have done. More than 20 of them take off for a round trip every morning at daybreak. Ballooning has become one of the greatest attractions that the region also vigorously uses for advertising for itself. And it all started so inconspicuously: 16 years ago, the operators of the former "Club Mediterranee" had the idea to offer balloon tours to their guests. The necessary equipment was bought right away, and two pilots were hired. There was a lot of excitement in the neighbouring communities. Many people were shocked by the huge unknown flying objects that were hovering above their houses. Most of them had never heard of hot-air balloons, and the hissing noise of the gas burners did not really increase their feeling of reassurement. Today the balloons are part of Cappadocia and except for the dogs, nobody feels endangered by them any more. When ten years ago the club facilities were sold, the two pilots started their own business and founded "Kapadokya Balloons". Up till today they have been running their business with great success. Other clever businessmen also noticed that a lot of money can be made with this idea. Thus today there are various providers who offer such balloon flights.

Ballooning in Cappadocia is something very special. Here you do not simply take off, soar across the landscape for some time and then come down again; here the flight rather resembles a permanent ropeway trip. The balloon basket with its passengers moves through deep valleys, over the peaks of the nearby mountains and through the treetops of green orchards. There is a steady rise and fall as if the vehicle were held by invisible rails. There is food, too, for the pilots ardently love picking fruits from the trees during the flight. Towards the end, the balloon rises to 1000 m. and allows a view over the entire rugged landscape. Winds from various directions make great movability of the balloons possible here in Cappadocia. The hillsides, which are warmed up by the rising sun, produce a thermal upwind that makes flying against the main direction possible. In the valleys the airstream adapts to the geographical conditions, and at higher altitudes there is often a different wind than near the ground. Thus the balloon can be easily steered in three different directions just by changing its altitude.

Ballooning is no cheap fun, though. The most inexpensive version is for about $180, and the most exclusive trip is $320 at the moment. These extreme differences between prices do not exist without any reason. The technical standard of the equipment and the pilot's aeronautical skill are decisive for them. In both aspects the suppliers differ considerably from each other. Evil tongues say that some of the balloon skins consist of old clothes bags from Europe. It is true that sometimes superannuated skins are imported from Europe, which is not entirely unhazardous. We were able to judge the differences in the pilots' abilities very well from our morning observation point. One balloon floated lazily over a chain of hills and down into the valley, then rose again and in agonizing slowness tried to return to its starting point during the rest of the one-hour trip. In this case the passengers had literally cast their money to the wind. Other balloons offered a little bit more and sometimes sailed through a complete valley. But here, too, the pilot did not show great interest in his job. Meanwhile some firms have even started making an intermediate stop to exchange their passengers.

But now the best supplier: His balloons jump over the hilltops, dive into various valleys, then regain great height in order to present another part of the landscape from the air. Even though this tour is quite expensive, one should not try to save in the wrong place here.

If you want to book one of those flights, you should do it well in advance, for the demand is quite great despite the respectable prices. You should also be an early riser, as the tours take place at sunrise. The price includes transport from your accommodation – about 1 hour before dawn – and the return transfer. Flight times are between one and one and a half hours, sometimes more. Especially in spring when the fields have been newly sown it is more difficult for the pilots to find a suitable landing site.

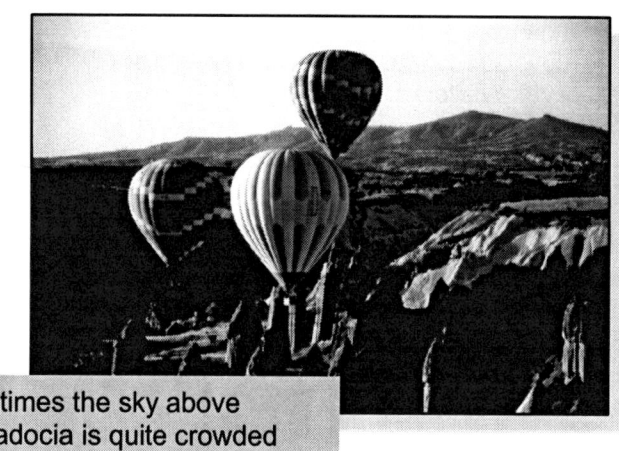

Sometimes the sky above Cappadocia is quite crowded

Finally, two more things: You should put on warm clothes, for temperatures can be quite low at high altitudes. And drinking coffee or tea before takeoff is not advisable to passengers who suffer from bladder weakness, as you will look in vain for any toilets up in the air.

Here now are the three biggest suppliers:

KAPADOKYA BALLOONS

First and best company on site. The agency is in Göreme, 150 meters from the centre, on the right side of the Uchisar road. The owners, Lars-Eric Möre and Kaili Kidner, have been running the business for more than 15 years, and both of them have more than 25 years of flying experience. Their air vehicles are always up to date, because security is very important here. Two versions are offered: The 1 hour flight in a wide-bodied basket for 20 passengers is $245, and you pay $322 for a trip in one of the two smaller balloons. There is only room for 8 passengers in them, but they are much more manoeuverable and the flying manoeuvres are much more spectacular.Two balloons mostly fly close together, so that it can almost be called an air show. Both pilots work together as an excellent team. This trip takes at least one and a half hours.

Phone.　0090 384 271 2442
Fax:　　 0090 384 271 2586
www.kapadokyaballoons.com

ANATOLIAN BALLOONS

The agency was founded in 2005 and presently helps making Cappadocia's sky become a bit crowded. By means of a large investment volume, 8 brand new balloons and a corresponding transport pool were bought. It remains to be seen whether in the course of time equally good pilots will be working there, too. The just about 1 hour normal flight is $210 and the 1.5 hour deluxe trip is offered for $315.

Phone:　 0090 384 271 2300
Fax:　　 0090 384 271 2588
www.anatolianballoons.com.tr

GÖREME BALLOONS

This company, too, has been roaming the skies over Cappadocia for more than 12 years now. The one-hour flight is $224 here and the so-called deluxe flight is $322. Children under 6 are free and up to the age of 12 only half the price is charged.

Phone:　 0090 384 341 5661 and 62
Fax:　　 0090 384 341 7245
www.goremeballoons.com

Cycling

Cycling is no big issue in Cappadocia. There are bike rental outlets for tourists at some places, but this kind of locomotion is mainly reserved for children by the Turks. Already the geographical conditions themselves do not make it any easier for the cycling fan. Additionally, there is the sun which often blazes down mercilessly from the sky and the infernal heat connected with it. The narrow and winding roads between the places and the heavy traffic on them will generally spoil the fun for you.

Cyclists are on the lowest position of the traffic hierarchy in Turkey, and cycle tracks are an unknown word here. It is only worth while exploring the country a little by mountainbike. But even this has its limits. The ride mostly ends in front of the terraced fruit orchards in the many little side valleys after a short while. So-called downhill routes for mountainbikers do not exist. The trails, which we have described in the chapter on walking, in their upper parts always lead through cultivated orchards. Bikers riding wildly downhill, plowing through the tomato plantations, are extremely unwelcome there. However, there are so-called 'offroad tours' offered by some local travel agencies. But those tours are only for very experienced mountainbikers, as the tracks are quite demanding for walkers already.

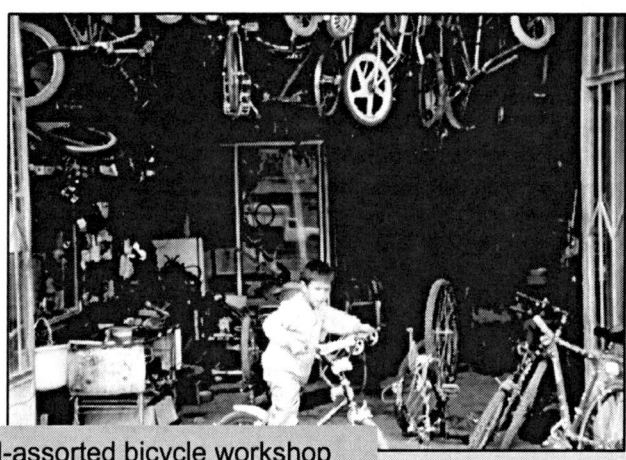

A well-assorted bicycle workshop

If you want to be mobile in order to move between the places, a rented scooter is the better thing for you, and for tourists who like to watch cycling sport, there is a trip round Cappadocia organized each year near the end of summer. The start and the finish are in Ürgüp.

Swimming

Swimming facilities in Cappadocia are very limited. There are some reservoirs and even a crater lake in the region, but all their shores are muddy and do not allow much fun to arise when swimming. For example, at the entrance of the Damsa reservoir you are charged 1 TL entrance fee per person, but swimming is nevertheless not permitted there.
The Kızılırmak River is another possibility. There are some places to swim about half a mile before the river reaches the town of Avanos. But they are quite hidden behind a strip of green and far away from the footpath. Behind the suspension bridge in Avanos you take the little road to the east along the river. A tunnel passes underneath the ring road and after 500 ms you take a field path to the right running past a ranch and through fallow land to the river. The water, however, is quite chilly throughout the year, and in spring you should absolutely refrain from swimming in the river because of the torrent. And never go for a swim behind Avanos, as the town has no sewage plant. As an alternative, there is the swimming pool of the Ada camping site. For an entrance fee of 10 TL the neat and tidy grounds can be used by everybody. Otherwise you should make sure in advance that there is a swimming pool when choosing your hotel or camping site. - Another bathing facility is described later on under the headword of "Bayramhacı".

Horseriding

Cappadocia is allegedly called the "land of the beautiful horses" (Katpatuka), but that seems to be quite a long time ago. There are some riding stables that have been established especially for tourists. The horseback rides which are available there are cross-country and off all paths through the landscape of Cappadocia. Trips of a day or a week can be booked there, too. But you should not expect any noble stallions there. It is more than 500 years ago that the Turks began to settle down. This is why horseriding is not so popular in the country any more, and the breeding results correspond to this. The horse is a sheer beast of labour to the Turks and is used in agriculture or for transport. The motorization of the past decades has contributed to making the horse become increasingly rare as a domestic animal. So, do not expect too much of those animals.

The somewhat rude behaviour towards the creatures might be a shock to Western animal lovers. Love of animals in our sense is not very widespread.

We want to mention two riding stables here:

Cecilia and Mehmet Sibik offer tours on horseback through Cappadocia which are entirely adapted to the needs and wishes of the customers. Anything will be organized from training lessons for beginners to 8 days' cross-country tours. During overnight excursions the participants camp in tents in the middle of the superb countryside and they are supplied with everything they need by Mehmet. There is no sportive riding, however. The horses and the riders are kept busy for 6 hours per day at a maximum, for Cecilia is a vet who knows what is suitable for the animals. A one-hour riding lesson is available for $10.50 and for longer excursions a price of $70 per day has to be calculated.

Mehmet and Cecilia Sibek – Cagatay Ranch, Avanos
Phone: 0090 535 238 8862
E-mail: cecilia.dervaux@laposte.net

Those who prefer a somewhat more sportive style should contact the « Kirkit-Voyage » agency, which also has its office in Avanos. With more than 40 horses it is one of the biggest horse-riding ranches in all Cappadocia. Weekend tours are also available there.

Kirkit-Voyage, Avanos
Phone: 0090 384 511 2135
Website :   www.kirkit.com

Pottery

The town of Avanos has pottery facilities in abundance. Along the main road to Kayseri or in the town centre there is one pottery shop next to another. Nobody there will discourage you from sitting down behind the potter's wheel. Quite contrary, you will be given a lump of clay and lots of advice and support. The wheel's headpieces are unfamiliar, as they are not over 15 cm in diameter. They are driven by a flywheel on the floor which is kept in motion by kicking it with your feet and which loses its momentum very quickly.

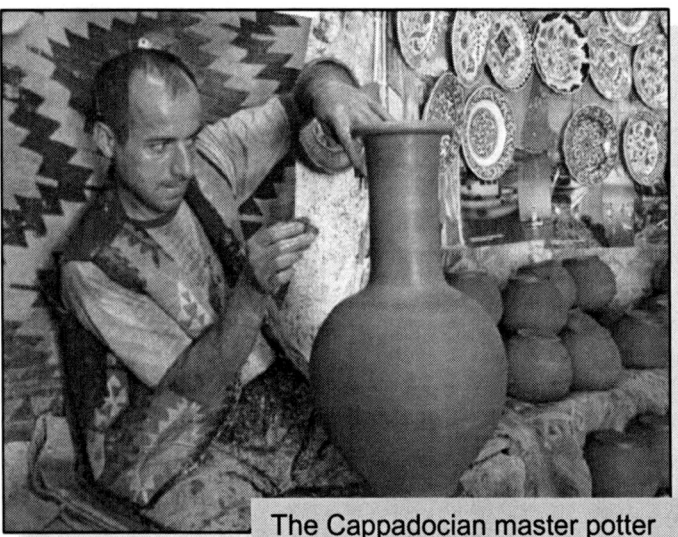

The Cappadocian master potter Gökhan Özgül at work

If you are interested in pottery on a long-term basis, you can book courses of several weeks. Prices include accommodation, meals and possible excursions through Cappadocia. Those potteries also have the pottery wheels familiar to us with bigger disks and electric drive. More about pottery on p.242.

Pottery courses over several days are offered by:

Chez Galip, the archetype among the potters who became involved in the tourist business. He has been part of it for more than 25 years now and offers a wide range of leisure activities. Meanwhile he even owns a little house for his guests. He has been in the Guiness Book of World Records for years for his international collection of women's hair: more than 10,000 curls and strands are hanging on the walls of one of his exibition caves, each with a little address tag on it. Thus, no female tourist gets away unshorn here.

Chez Galip, Avanos
Phone: 0090 384 511 5758
www.chez-galip.com

Erdogan Gülec, « Bei Kaya » runs his little studio right in the town centre, far away from the streams of tourists. He has specialized in the production of so-called relief pictures on glazed tiles and also offers pottery courses of several days for groups. They are in combination with day trips through Cappadocia.

Erdogan Gülec – Bei Kaya, Avanos
Phone: 0090 384 511 3464
www.katpatuka.org/beikaya

Taking Photos

Fans of romantic landscape photos will find eveything they need in Cappadocia. Especially towards evening, when the setting sun bathes the bizarre rock formations in deep red, it is worthwhile scrambling through the extensive hilly landscape with heavy photo equipment. With a tripod, a long exposure time and a high number (small aperture) f-stop you will now be able to take the most atmosheric pictures. Those who prefer working around noontime should use a polarizing filter, as the strong direct sunlight makes the normally colourful rock formations look somewhat pale at this time of day. Also, strong contrasts in brightness and shadow are to be expected at noon.

On the subject of portrait photography or photographing Turkish people, we would like to remind you that Turkey is an Islamic country and that making portraits of people is forbidden for religious persons. Therefore, an Imam will not like to be photographed at all. The same applies to elderly people and in remote villages. But apart from this the Cappadocians are not camera-shy. On the contrary, you are often positively invited to take a picture. The reason for this is that cameras are very expensive and therefore very rare in Turkey. Thus many Turks will see a chance to come by a photo of themselves and of their family this way. A print of a photo sent to them after the end of your holidays is always a most welcome additional present. But in this era of the photo cellphone, this could very soon be over.

If no real invitation to take photos is obvious, then politeness demands asking for permission beforehand - actually this should be a matter of course in the whole world, which, however, is frequently forgotten.

Can I take a photo of you? > foto cekebilir miyim?

If you want to take really good photos of people - and if you are a man - ask your female partner to take the camera and do it. Female photographers have much easier access to all areas of life and therefore also to the milieu of Turkish women. And please, do not snap at people suddenly and unexpectedly, but start a short conversation with your "victim" before. By doing this you can increase the people's readiness to serve as a model for you.

If you have not joined the world of digital photography yet, you should bring a sufficient number of camera films with you, for it is hard to get good films that will not be too old or have been lying in the sun for ages. You should especially refrain from buying films at the many souvenir kiosks. Besides, films are very expensive here, and slide film is not available at all. Please remember to take a couple of extra batteries or enough storage media with you, because they are anything but cheap here.

It is recommended to transport your camera in a protective cover, as Cappadocia is rather dusty. A camera that is aways exposed to the climatic conditions can lose its function very soon.

If your expectations are not too great, you can have your films developed in the local photo shops. That is also where you should buy any missing films or forgotten memory cards.

Tourists taking photos have been a common sight for years in Cappadocia now and actually there is almost nothing here that has not been documented on a photo by somebody. The only thing we would strongly advise you not to do is to take photos of military institutions. The military treats this very seriously and does not see it as fun at all.

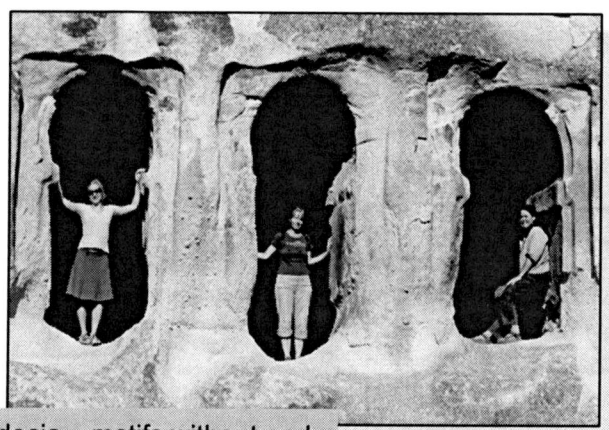
Cappadocia – motifs without end

Hamam

To the inexperienced tourist the hamam follows right after the word harem, as far as exoticism is concerned. Even though both words begin with an "H", their functions are nevertheless very different. While the harem excludes people – it does not let women out and does not allow men in – the hamam is regarded as a social meeting place. A strict separation of the sexes exists there, too, but it is also an ideal place for chatting, talking and calmly discussing problems without being disturbed. Many a marriage was contrived here, wrapped in the cozy warmth and the mist of the hot steam, by the mothers of the future bridal couple. And many disagreements between families became possible to be resolved by the husbands during their phases of dozing on the hot stones.

However, the hamam is no Ottoman invention. During their advancement towards Constantinople and their conquest of Asia Minor, the Ottomans got to know the advantages of the antique Roman baths and carried on their tradition.

Cappadocia does not possess many Turkish baths. Those institutions were mostly reserved to larger towns. There is one in Nevşehir, shortly below the big main mosque. Another one is in Ürgüp, directly in the town centre, and in Avanos a new one was built some years ago. The hamam of Avanos was built mainly for tourist reasons. In it, there is no separation between the sexes. This also refers to the bath attendants, and so women have to tolerate being washed or massaged by completely strange men. An ideal place for bringing on busloads of tourists, with prices being accordingly steep, no Turkish woman would ever come here.

But the baths in Nevşehir and Kayseri are old traditional institutions. As they are not very large, they have no special areas for men and women. Instead, there are appointed times for men or women. Thus you will never be able to attend an old traditional hamam together with your husband, except if you go to Ürgüp. The bath there was privatized some years ago and the segregation of the sexes was abolished.

What, then, is such a traditional Turkish bath like? First you enter the reception hall, to which the changing rooms are connected. Here you take your clothes off and are given beach slides and towels; one big towel is wrapped around the thighs as a substitute for your shorts. Women always keep their underpants on! If you have any valuables with you, you can deposit them at the reception. Now you enter a little room that separates the entrance hall from the real bath. It is getting somewhat warmer here already. Often the toilet rooms branch off here, which are always a little smelly because of the heat. Then there follows the main room, from where heat and moisture gush towards you. In the centre there is the large hot stone which takes up most of the space. Along the walls there are wash basins with faucets for hot and cold water. There are small cubicles in the four corners of the room. There you can wash those body parts that other bathers are not allowed to see. The whole room is vaulted by a huge dome with small coloured lighting orifices in it, which allow the light to filter through the mist in thin rays. Your first job is to go to a wash basin and to splash yourself properly with water. Little bowls have been prepared for this purpose, with which you have to mix the hot and cold water from the faucets yourself. Often the warm water is much too hot at first. After that you wash thoroughly as usual at home. Then you lie down on the central hot stone for a proper sweat. Be careful, for at that point you can easily fall asleep. The whole atmosphere contributes to this: Often only the splash of water can be neard. The voices of the other bathers are muffled and die away in the cupola. In between you always hear the dripping sound of the water drops which, having condensed in the dome, fall down and burst on the hot stone.The stiffling humid air adds to the effect. The skin opens its pores and the sweat transports the remaining Anatolian dust to the surface. Now you rinse yourself thoroughly with water and a feeling of intense cleanness begins to spread. But that is deceptive. Now the washerman has his big moment. He orders you to lie down on the stone again and begins his procedure. First you are covered with lather again with a sponge until you cannot see anything but an ocean of white mountains. Afterwards you are showered mercilessly with floods of water to remove the lather. Then the washman starts scrubbing you with a coarse piece of cloth. This is the moment of truth, which always makes us blush with shame, too. Especially on your arms and legs, pitch black little fragments of skin are rolled off your body. The dead skin is scrubbed off in the hamam, and only after this you can be called 'clean down to the pores'. Even if you take a shower every day, you are by far not clean in the sense of the Orient.

When once we visited the hamam with a friend, we had a fortnight of concrete work behind us. We had had a good scrubdown in the shower every day after work. In the Turkish bath however, the same tiny rolls of skin appeared, this time in the greenish gray colour of freshly mixed concrete.-

Finally, you should take a rest again on the hot stone to get over the shock. At the exit, freshly warmed towels are waiting for you, which are skilfully wrapped around you. There is often a chillout corner in the reception hall, where you can slowly get used to normal temperatures again and have a cup of tea. Women will then dedicate themselves to epilation. If two hours have passed during the procedure, that is absolutely normal.

In other baths in larger towns there is also a barber and a shoe-shine with it, which complete the cleansing program. We want to warn you of the massage; it is not for everybody. It is rather violent and demands a certain amount of masochism. Especially with tourists the massagers like to show sadistic tendencies: they dislocate your vertebrae or trample about on your back.

Another possibility of relaxing in warm water is at the 'Bayramhacı' (see in that chapter p.250).

The baths in detail:

Ürgüp:

Situated at the central square opposite the mosque, open daily from 7.00 a.m. to 9.00 p.m.. Unfortunately, tribute has meanwhile been paid to tourism and the separation of the sexes has been abolished. Women can only be with each other undisturbed on Sundays between 12.00 noon and 4.00 p.m. 20 TL entrance fee, washing and massage included.

Avanos:

Turkish bath which was rebuilt on the foundations of a bathhouse of the Seljuk era. Today it is totally aimed at tourists and there is no segregation of the sexes. A sauna is combined with the bath, which is not found in traditional baths. On the whole it seems to have been built totally adapted to the ideas of the tourists. The bath is open from 8.00 a.m. to 2.00 a.m. at night, and reservation is necessary. The price is 40 TL per person, with everything included.

Göreme:

In the spring of 2008 this little bath combined with a Finnish sauna opened its doors for the first time. Although at first glance it does not look like it, it is a new building in the old Ottoman style. You will not find segregation of the sexes here, either, as it was built especially for the many tourists who stay here in Göreme. The fee is 35 TL.

Nevşehir:

Traditional Ottoman bath at the Ibrahim Paşa Complex, near the main mosque. Open daily from 5.00 a.m. to midnight. Admittance for women only on Saturdays between 10.00 a.m. and 4.00 p.m. Separation of the sexes is maintained here. Fee: 15 TL including washing and a massage.
Another, newer and more often frequented hamam is directly next to the terminal of the local bus lines in Lale Caddesi. Here, too, entrance, massage and washing in combination are 15 TL.

Kayseri:

Also an old Ottoman bath with strict separation of the sexes. Open 24 hours daily. Bathing time for women is from 6.00 to 10.00 a.m., the rest of the day is reserved for men. Entrance fee: 7 TL, massage or washing are 4 TL more. Like in Nevsehir, the historic bath belongs to a complex of the mosque and the Madrasa.
A second hamam, with the same opening hours and prices, is situated south of the town centre.

Souvenirs and Carpets

There are countless opportunities to buy little souvenirs for yourself and for your friends at home. Numerous souvenir stalls have been put up around the entrance sections of the tourist sights, and there literally is no escape from them. Even at the most beautiful lookouts whole villages of hastily built huts of corrugated iron have been put together. While only 20 years ago there were only cultivated fields, today one stall follows another and one tourist bus is parked next to another. The supply is in fact not very manifold. There is often a limited supply of cheap knick-knacks, from miniature plastercast fairy chimneys down to frail tin products whose premature death due to rust is already foreseeable. Especially the electric tin samovars must be regarded with extreme scepticism. They are only for people who intend to refurbish their little family home by means of fire: water, faulty insulation, electricity and cheap corrosive tin add up to a sparkling mixture. A large part of the offered products consists of onyx items, pottery (which sometimes is only made of plaster) and the usual holiday textiles. But if you have a penchant for beautiful scarves or wall carpets, you can get your money's worth here. And do not forget to bargain, as many prices are rather exaggerated at first and can be corrected downwards at about one third. If you are after something special, you should look around the antiques shops in some of the town centres. They partly offer the usual items, too, but among those you can discover some little hidden treasures. The vendors are well-informed of the prices, however, so real bargains are very rare. If you discover a rarity, however, make the seller give you a receipt with the price and specification of the object on it. Thus you have a proof for the customs when leaving the country. Great care is recommended when buying carved stone and ancient clay pottery. You are better to abstain from purchasing such objects. Some years ago there were newspaper reports about thieving tourists who smuggle Turkish cultural treasures out of the country, and they were hard to ignore.

Just a few remarks about the offered "onyx" products. They are not made of real onyx, but of so-called onyx marble, a mineral which contains neither onyx nor marble and which bears its name because it closely resembles real onyx , while the term 'marble' only refers to the chemical composition. Genuine onyx is much harder and is not available in sufficiently large quantities to produce all those beautiful souvenirs from it. But this should not prevent anybody from buying such a souvenir. If these products were made of the genuine semi-precious stone, they would be almost unaffordable.

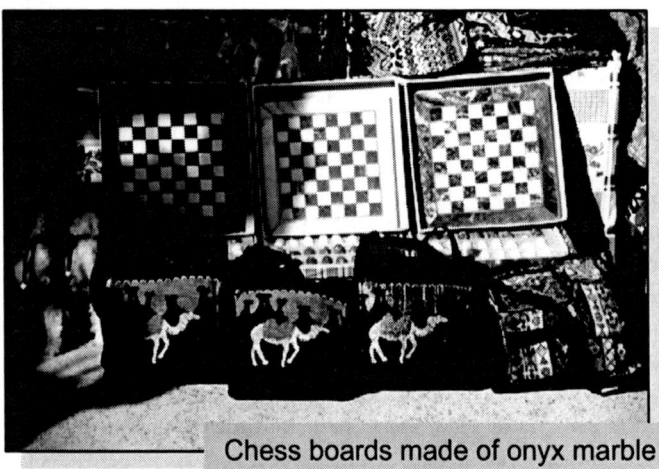

Chess boards made of onyx marble

No tourist escapes the rug dealers unscathed. This is of course not absolutely necessary. If you like Turkish carpets, you should let them be shown to you. But you should be fair and let the dealer know before that you are only toying with the idea of buying one. The demonstration will not be any poorer because of that, as it will incite the rug dealer to show off his art of persuasion. He will pull all the stops to talk you into buying something. If the rare case occurs that the tourist does not buy anything, the dealer will not be angry about this anyway. Even after an hours-long demonstration of the products and several rounds of tea you do not need to have a guilty conscience about leaving the shop without a rug.

If you are seriously interested in buying a carpet we recommend looking for comparative offers also in other shops, because bargaining is called for with carpets, too. The prices in Cappadocia are not necessarily lower than in Europe, but there is a considerably larger choice. It starts with a small Kilim for $25 and perhaps ends with a large sized silk carpet for $25.000.

Your excuse that you have not got enough cash with you will be answered with great complaisance by the dealer: he will propose to mail the item to your country so that you will have to pay at home. Do not get any crooked ideas now, for there is a man of his confidence in your country, who only delivers the item to your door against cash.

If you have bought a carpet you will be given a receipt by the dealer with a specification of the item and the price on it. The Turkish customs is not interested in the number of rugs you are exporting, but in the question whether there is a rarity from a sultan's palace among them. But never fear, the little Cappadocian rug dealers will never get hold of such items. The European customs will be more interested in the question whether you want to start an international carpet business yourself.

Three completely different types of carpets must be distinguished. First there is the "Kelim", which is a thin and light flat-woven rug. Then there is the "Cicim", which consists of a unicolour piece of fabric which has been embroidered with images. It is also used as a wall carpet, or you can also find it as a large embroidered camel bag which, having been filled with soft material, is used as a cushion. The third in the bunch is the "Halı", which is a carpet produced in the fashion best known to us and consists of tied knots. As its production is very laborious – a carpet weaver works on such a work of art for several months – a knotted carpet is mostly more expensive than a Kelim or a Cicim. A small Kelim fits into any baggage and is a beautiful souvenir; a real piece of art handicraft which will remind you of your holiday in Cappadocia for a long time after it is over.

However, we have to inform you of some excesses that have taken root in the carpet industry in recent years. Thus for example, some big companies offer up to 40 % of commission to anyone who recruits a paying customer. It need not be said that you as the customer in such a case would have to pay for a grossly overpriced product in the end. Sometimes it is even more profitable for many little rug dealers to recruit well-to-do customers for a big competitor than selling their own products. Often the inexperienced holidaymakers are told the story of the state-supported local carpet weaving school. You are led into a room where a group of young women is sitting at their looms weaving carpets. All this serves the purpose of making the customer believe in the integrity of the business and of making him feel safe as well as setting one's firm in a favourable light. You are not only expected to buy something, but also to be willing to help and to support a carpet weaving school with your purchase. Carpet dealers could not act more perfidious. The truth is:

There are no carpet weaving schools in Cappadocia !

They are fighting with no holds barred in the carpet industry, and the tricks of the traffickers are not recognizable to the visitor. The biggest packs of lies are presented for this purpose. Once some young man pretended to be a plain clothes tourist policeman who allegedly wanted to guide us to the only reliable rug shop in the area. Common sense and good judgement are necessary in this case. Firstly, there is no tourist police in Cappadocia and secondly, a plain clothes officer of such a police would not make much sense. How would an inexperienced visitor be supposed to recognize him, if not by his uniform?
If a local acquaintance or tour guide makes too much promotion for a certain firm, simply just choose a competitor. Do not let yourself be taken in, this will only make the goods more expensive than necessary.

Another beautiful souvenir of a holiday in Cappadocia is the Oriental amulet "against the evil eye", a stylized eye made of blue glass that is believed to protect people against bad influences everywhere in the Orient. It is worn by children as a necklace or as a miniature badge on their clothing; it is hanging above doors or from the rear-view mirrors of cars. You will find those amulets for little money on all markets and in all sizes. It is also said to protect you against envy and resentment – a suitable gift for your loved ones back home.

Cappadocian Carpets

- a Rare Nomad Furniture

by Ali Fuat Illeez

As with every nation of nomadic origin, the Turkmens have maintained the tradition of carpetmaking and have kept it up until today. Although the people here in Cappadocia are not wandering through the country with their herds of animals any more, carpets still play an important role in their lives. An empty house draped only with carpets is already regarded as a habitable home. This is not very surprising as, until recently, domestic life used to take place on the floor of the room.

Carpet weaving has always remained a woman's job by tradition. Young girls especially were engaged in weaving very early, as they had to contribute at least 5 carpets as an endowment for their future marriage. For men wanting to get married it was easier.They only had to contribute one carpet – if any – to the household, and that one was made for them by their mother or sisters.

As a rule, the work started in spring when the sheep were shorn. After this the wool was washed, combed through, spun and dyed. Local plants were used for dyeing them. Shades of brown were made by decocting (boiling down to a concentrate) walnut shells. Yellowberries, as their name implies, gave the wool a yellow colour, and blue and green were produced with indigo, which had been introduced to Asia Minor very early by the Arabs. Spinning and colouring took place outdoors in the summer, so that there would always be enough material ready for the long winter evenings.

Cappadocian carpets have various colourful names, which refer to their future use or their design. But some techniques or designs go back to special periods of life. Thus the first months after the marriage are called the 'cicim' period. As in former times the parents used to arrange the marriage and the marriage partners did not know each other, a more intimate contact between them did not develop until this period. The bride would then embroider images on the woven cloth which symbolized her expectations of life and of her marriage. Thus, this type of carpet is called "cicim" (darling, sweetheart). But often you will also find symbolic images against malevolence, envy and resentment or even against the "evil eye", or so-called "muska", amulets with sacred texts, are woven into the carpet.

Another frequently used image is the tree of life. This symbol requests the young couple to beget children and to keep up the family tree.

If in our days you are looking for a Cappadocian carpet in the shops, you must be very patient, as they have become rare. For many years, hardly any of them have been produced any more. Tourism is to blame for this. The women from the area noticed very soon that more money can be made by producing colourful pullovers, scarfs, and, as in Soganli, little dolls; and all this with less effort. But also the former monopoly position of the local rug dealers helped to decrease production. Trading wool, colours and the finished products put the dealers in a position which enabled them to control the prices. But the women, who spoiled their eyesight and crippled their backs during weeks and months of labour, always only received a pittance in the end. Thus, real Cappadocian carpets are rarely produced today and have had an enormous increase in value for this reason.

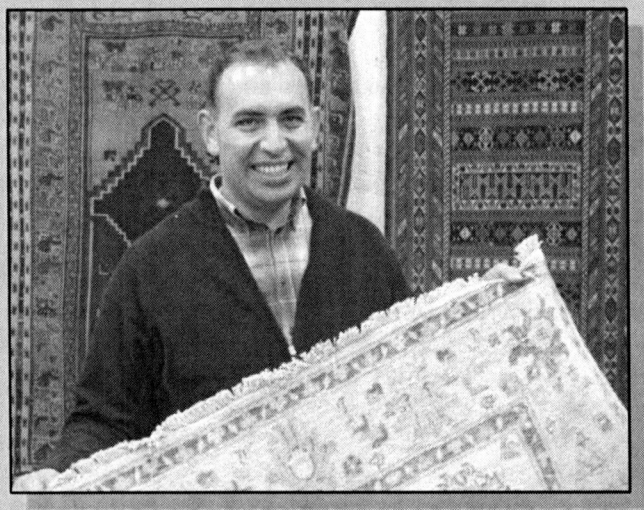

Ali Fuat Illeez runs a carpet shop in the town centre of Avanos together with his brother Ertan. Having specialized in exclusive and valuable products, he presently supplies an international clientele. The "Yörük Gallery" is in the Sere Sok. 31. Avanos – Nevşehir.

E-mail: galeriyoruk@yahoo.com

Museums

Several places in Cappadocia maintain small museums which mostly exhibit archeological finds from the neighbourhood or present objects of daily use from Ottoman everyday life. Unfortunately the exhibits on show in their glass cases are often sparsely labelled. Modern forms of presentation, as they are known from European or Western museums, are not found here. Explanatory signs, short videos or even illustrating models have not yet reached the museums in Cappadocia. Nevertheless you should not let yourself be kept from admiring the artefacts of the great handicraft art left behind by the many nations of Asia Minor. The oldest finds go back to the eighth century BC, a time when we Europeans were still living in draughty caves and agriculture was only just coming into existence. The Ethnological museums in Ortahisar and in Kayseri are recommended in any case. They illustrate the people's former everyday life graphically and by means of life-size representations in historical rooms.

As a general rule, state-owned museums are closed on Mondays. Only the open air museum in Göreme is open every day, like the private museums are.

Göreme - **Open Air Museum:** Cave churches and monastic buildings with their excellently preserved frescoes

Nevşehir - **Archeological Museum:** from prehistoric finds up to Ottoman objects of daily use

Ürgüp - **Archeological Museum:** finds from the Roman period and Ottoman objects of daily use

Ortahisar - **Ethnological Museum (private):** Representation of traditional Cappadocian life (closed from 12.00 noon to 5.00 p.m.)

Kayseri - **Archeological Museum:** Mainly finds from the Hittite and the Roman periods

- **Ethnological Museum:** Life of a wealthy Ottoman merchant family

Clothing

If you plan to visit Cappadocia in winter, you should take your winter clothes with you. Freezing cold with temperatures of up to -20° C (- 4° F) – and that for weeks - is not uncommon here, and the central heating in Turkey is notoriously unreliable. But most visitors come here in the warm season. Then light cotton clothes, which possibly should not be skin-tight, are the order of the day. Light and loose clothes allow the necessary cooling of the body. Do not wear shorts or tank tops – not only to avoid sunburn; it just would not be decent to be dressed like that here in Central Anatolia. You will not meet a local person dressed in shorts, only tourists can be identified by this from miles away. Also black or white clothes should be avoided, as Cappadocia is a very hot and dusty region. Black clothes will be heated up too much in the blazing sun, and white ones will adopt the colour of the landscape within hours. Hikers should wear hard-wearing trousers, as in some routes there are passages which can only be overcome on the seat of your trousers. Sturdy shoes should also belong to your gear. This applies to everybody who is on his way inside Cappadocia. Even when sightseeing at certain historical places, unpaved paths or smaller obstacles have to be expected. Sturdy shoes are also advantageous for people who intend to rent a motorcycle. Wearing sandals should be limited to strolling along the streets of the town in the evening. A head covering is an absolute necessity. First, the sun shines down more vertically in Cappadocia than at home, and second, the countryside is situated at 1000 m above sea level. Therefore the solar radiation should never be underestimated. Sunstroke is a very nasty and dangerous affair. You should also remember to take a tube of sun cream with you for your face. We recommend bringing one set of warm clothes for cooler evenings to guests who come in spring or in autumn. Women should always have a large and light scarf with them. For visits to Islamic holy places, and mosques belong to these, a headcovering is absolutely necessary. Men and women are also obliged to wear long-sleeved clothes on such occcasions.For transporting your excursion utensils a small rucksack, a so-called day-pack, is most useful. Whether you are on a walking tour or on a motor scooter, nothing is more effective than a piece of luggage that can be buckled on your back. And nothing is more impractical than a handbag that has to be put aside all the time, with which you get stuck and tear all kinds of things down.

Post Offices

They can be recognized by a yellow sign bearing the letters **PTT**. Here you can buy stamps for your postcards, and the letterbox is also here. All letters and postcards must have the name on the destination country on them in clear large letters. You will have to expect your friends at home to be a little annoyed because allegedly you did not write to them. Unfortunately, your picture postcards will arrive in your home country only several weeks later.

Besides this, you can mail packages, send telegrams and transfer money from here. Parcels and money can also be received poste restante (general delivery) from your home country to here; the remark POST RESTANTE must be written on the envelope. On showing the passport the item is handed over to the addressee. Additionally, you can purchase telephone cards and telephone abroad very cheaply from the local post office.

Opening hours:
From 8.30 to 12.30 and from 1.30 to 5.30 p.m.
The offices are closed on Saturdays, Sundays and on public holidays.

Internet

Meanwhile there exist internet cafés in various places in Cappadocia. But the term 'café' is not quite correct here, as those institutions are rather used as gambling houses by the younger generation and the noise level is often quite high in them. Working quietly and undisturbed is often impossible. But it ought to be sufficient for a short look at your mailbox or for sending some E-mails. The internet shops are technically well-equipped and the prices are moderate. The only problem is the Turkish language setting of the computers, but the layout of the toolbar is the same all over the world. About the keyboard it is important that the (normal) letter "I" is in the right corner of the middle row of keys. If you hit the "I" above the letter "K" as usual, your friends at home will see a "Y" on their screens. The word "**initiative**" would thus look like this: "**ynytyatyve**", which would be quite confusing.

Electricity

In Turkey electrical devices are operated with 230 V alternating voltage as in Europe and in general Euro plugs fit into Turkish sockets. Meanwhile, more and more so-called PG contact sockets are used. But be careful: this does not necessarily mean that a grounding cable is connected. Especially in older buildings this standard is not always available.

Power blackouts hitting a whole town or town quarter must still be expected now and again, unfortunately. But in most cases this problem will not last very long. While 20 years ago those blackouts used to happen almost every day, they have become rare today and are tolerated by the locals with a shrug. The only ones who will not find this funny at all are tourists who are just visiting an underground town and who have forgotten their torches.

Telephone

Telephoning has become a lot easier in recent years. The privatization of telecommunications has played a big part in this. Today there are numerous telephone shops which provide good and fast connections. You can ask to be connected or can dial yourself and pay afterwards. Prices are very moderate. For international calls you have to go to the cubicles with the **International** sign. A telephone card is another option; it is also available at the telephone shop or in other shops selling entertainment media. A card for 4 TL contains 50 units, for which you can call Europe for at least 15 minutes from a public telephone. The card is especially recommended for people who want to make calls at night, for then the telephone shops are closed.

The cheapest way of making a telephone call is directly from the post office, where you find several telephone sets. Calls of several minutes to Europe only cost a few kuruş from here. Unfortunately the post office is closed from 5.00 p.m., a time when most relatives at home are just returning home from work. If you want to make a call to Great Britain, dial **0044** and then the town code (without the initial "0") followed by he individual number, to the USA and Canada, **001** etc., to Australia, **0061** etc. Turkey itself can be reached under the number **0090.** Most foreign cellphones work in Turkey, too, via the local Turkish net provider, who will welcome you when you switch your cellphone on. However, international calls are extremely expensive, the same with arriving calls. Ask your net provider for information on the conditions for international calls before you start your journey.

Scanning your mailbox or sending photo or video messages from your mobile phone is a really costly affair.

Taxis

You can identify taxis by their yellow colour and by a black and white chequered band around the body. On the roof there is a sign with the word "**taksi**" in big letters. Everything else is done in the usual way. You get in, state your destination, the driver switches the taxi meter on, and off you go. If the driver does not start the meter you should insist on it, because otherwise there could be a bad surprise with much hue and cry at your destination. If you are told that the taxi meter is out of order, just hire another taxi. Sometimes you can also negotiate a fixed price before starting, but this is only recommended if you have done the route before and thus know the usual price. An augmented rate is valid at night-time. The price for the 60 km from Göreme to Kayseri airport for example increases from 120 TL to 180 TL at night.

But on the whole, little tricks like driving detours or charging exorbitant prices belong to the past. Taxis are especially useful for walkers who want to reach their point of entry above a valley. You can save yourself having to walk along the heavily frequented roads, which, especially at noon, often seem to be boiling under the mercilessly blazing sun.

Toilets

To the experienced traveller in the Orient the following chapter will be old hat. But we want to save the newcomer from embarrassing situations. As far as tourist facilities are concerned, you can expect the usual Western standard. The sanitary facilities are modern and in good order. In small and inexpensive boarding houses the ambience is perhaps somewhat plain and simple, but there should be no problems either. Public toilets often present a totally different picture. They are situated at bus terminals, resting places and in town centres. Their condition can only be appropriately described as dirty, decayed and unacceptable. In addition, there are the unaccustomed 'squat toilets', which may only consist of a hole in the ground over which you squat down. Because of the poor hygiene we are very fond of this toilet version, as, apart from the shoes, there is no physical contact with it whatsoever. In spite of the mostly pathetic care and maintenance conditions, one is charged a small sum of money at the entrance. You will also find napkins there, which are for drying your hands. Take some of them with you under all circumstances, as toilet paper is not customary in the Orient. Once it happened to me that I accidentally forgot to think of it. The only thing I carried with me which at least partly consisted of paper was my passport. Thus, the two central pages, which I tore out cautiously, had to serve as an emergency solution. But I would not recommend anyone to imitate this. Apart from the paper being quite hard, a missing entrance stamp always contains the potential of a lot of trouble at the exit. Besides, your passport is the property of your national government, and damaging it could be an indictable offense.

Any Oriental would not have got into such a dilemma at all. With the help of water from a small tap close to the floor, he simply cleans himself with his left hand after having done his business. Left-handed persons, incidentally, should think about which of their hands they use for shaking hands or for eating.

Next to the toilet there is always a small waste basket. This is where used toilet paper belongs. Please do not throw it into the toilet, as the sewage systems in Turkey are not suitable for disposing of paper and will be blocked after a short time. Sanitary pads, especially, have driven many a hotel owner into ruin.

In order to avoid a big hue and cry, men should look for the door marked ***Erkek*** or ***Bay*** (man, gentlemen). Ladies' toilets are labelled ***Bayan*** or ***Kadin*** (lady, woman).

Garbage Problems

One-way packages have also reached Central Anatolia in recent years, with their associated environmental problems. Unlicensed garbage dumps, plastic packages washed ashore by wind and water and roadside ditches strewn with empty plastic bottles have been the consequences. The older ones among our readers will possibly remember the time when the first plastic detergent bottles and margarine boxes appeared on the market. In those days, too, the unlicensed garbage dumps rose up to the sky. Central Anatolia is just now going through this development, and the ecological awareness of the population has still to be raised. Even today in the poorer areas of some towns you can see people dispose of their household garbage by throwing it over the wall of the yard and into the nearest ditch or on a hillside. Twenty years ago this was not a problem yet, as it used to be biodegradable garbage which would either rot or be eaten by animals. Unfortunately it has not yet got around among all inhabitants that plastic packages have a considerably longer lifespan or that batteries contain poisonous substances which may contaminate the groundwater.

Also returnable bottle systems are practically unknown in Turkey, for which reason e.g. empty water bottles are thrown carelessly into the countryside. After this, the wind takes care of distributing this garbage evenly all over the area. The Efes beer company is the only one which has an efficient bottle return system.

But even if the garbage is disposed of correctly in garbage bins, it will nevertheless wind up in some little Cappadocian side valley that has been declared a garbage dump. Waste separation or even recycling are still years away in this country. Quite the contrary, controlled torching of such garbage dumps is unfortunately still part of everyday life.

But we, the tourists, should not turn up our noses at that too much, as our own recycling problems have been solved quite reasonably only a few years ago. And those who complain of possible garbage on the streets should sometime take a look at their own Western roadside ditches in winter. They will be amazed at what all they will find there.

Time

As Turkey is situated in Eastern Europe, you have to put your watch to GMT plus 2 hours (GMT plus 3 hours between the last Sunday in March and in October) when you arrive and you reverse this procedure when leaving the country. If you enter Turkey by car from Greece, you should adjust your watch already there, because Greece is in the same time zone. The change from daylight saving time to normal time takes place on the same day as in all other European countries.

Do not be surprised that on Summer evenings it gets dark earlier than in Western Europe. Cappadocia is situated between the 38th and the 39th degree of latitude. Munich, for example, is on the 48th degree of latitude. This difference of ten degrees causes the difference between day and night to be less extreme. Unfortunately, the twilight at dawn and at dusk is shorter, too, because of this.

Hitchhiking

Hitchhikers will have a hard time in Turkey, at least on long distances. Buses and railways are just too inexpensive for this in the country. And lorry drivers do not need any passengers for their entertainment, as they mostly have a co-driver or even their wife and children with them. But this is different on short distances. You often see local people coming from their work in the fields standing by the roadside and asking for a ride. You do not raise your thumb for this purpose as we do, but you hold your hand horizontally towards the roadway. Then the hand is moved slightly up and down, with the back of the hand upwards. You can do this also as a tourist for short distances. Some patience is necessary, however. If you have missed your last bus in the evening you will find even greater compassion from the drivers and will almost always get a ride.

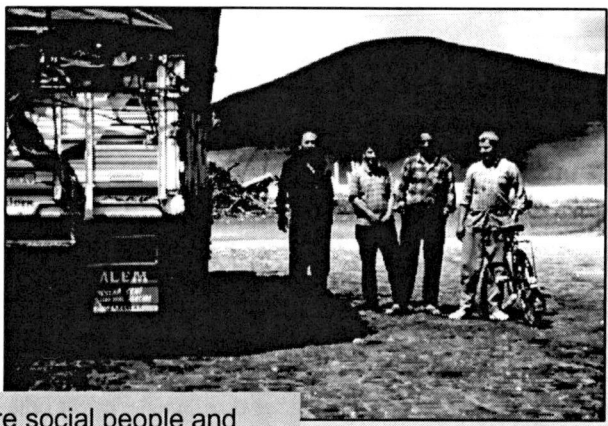

Turks are social people and like to offer a ride to others

Parking Taxes

Since some years ago it has become a habit in Cappadocia to collect parking taxes from car drivers in front of the tourist sights. Even though some people might be upset by being pinched for 2 or 3 TL for each dusty car parking space, this regulation is quite understandable from the local council's point of view, as they do not profit from the entrance fees because those all go to the Ministry of Culture and Tourism's cash box. At the same time the local councils have to keep the infrastructure around those places in order. Thus it is quite understandable that the villages and towns want to cut off a piece of the big cake for themselves to be able to fulfill their duties. So, please remember that you are helping to keep the road you have just used in good order by means of your car park ticket.

Finally, it could also be worth mentioning that Avanos is the first municipality in Cappadocia which collects parking taxes everywhere in the town centre. For one Turkish Lira you are allowed to park your vehicle there for an hour.

Maps

Finding maps of Turkey or even of Cappadocia is not easy. Atatürk's military success against the Greek invaders in 1922 was based for the most part on the fact that his troops had the better maps. Therefore, the Turkish military have been guarding their maps like gold until today, despite modern satellite intelligence. Maps with a scale of 1:200,000 and 1:100,000 are only sold by the generals for many hundreds of dollars. However, maps with a scale of 1:50,000 and 1:25,000 are classified top secret. So it is no wonder that no usable hiking maps for Cappadocia exist.

Since 2009 the Tourist Authority has distributed a map of the region and the province for free. It is available in Turkish and in English at all Tourist information offices, and is entirely sufficient as a rough guide.

If you want to travel to other parts of the country you should in any case buy a general map of Turkey already before in your home country. The available local maps unfortunately often turn out to be very inaccurate and incorrect.

If such a map is not available in your native language, we recommend buying the Turkey map of the ADAC (German Automobile Club), since its legend is multilingual.

ADAC – Map of Turkey: Scale 1:800,000, summer 2009
ISBN 978 – 3826418747

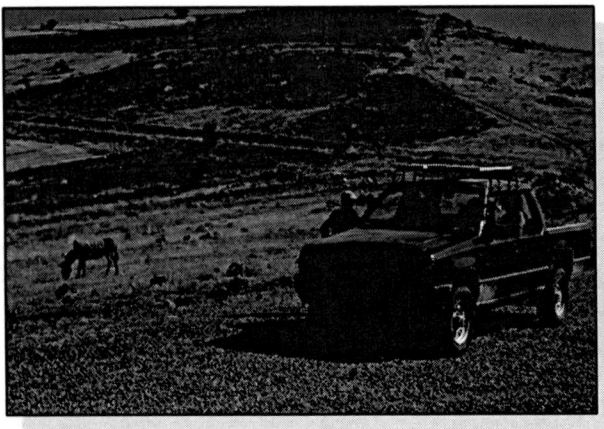

Important Addresses and Emergency Telephone Numbers

Here is a list of the most important addresses and numbers which hopefully you will never have to use in Cappadocia as a tourist:

Police:	155
Militray police:	156
Medical service for Emergencies:	112
Fire brigade:	110
Forest fire alarm units:	177
Turkish Touring and Automobile Club (Ankara):	0312 229 3806 or 3807

Addresses of Embassies:

For US Citizens:

AMERICAN EMBASSY ANKARA
Atatürk Bulvari 110
06100 Kavaklidere
Phone: 0(090) 312 455 5555
Facs: 0(090) 312 467 0019
Email: webmaster_ankara@state.gov

For British Citizens:

BRITISH EMBASSY ANKARA
Sehit Ersan Caddesi 46/A
06690 Çankaya
Phone: 0(090) 312 455 3344
Facs: 0(090) 312 455 3352

For Canadian Citizens:

CANADIAN EMBASSY ANKARA
Cinnah Cadesi 58
06690 Cankaya
Phone: 0(090) 312 4092700
Facs: 0(090) 312 4092811
Email: ankra@internationa.gc.ca

For Australien Citizens:

AUSTRALIAN EMBASSY ANKARA
MNG Building - Ugur Mumcu Caddesi 88, 7th Floor
06700 Gaziosmanpasa
Phone: 0(090) 312 459 9500
Facs: 0(090) 312 446 4827
Email: consular.ankara@dfat.gov.au

For New Zealand Citizens:

NEW ZEALAND EMBASSY ANKARA
Iran Caddesi 13
06100 Kavaklidere
Phone : 0(090) 312 467 9054 /6 / 8
Facs: 0(090) 312 467 9013
Email: nzembassyankara@ttmail.com

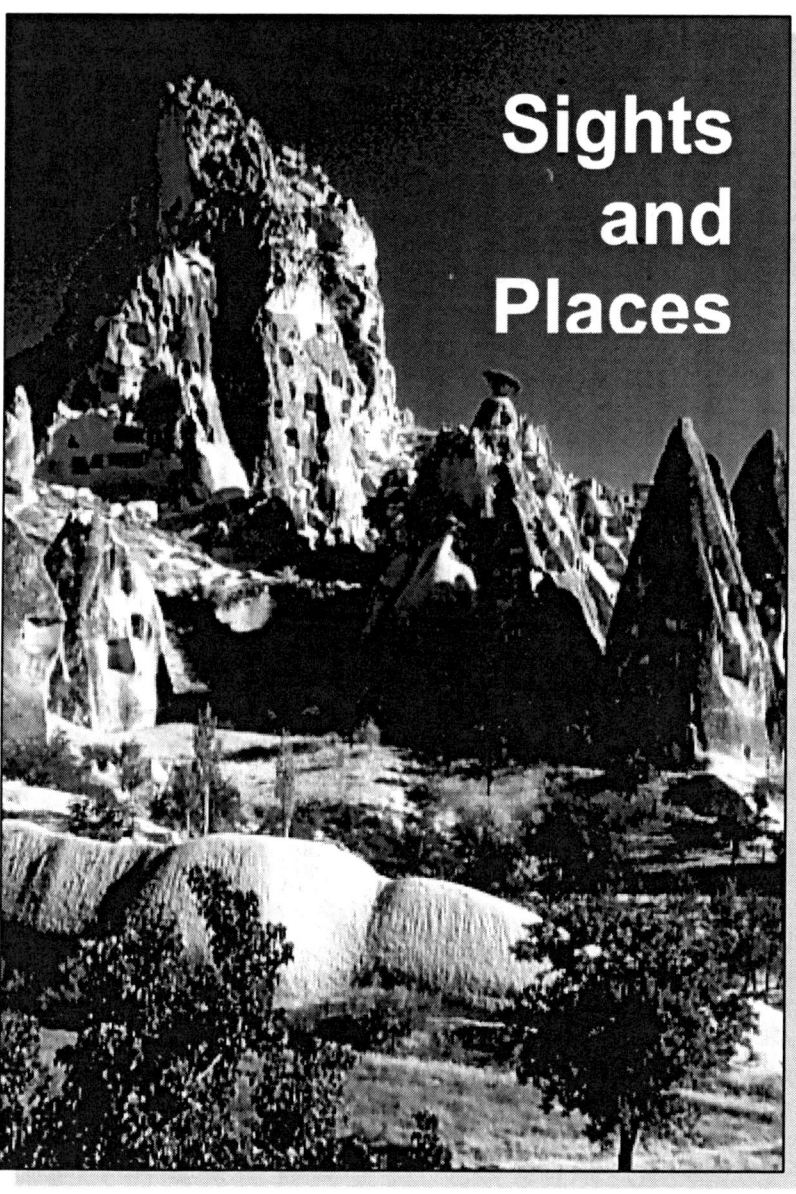
Sights and Places

Some Words in Advance

In the third part of this book we will finally go on our trip through Cappadocia. The places and the sights of the region are described here. We have listed the tourist attractions under geographical aspects, so that it will be easier for the traveller to put his day trips together.
Most descriptions of places are followed by a list of accommodations, which, however, is not complete, as this would go beyond the scope of this book. As we, the authors, were always travelling by camper van, we cannot give any information on the service or the courtesy of the personnel. On our visits we always had to depend on the first impression and on the outward appearance. For a future edition of this travel guide it is therefore essential that you will inform us about your experiences, no matter if they are positive or negative, so that we will be able to eliminate the black sheep and to include any good accommodations that we, the authors, have accidentally overlooked.

And now, we wish you a safe journey and a pleasant stay in Cappadocia.

Uçhisar

Uçhisar's landmark is the 1460 m high rock which towers above the place. From there you have a great view far over the Göreme valley to the Erciyes volcano which is 80 km away and often snow-covered. Centuries ago, the rock, which is affectionately called the 'Kale' (castle) by the locals, was used as a refuge from foreign invaders by the inhabitants. Today the many corridors and rooms, which in former times traversed the mountain hidden inside the rock, can be easily seen from outside. The rock of Uçhisar is one of Cappadocia's greatest tourist attractions today and is therefore very well-frequented. The turmoil is limited to the area round the 'Kale' and the main road from Göreme to Uchisar at the foot of the mountain. The rest of the place appears rather sleepy. Some decades ago, a new town quarter developped to the West of the 'Kale', as the old town centre in the East was gradually decaying – a problem which all places here in Central Cappadocia have. But here, on the Eastern slope below the rock, the picture has begun to change since some years ago. Among the ruins of half-decayed traditional dwelling houses, more and more restored and maybe a bit too stylish new buildings can be found. As the local inhabitants cannot afford this expensive and intensely regulated refurbishing work, more and more investors have been putting their money into the acquisition of building sites and are building hotels of a more exclusive style. Thus, the last remnants of village life are slowly disappearing and are making room for tourism. And there are still many buildings under construction on the Eastern slope. But there is no mass tourism here, due to the high accommodation prices and the closing of the main road to coaches and heavy transport. The location here on the hillside is fantastic. The heavenly peace and the incomparable view make Uçhisar one of the most beautiful places in Cappadocia. And additionally, you are not isolated from the world. A minibus leaves for Nevsehir every 30 minutes, and the place has a good infrastructure. A post office, a bank and some small shops for people's daily needs make the place a good address for the individual tourist. In any case, climbing on the 'Kale' is worthwhile (fee: 3 TL).

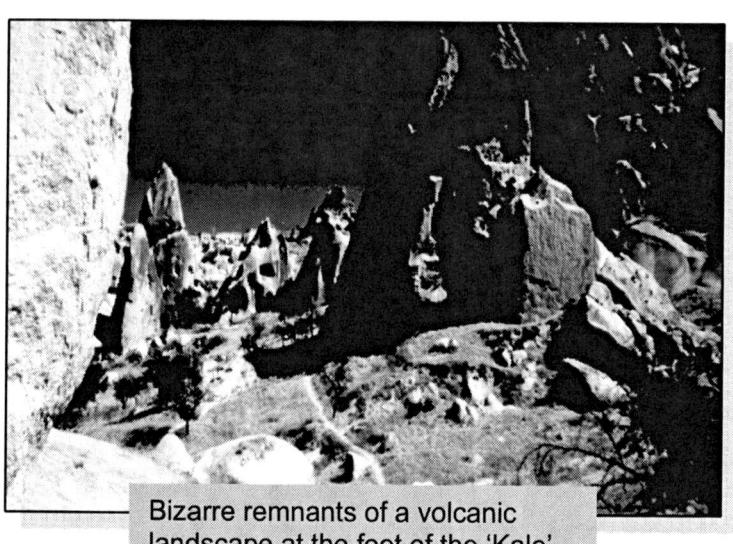

Bizarre remnants of a volcanic landscape at the foot of the 'Kale'

194 Central Cappadocia

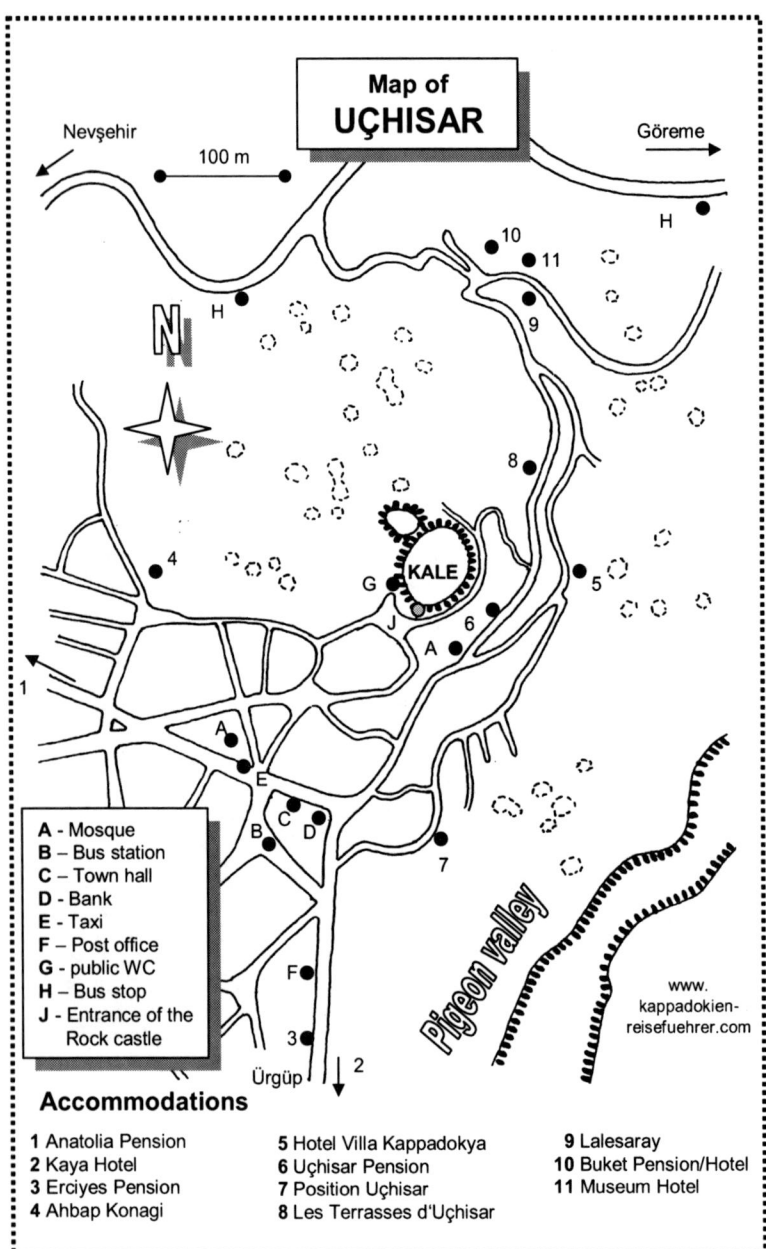

Accommodations in Uchisar

➢ ANATOLIA PENSION
Small boardinghouse, located very quietly in the new part of the town and therefore unfortunately without the magnificent view which most houses in the town have.The owner seems to be very dedicated, however, he drives his guests to the starting points of their walks and collects them afterwards. The new annex in the back has been constructed in the traditional vaulted style. A little green orchard invites you to relax.

1	60 TL	14	E – F	▼ ⦿	①⑤⑦⑧

Phone: 0384 219 2339   www.anatoliapension.com

➢ KAYA HOTEL
Large hotel situated at the edge of the Pigeon Valley. It is the oldest tourist hotel here in Cappadocia and was first opened in 1968. It does not look its age, however, as it was run and well maintained by 'Club Mediterranee' for almost 30 years.This is partly the reason why many people speak French in Uchisar.The then Mayor of the town was very clever and connected the hotel licence and the building permission with various conditions, e.g. that the staff had to be from Uchisar, and that they had to be employed also during the winter.Thus it happened that staff members were flown to France or to Switzerland in winter at the expense of the Club in order to work there. A hotel that leaves nothing to be desired but spreads a somewhat formal atmosphere.

2	220 TL	72	E – F		①④⑤⑥⑦⑧

Phone: 0384 219 2007   www.uchisarkayahotel.com

➢ ERCIYES PENSION
A real alternative for the limited budget and situated 100 m south of the town centre on the road to the south. A genuine small familiy business in which you still take closely part in traditional village life. The rooms are simple but very clean, and in the shady orchard you can watch the landlady prepare Pekmez (grape juice) for the winter with her neighbours. You are right in the middle of Cappadocian daily life.

3	45 TL	6	TR	▼ ⦿	①②③④⑤⑥⑦⑧⑨

Phone: 0384 219 2090   erciyespension@hotmail.com

➢ AHBAP KONAGI

As the word Konak (palace or little castle) suggests, this is a somewhat larger complex. Very nice location with a great view on the 'Kale' glowing red in the light of the sunset. The guesthouse was opened in 1999 and is situated as an alternative to the lodging houses on the eastern slope of the old village. The complex is situated directly next to the village population on the West side of the great rock. The owners do not cook the meals themselves in the connected restaurant, but have hired their neighbour for this purpose, which is perhaps a reason why also guests from other hotels sometimes come here for supper. Architecturally, the lodging house is just a dream, and the quietness here is out of this world.

4	140-220 TL	17	E – F - I	⌶ 🍽	①③④⑤⑥⑦⑧

Phone: 0384 219 3020 www.ahbapkonagi.com

➢ VILLA CAPPADOKIA

A hotel which is also located very quietly with a great view all over Cappadocia. Beautiful architecture, as the complex consists entirely of restored ancient houses. A shady green orchard on the hillside is balm for the soul and the rooms, each with an open fireplace, are equipped with lots of love. In winter the hotel can be opened especially on demand for larger groups. A public cave restaurant is connected with the hotel.

5	200 TL	9	E	⌶ 🍽	②③⑤⑥⑦⑧

Phone: 0384 219 3133 www.villacappadocia.com

➢ UÇHISAR PENSION

Inexpensive and simple family boardinghouse on the paved road on the Eastern slope. Unfortunately the house only has a very narrow inner yard. More room is available on the roof terrace with a wide view, where a rich and tasty dinner is served in the evenings.

6	70 TL	8	E – F	🍽	②③⑦⑧

Phone: 0384 219 2662 www.uchisarpension.com

➢ POSITION UÇHISAR

A small and inconspicuous inn which has hidden qualtites. If you are culturally interested, this will be the right place for you. Mrs Almut Wegner, the German owner, is familiar with all fields of art. Whether it is drawing lessons, dances or music soirees – you can let off steam endlessly as an artist here. Several musical instruments are at your disposal and if you want to capture the magic landscape of Cappadocia on the canvas you can just rent a scaffold with everything. There is practically nothing Mrs Wegner cannot arrange. Just ask her! The excellent location is another advantage: very quiet and with a fantastic view.

| 7 | 120 TL | 8 | E – F – D - I | 🍴 | ①②③⑥⑦⑧ |

Phone 0384 219 2172   www.projekt-uchisar.org

➢ LES TERRASSES DE UÇHISAR

French-run family business with a large lounge and a beautiful terrace on the top floor. On the ground floor there is the lunchroom with a great atmosphere, and on the whole this guesthouse offers a good price-performance ratio. The good cuisine, which is run by the landlady and her daughter, is said to be well-known in more than the region only. Alright then: Bon appetit!

| 8 | 80 TL | 14 | E – F | 🍴 | ②③⑤⑦⑧ |

Phone: 0384 219 2791   www.terrassespension.com

➢ HOTEL LALESARAY

This hotel is a good piece of luxury which is something special because of its arches made of black basalt. Some rooms are very large, furnished with great taste and with an open fireplace each.

The spacious bathrooms are equipped with huge whirlpool bathtubs. The whole complex is a masterpiece of architecture and the view from the terrace is gorgeous. A dream hotel where now and again one can also enjoy some traditional live music.

| 9 | 180-500 TL | 14 | E – F | 🍴 | ①②③⑤⑥⑦⑧ |

Phone: 0384 219 2333   www.lalesaray.com

➢ BUKET PENSION AND HOTEL

Large complex with boarding house, hotel and restaurant service. As they are separated by a large garden, one does not get in the other's way. Whereas the boarding house rooms are quite simple, they have put themselves out with the cave suites. The furniture and the doors are made of fine wood, and all rooms have an open fireplace and a bathtub. The complex has had a new owner/proprietress since only 2008.

| 10 | 50-160 TL | 13 | E | 🍴 | ①②③⑤⑥⑦⑧ |

Phone: 0384 219 2490   www.bukethotel.com

➢ MUSEUM HOTEL

If you have won first prize in a lottery or if you are rich and famous, this will be the right place for you. A hotel of superlatives when it comes to equipment and architecture, but prices, too. You do not see from the outside what kind of luxury the house offers. The only thing you can see from outside is the lobby. The terrace, the pool with a view over the landscape and the first-class restaurant are hidden from the eyes of all strangers. The highlight, however, is the cave rooms in the rocks underneath the whole complex. Large spacious cave suites guarantee a breathtaking view of the Cappadocian landscape and are unique in the region. A dream in tuff!

| 11 | 180-1700TL | 30 | E – F - D | ⊤ ⦿ | ①②③④⑤⑥⑦⑧ |

Phone. 0384 219 2220   www.museum-hotel.com

Göreme

No sooner have you begun to think about the sights of the town, than inevitably you come to a halt: well, what have we got there? All right, there is a rock cone in the town centre with a Roman tomb in it high above, of which you can still see the remains of some columns clinging to the ceiling. That is about all there is to be said about it. – No, not quite so. If you follow the canal in a south-western direction, after a hundred yards you will find signs to the Yusuf Koç Church on the right-hand side. After a hundred yards more you will find the small chapel, which once again shows the visitor that its broken columns did not have to support much weight in reality. The Kadir - Durmuş Church is a lot more interesting, however. Where the road forks for the Yusuf Koç Church you walk straight on along the canal to the next junction. A paved path leads to this special church. It is one of the very few from the time of early Christianity. There are no colourful frescoes waiting here, but masterly sculpture work arouses the visitor's amazement. The most conspicuous aspect of this historic church is the ambo, the pulpit neatly carved from the existing rock in the centre of the room. You will seldom meet any visitors here. An ideal place for taking a short time out from the hurly-burly in the town centre.

Göreme must once have been located romantically among the many rock cones – the present onrush in the town cannot be explained in another way – for the small town is simply the absolute tourist centre of all Cappadocia. With its more than 70 lodging houses, countless restaurants and its many souvenir shops there is everything in Göreme that pleases the visitor's heart. Around the bus terminal in the town centre, owners of mini-scooters are waiting for customers, and the travel agencies offer all kinds of day trips and other rentals. Bus tickets to every part of Turkey can be bought here, and in the early evening, even the bus to Damascus stops here. In a larger circle round the terminal there are the numerous restaurants and teahouses, which have to share the narrow space with an equally large number of souvenir shops. A second circle is formed by the hotels and boarding houses, which finally leave hardly any space for the ordinary population. Thus entire rows of houses have sometimes been bought up and turned into luxury hotels. This vast but repetitive choice is an advantage for the tourist, as here you can compare prices very well and there is also a high competitive pressure on the suppliers. In the pre- and off-peak season, bargaining is always profitable; especially with car rentals, there are considerable differences in prices. In any case you should book or rent items directly from the supplier, as otherwise a go-between will earn extra money, which makes the price increase considerably. Especially in the high season, Göreme is anything but a quiet place, but if you like long party nights, you are in good hands here, as there exists some nightlife in the town. Some bars in the town centre are open until early morning and are an ideal hangout for night owls. Those who are rather looking for peace and quiet should therefore make sure that their accommodation is near the edge of the town. The nightly activities diminish greatly in the off-peak season, however, and then also the town centre becomes a little quieter.

Finally, a few tips for the day trips offered by the local agencies. You should make sure that lunch, an expert guide and reduced entrance fees to the museums are included in the price. Here, too, the price margin is different and partly negotiable according to season. As already mentioned, it remains a mystery why Göreme among all others has been able to focus so much on tourism. Perhaps its original name, "Avcilar" ("hunter" in English), already explains everything.

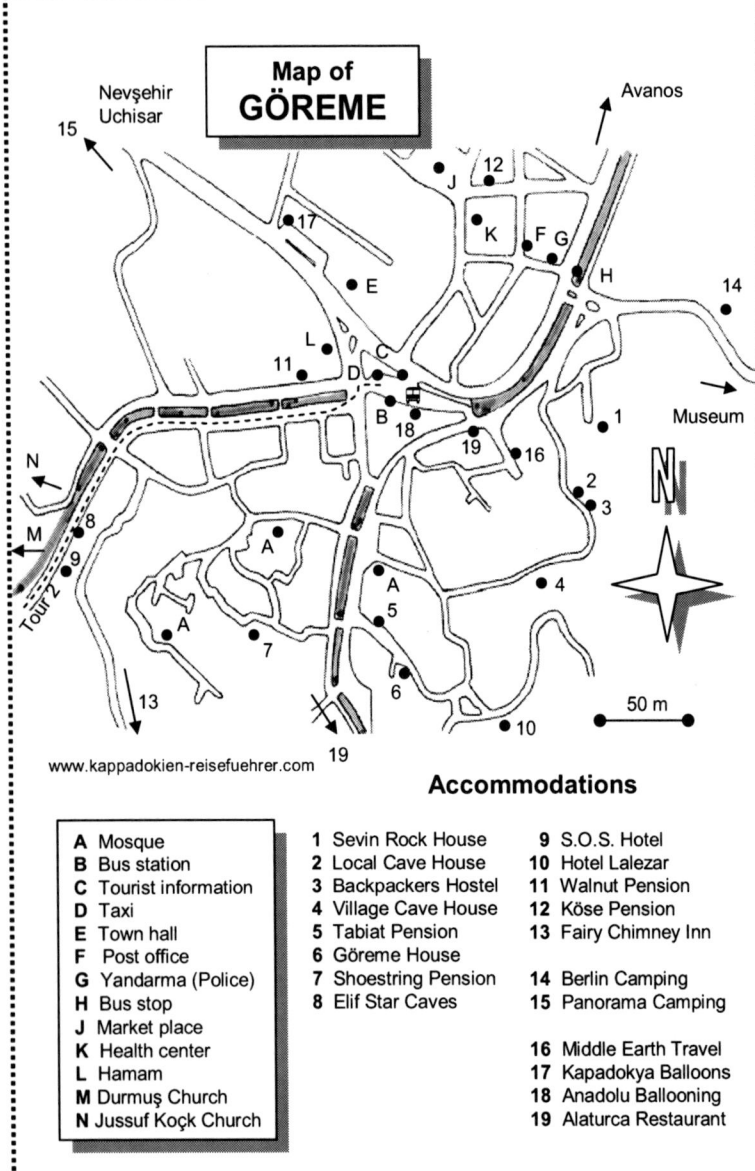

Accommodation in Göreme

At the bus terminal in Göreme there is a large sign on which the hotels and boarding houses are listed on a town map in accurate numeric order, from 1 to 60. But the local inhabitants confirm that it is five years old and that meanwhile the number has risen to at least 80. It would be too much to list all of them in this book, and not every lodging house in the town deserves a recommendation. This is why we decided to present only a limited choice. We would welcome any information from our readers regarding their experience with their accommodation with great pleasure, as we, too, are not always able to see behind the scenes of such a lodging house. On the whole, the large number of hotels and pensions has led to the fact that accommodation prices in Göreme have remained quite moderate.

➢ SEVIN ROCK HOUSE
A family business situated somewhat out of the way, offering some simple cave rooms. There is a large open-air area round the building where camping is possible. The beds made of tuff and the pool in the garden are the attractions of the house.

1	40-60 TL	7	E		①③④⑧

Phone: 0384 271 2462   sevinrock@hotmail.com

➢ LOKAL CAVE HOUSE HOTEL
Rather new complex with rooms arranged on 2 floors around a pool. Everything is designed pleasantly and invites you to a couple of lazy days with a constant change between water and cozy corner seats.

2	100-140 TL	9	E – F – NL	⛾🍽	①②③④⑤⑧

Phone: 0384 271 2171   www.lokalcavehouse.com

➢ BACKPACKERS CAVE HOSTEL
Situated directly next to the one before, with a green and shady garden and Turkey's smallest swimming pool. Single beds in the dormitory are available form 13 TL. Kept simple, but neat.

3	45-60 TL	11	E	⛾🍽	①②③④⑤⑧

Phone: 0384 271 2   www. backpackerscave.com

➢ VILLAGE CAVE HOUSE HOTEL

Beautiful historic old building which is kept meticulously clean by the proprietress. Unfortunately, no foreign languages are spoken, but there is a magnificent panoramic view over the town and the surrounding area.

4	65 TL	9	E	🍴	①②③⑧

Phone: 0384 271 2182　　　　　　www.villagecavehouse.com

➢ TABIAT PENSION

The pension hides behind the mosque and is only accessible by a narrow entrance door. The large inner yard is designed with love and equipped with old wooden chairs. Lots of green in the yard and the quietness there are balm for the nerves. The rooms and the lounge are furnished simply and traditionally and not over-modernized. Good breakfast and the atmosphere make this inn a hot tip.

5	40 TL	8	E		②③⑧

Phone: 0384 271 2267　　　　　　tabiatpension@yahoo.com

➢ GÖREME HOUSE

A slightly better place situated high up on the edge of the town. The rooms are nicely furnished and the whole complex looks rather classy. The courtyard is furnished with cozy corner seating units and has shady trees. A library and a good breakfast round out the positive impression of the hotel.

6	120-190 TL	13	E – F	🍴	①②③④⑤⑥⑦⑧⑨

Phone: 0384 271 2060　　　　　　www.goremehouse.com

➢ SHOESTRING PENSION

What a contrast, for there is always something going on here. The inner yard looks like a little tuff valley itself, with the rooms of this backpacking hostel arranged round it. Tourists looking for peace and quiet should not stop here in the peak season. As in the old days, backpackers from all over the world come together here. The pool, which is high above the house, is really out of this world; it is so crowded with visitors in the summer that there must be hardly any water left in it. A 'must' for everyone who wants to experience Göreme as it used to be 25 years ago.

7	50 TL	16	E	🍴	①②③④⑤⑦⑧

Phone : 0384 271 2450　　　　　　www.shoestringcave.com

➢ ELIV STAR CAVES

A renovated cave complex with nice old cave rooms which have not been over-renovated. The guests on site praised the hotel and the management to the skies. The yard and the rooms were immaculately clean and the view over the Cappadocian tuff cone scenery is magnificent.

8	90-100 TL	7	E - D	♈ ⦿	①②③⑤⑦⑧

Phone: 0384 271 2479   www.elifstar.com

➢ S.O.S. HOTEL

It was rebuilt in 2005 and equipped with well-lighted and pleasant cave rooms. Lots of flowers and a magnificent panoramic view make the large terrace a cozy lounge. The highlight is a so-called honeymoon room with a large whirlpool bath and a private balcony with a view over the rocky countryside.

9	60-120 TL	17	E – F - D	♈ ⦿	①②③⑤⑥⑦⑧

Phone: 0384 271 2134   www.soscavehotel.com

➢ LALEZAR HOTEL

Situated at the far end of the town, this new hotel extends up the hillside with its 5 floors of rooms and terraces. The rooms are furnished with taste and are rather large.

10	40-80 TL	13	E – D - NL	♈ ⦿	①②③⑤⑥⑦⑧

Phone : 0384 271 2298   Fax : 0384 271 2679

➢ GÖREME WALNUT HOUSE

Although not more than 100 m from the bus terminal, this hostel is situated a little out of the way; it offers comfortable rooms in the historic vaulted style. In 2006 the owner had a new house built in the garden, which represents a very tasteful new part of the resort in the old Cappadocian style. Vaulted rooms built of natural rock and underfloor heating form a combination of tradition and modern conveniences.

11	40-80 TL	12	E - D	♈ ⦿	①⑤⑥⑧

Phone: 0384 271 2235   www.walnuthouse.com

➤ KÖSE Pension

Here there still exists the system where there are self-service drinks, tallied to your account at the end, as in the old days. Situated in the new part of the town at the marketplace and in the middle of a housing area, this inn can be seen as a real alternative. The large selection of breakfast options is worth seeing, and the large garden with its pool justifies the price, which is rather high for backpackers.

12	60 TL	18	E	⊤ 🍽	①④⑦⑧

Phone: 0384 271 2294   www.kosepension.com

➤ FAIRY CHIMNEY INN

In 2005, Andus and Gülcan Emge opened their boarding house in a rock cone at the end of the town. Lovingly furnished rooms and a very special ambience in the outside area make this inn an oasis of tranquility. A good description would be "guest house of the Kappadokya Academy" - the visitor who is interested in culture is completely at home here. The German owner, Dr. Andus Emge, has engaged for years in the culture, social services and history of the region and has finally written his doctor's thesis about it. He will be pleased to answer all questions about these topics.

13	110-220 TL	6	E - D	🍽	②③⑤⑥⑦⑧

Phone: 0384 271 2655   www. fairychimney.com

Restaurant tip: ALATURCA RESTAURANT

If you have a very special reason to celebrate and want to go out for a first-rate meal, we can recommend the "Alaturca Restaurant" to you. This restaurant distinguishes itself by far from all others in town by its supply. The prices are a little different, too, but they are not exorbitant. Some historic recipes from the Sultan's court are on the menu here, too.

The terrace in particular, with its view over the busy town centre, guarantees a successful evening. So, do not be surprised if suddenly the provincial governor, together with his entourage, is seated at the table next to yours.

Phone: 0384 271 2882

Göreme Museum

This is a must for everybody who comes to Cappadocia – at least in the opinion of the big tour operators. And therefore, busloads of visitors are put through the open air museum every day. If you want to take a look at the complex without hurrying, this will not be easy. Especially if you get caught among two groups of tourists, it will get rather dark and much louder instead in the narrow church rooms. A religious atmosphere cannot be expected then. The price policy and the ticket sale conditions make you feel a little strange, too. For example, there is no single ticket for the "Tokalı Kilise", a church a little outside the museum area, so that you can only see it if you buy the ordinary ticket for 15 TL and pay an extra 8 TL for this single church. Inside the area of the museum, there is another ticket counter for the "Karanlık Kilise", where they want you to pay another 8 TL again. At the entrance the visitor is told by a sign that all this money is applied for the preservation of the old cave churches in Cappadocia. It is annoying if then, only a few yards outside the museum area, you step into church rooms which are on the brink of collapse, which are full of garbage and – we beg our readers' pardon – sometimes full of excrements. Other marked churches are closed, or you are asked to pay more than once for visiting a half-decayed little chapel. All this really makes you feel rather thoughtful.

A little tip for your tour round the museum: start your tour of the area with the "Çarıklı Kilise". This way you are moving contrary to the flow of the large groups and will perhaps get a chance to look at the cave churches without hurrying. On the other hand you might meet an English-speaking group, which you can join discreetly and then listen attentively to the explanations of the tour guide.

St. Basilios Church (1)

The picture of St. George fighting the dragon is most conspicuous here. Like in most of the other churches, there are burial places in the side walls. The basic structure is covered by a barrel vault, and there is a side section separated by pillars (narthex). The building is from the 11th century and the paintings in it also show St.Theodorus and St. Mary with the child besides St. George.

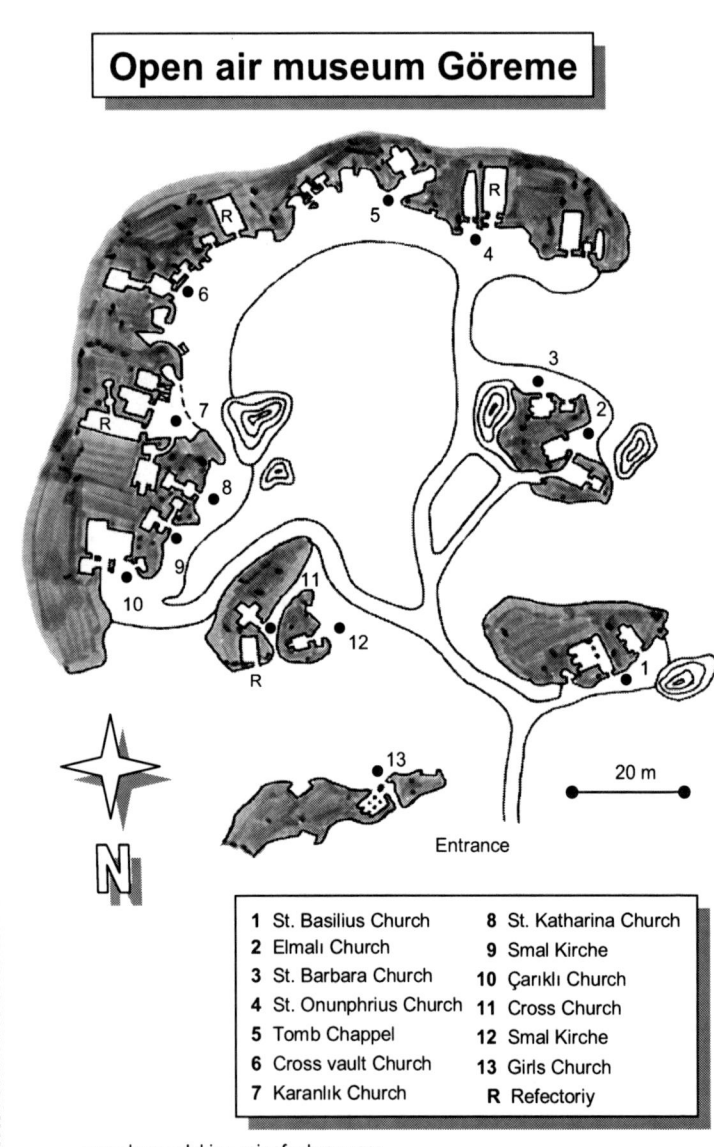

Elmalı Kilise (2)

This 'Church with the Apple' has a cruciform layout with four small central columns, which do not need to support the nine small domes, however. There are three apses opposite the entrance. This church is believed to be the most recent in the museum area and is dated to the 12th century because of its wall paintings. Even though the iconoclastic controversy was over then, two different types of paintings can be distinguished: simple ornaments painted directly on the rock, and from later on, figural images painted on plaster on top of the old ornamental decoration.

St. Barbara's Church (3)

Here, too, the layout is cruciform, but some sections of the ceiling have been constructed as barrel vaults. The church is famous for its well-preserved ornaments, but also for its images, which almost resemble naïve art or children's drawings. In any case those paintings leave much room for speculation and interpretation for the world of professional church historians. We were reminded of a children's prank by some of the images and, on the whole, the building seems rather unfinished. This may also be due to the painted imitation brickwork in the barrel vault sections.

St. Onunphrios Church (4)

This building is also called Yılanlı Kilise (Snake Church) because again of St. George fighting the dragon, which is this time represented as a serpent. The portrait of St. Onunphrios, who is shown in the nude with concealed pubic area and female breasts plus a beard, is much more interesting, however. He is said to have been called Onunphria before, originally having been an unchaste woman who could not save herself from the advances of the men. She asked God for help, who made her grow a nice big bushy beard, so that she was able to withdraw to seclusion and to lead a God-fearing life from then on. Perhaps this is the first sex transformation in the world documented by a human being. At least it is a dubious story that some tour guides are fond of telling. Besides, a portrait of Emperor Constantine and his wife, Empress Helena, can be discovered here. Both are said to have supported the Christian communities here in Cappadocia.

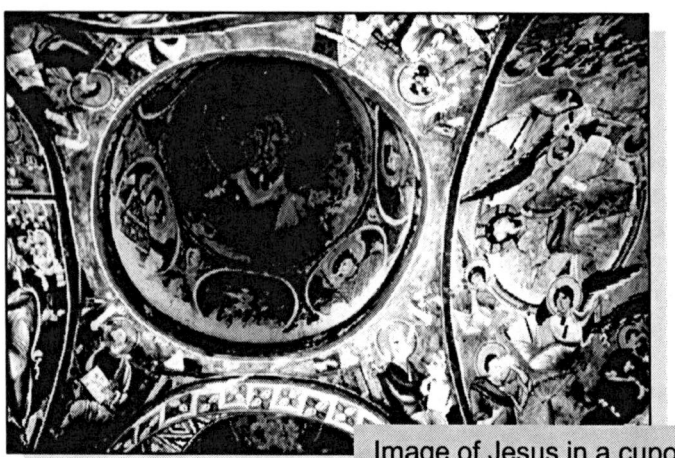

Image of Jesus in a cupola

Karanlık Kilise (7)

It is also called the 'Dark Church' because only a minimum of light enters through a narrow opening in the narthex. As a consequence, the colours of its splendid paintings were excellently preserved. You enter the building by a narrow winding staircase and a vestibule. Here, too, the classic cross-shaped layout with its domes and apses is to be found. The wall paintings show almost all stages of the life of Jesus, with the Son of God shown as the pantocrator (ruler of the world) in the central dome. In this cave church the visitor is able to find some tranquility after the turmoil of the rest of the museum area. The travel groups seem to avoid the extra 8 TL for the walkthrough.

Çarıklı Kilise (9)

The footprints which are visible below the picture of the Ascension of Christ have given this church its name, 'Sandal Church'. Today it is only accessible by an iron ladder, as the old stone steps were destroyed by erosion a long time ago. Here, too, the life circle of Jesus is shown. As well, there is a representation of Abraham's hospitality and the 12 apostles with their names can be discovered in the vault.

Churches in the vicinity of the Open Air Museum

There are many other sacred rock buildings outside the fenced-in museum area, but often there is not much left of them. Erosion and the utilization as sheep sheds have done a lot of damage to the fragmentary buildings, and often chapels listed by travellers in the past cannot be located at all any more. Here we want to mention some of the few remaining cave churches worth seeing.

The Tokalı Kilise

This is on the way between the car park and the entrance to the museum, on the other side of the road. The name 'Buckle Church' was given to it, as with most churches here in Cappadocia, by common usage. There is said to have been a buckle-shaped lamp hook in its ceiling in the past. It belongs to the largest rock churches of the region and it is famous for its colourful paintings and its rich decoration with columns. Here, too, a long period of darkness was the reason for the colours being preserved so well. The large quantity of blue in the paintings, which makes these frescoes unique, is especially remarkable. The entire complex consists of an old church, which seems like a narthex today, the new large church with a crypt, which is not accessible any more, beneath it, and a northern side chapel. The representations in so-called friezes, series of relief paintings on the walls, and the rich decorations in the form of pilasters, arcades and cornices are another specialty. The Tokalı Church belongs to the most impressive sacred buildings in Cappadocia and visiting it is actually a must.

St.Mary's Church

This is situated hidden in the rocks a little above the Tokalı Church. From here you have a magnificent view over the Kiliclar Valley (Valley of the Swords). The church owes its name to the many images of St. Mary on its walls. It can only be entered in a stooping position through a narrow entrance. A millstone rock next to the entrance door shows how important a possibility of defence was at the time of its construction. This is proof that the complex must be rather old.

210 Central Cappadocia

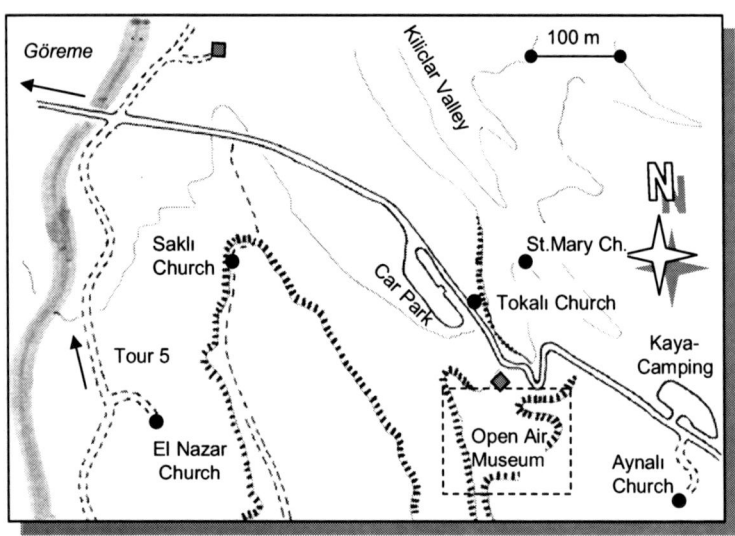

Ayanlı Kilise and Firkatan Kilise

This small church complex is situated about half a mile above the Göreme museum, opposite the Kaya Camping ground. One is a little confused at first, as the complex is hidden behind large trees and one does not know exactly where to go. But Süleman, who has been working here for 15 years and who speaks a little English, will certainly guide the confused visitors to the right place. Those churches originated in troubled times, which can be seen from the way they were built. Narrow tunnels lead to the upper floors, which could be secured by several millstone doors. Süleman does not only collect 2.5 TL of admission fee, but also distributes electric torches. Without these, entering the tunnels and passageways would be quite dangerous. A steep and unsecured climb-down shaft leads downwards from one of the upper rooms. Try to climb it, simultaneously holding the torch, then you will understand

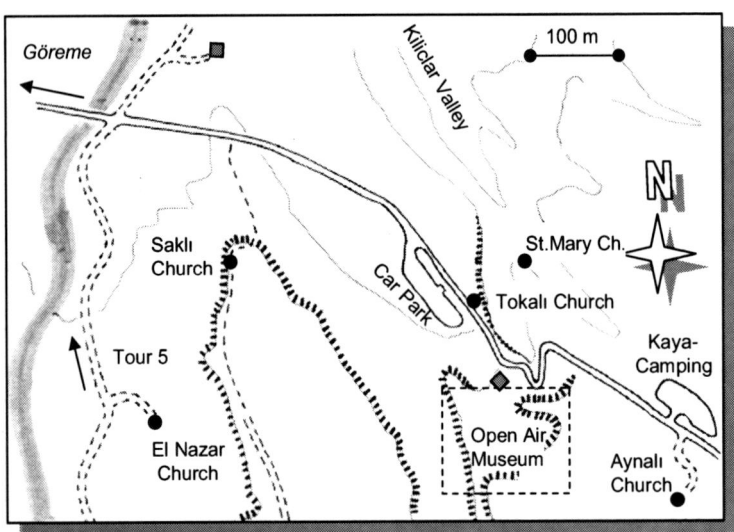

how well those shafts could be defended. You will also often still find the ancient communication shafts which connected the separate floors. In cooperation with your fellow travellers, you should test their acoustic qualities. Süleman takes a winter break from October to April, and the complex is closed then.

Saklı Kilise

After 300 m from the museum towards Göreme, this church is marked on the left. Beside a teahouse, the path leads about 10 m up the hill, where you will find the entrance of the "Hidden Church". Its entrance had been buried under rocks for centuries, until the complex was finally rediscovered in 1956. The church displays some untypical features. There are two rectangular pillars in the centre, and it has a flat ceiling. But the paintings, too, are different from those of the other churches of Göreme. They must be the work of some local artist, as there are images of trees, birds and also of rock cones which dominate everything in this region. Also the classical animals, the ox and the donkey, are missing in the image of the birth of Christ. From outside the door you have a splendid view of the El Nazar valley, where another sacred building awaits the interested visitor.

El Nazar Church

This was carved into an isolated rock cone in the 10th century. It actually consists of two church rooms above each other in the cone. The rooms and their frescoes were exposed to the open air for decades, as part of the cone had collapsed. When in 2007 the church was renovated, the cone was closed again. If you are doing walk No. 5 (p. 324) through the Zemi valley and if you are not shocked by the admission fee of 8 TL, you should make the short detour and visit this church by the roadside.

Between Ecstasies and Asceticism

- early Christian Communities in Cappadocia

by Bernd Junghans

If you want to get an idea of the community life of those early Christian communities, you have to say farewell to the conception of the present Church. Without the guidance of a superior ecclesiastic authority, a great variety of explanations and interpretations of the idea of a God-fearing life developed in the young Christian community within a short time. The retreat to a hermitage was a very widespread form of religious devotion. The 40 days which Christ was said to have spent in the desert were a model to many believers to choose a life in seclusion and asceticism for themselves, too. The remoteness of the Cappadocian valleys seemed to be almost ideal for this way of living. The soft tuff rock enabled the hermits to dig little cave dwellings into the rock, and the gardens at the bottom of the valleys secured their subsistence. Not infrequently the 40 days thus became many months. Some of the hermits even went so far as to have themselves walled in, or they did not leave their rock cones for years. However, most of the early Christians seem to have strived for community, and from the casual coexistence there developed the first monasteries. St. Basil, the bishop of Caesarea, gave the new communities a fixed set of rules of how human community life had to be lived in the Christian way.

The first large Early Christian assembly rooms kept closely to the classical market hall and were used for all kinds of meetings, as the modern distinction between religion and worldly life did not yet exist. Those public assembly halls later were to develop into what we call a church today. But here, too, we must first say goodbye to the familiar concept of a house of God. As in the ancient temples, such rooms were anything but places of silence and tranquility. Their architectural origin itself makes a busy life inside their walls seem probable; after all, this type of building had been known already before the birth of Christ and had been used as a market hall or for other public events.

The Kadir-Durmuş Church in Göreme is the best example of such a hall in Cappadocia. The decoration of the room with embossed columns and round arches reveals a strong Oriental influence. Additionally, there is a large ambo, a two-step pulpit which is accessible from two sides, in the centre. Besides, the room is open on the long side, so that it could be entered by all members of the community at any moment. Those architectural characteristics suggest a rather democratic coexistence in the early Christian sense. Social and gender differences were disregarded in those days, according to the words of the Bible that "All human beings are equal before God". During the further development of church architecture the ambo, as a platform for everybody, was to disappear in favour of a pulpit which was relocated from the inner church room to the back or to a higher position. Now, only one person has the final say, and the main axis of the church moves towards the longitudinal direction, so that it became possible to establish a strict seating and ranking order. Councils and Patriarchal edicts changed the architecture and in the course of time created the concept of the institutional and architectural structure of the Church that is known to us today. The realization of those ecclesiastic edicts often took place contrary to the religious views of the majority. Groups who did not adapt to their superiors were prosecuted as deviationists or heretics and had to seek shelter in the remote valleys of Cappadocia.

Some of those groups displayed rather strange rites. To some of them, the human body was an enemy of the soul which had to be controlled by scourging, fasting or sharp freezing. Others had themselves killed after being baptized as adults to enable their soul to ascend to heaven without blemish. They had themselves buried openly high up in the rocks, so that at least the birds would be able to profit from their sinful bodies. Here it becomes clear how closely the early Christian belief was sometimes amalgamated with ancient habits and religions, as this form of burial originates from the old Perisian fire cult of Zarathustra. Most unusual from today's perspective, however, appears a religious belief which sought salvation and God's blessing in permanent sexual ecstasy.

If you want to undertake a historically well-founded guided tour of the church region of Cappadocia in order to explore many hidden treasures, you can contact the German "itinerant charismatic", Bernd Junghans, and arrange excursions and walking tours. He will guide you along narrow paths and to the most extraordinary early Christian sites. However, you should be a good walker and have good fitness. More information is available under: **www.berndputz.de**

Çavuşin

This place is situated on the road between Avanos and Göreme. Although it lies in the centre of Cappadocia, it looks very sleepy. If you let the minarets disappear and add some dry tumbleweeds rolling along the road in your imagination, the dreariness of a Mexican siesta arises. The contemporary buildings, of which the town almost completely consists, do not make it any nicer, either. The reason for this becomes visible when you see the destroyed old town on the mountainside at the end of the town. The great earthquake of Erzerum in 1939 had negative effects to as far as Cappadocia (at a distance of 700 km), where Çavuşin was hit hardest. The village was not immediately destroyed completely, but the basic structure of the rock was destabilized so fundamentally that under state pressure the slope had to be given up as a dwelling place for good in the sixties. Only some houses opposite the mountain remained intact and continued to be used as dwellings. Here, at the foot of the mountain, you will also meet tourists again. They are either brought here by bus, or they come through here at the end of a walk. But compared with the rush of visitors in Göreme or Ürgüp, things are quite leisurely here. The village square is only surrounded by a few souvenir stalls and small cafés. The horses and carts in front of the houses are not for decoration, but are still used every day. Çavuşin is a place for peace fanatics, also because the road from Göreme to Avanos, although rarely used, runs past it at a great distance from the village centre. And if at daytime you pass by the café next to the mayor's office and watch the old mans discuss and argue in front of it, a somewhat archaic feeling begins to develop indeed.

Apart from the aforementioned slope of the old town, which can be climbed, there is also a church by the road at the edge of the village that can be visited. It was carved out of the rock during the years between 963 and 969 AD and was dedicated to the Byzantine Emperor Nikephorus Phokas. Unfortunately the vestibule collapsed many years ago, so that only a painted wall is visible from outside. Parts of the monastic complex belonging to it have also been missing for a long time, so that the entrance passages to some of the rooms end in the void of an abyss. On the whole the church is in rather desolate condition. There can be some doubt whether the exorbitant admission fee of 8 TL is justified. The paintings in the large apsis which used to be described in the old travel guides have crumbled from the wall almost completely, and wide cracks in the ceiling of the church building give proof of its continuing

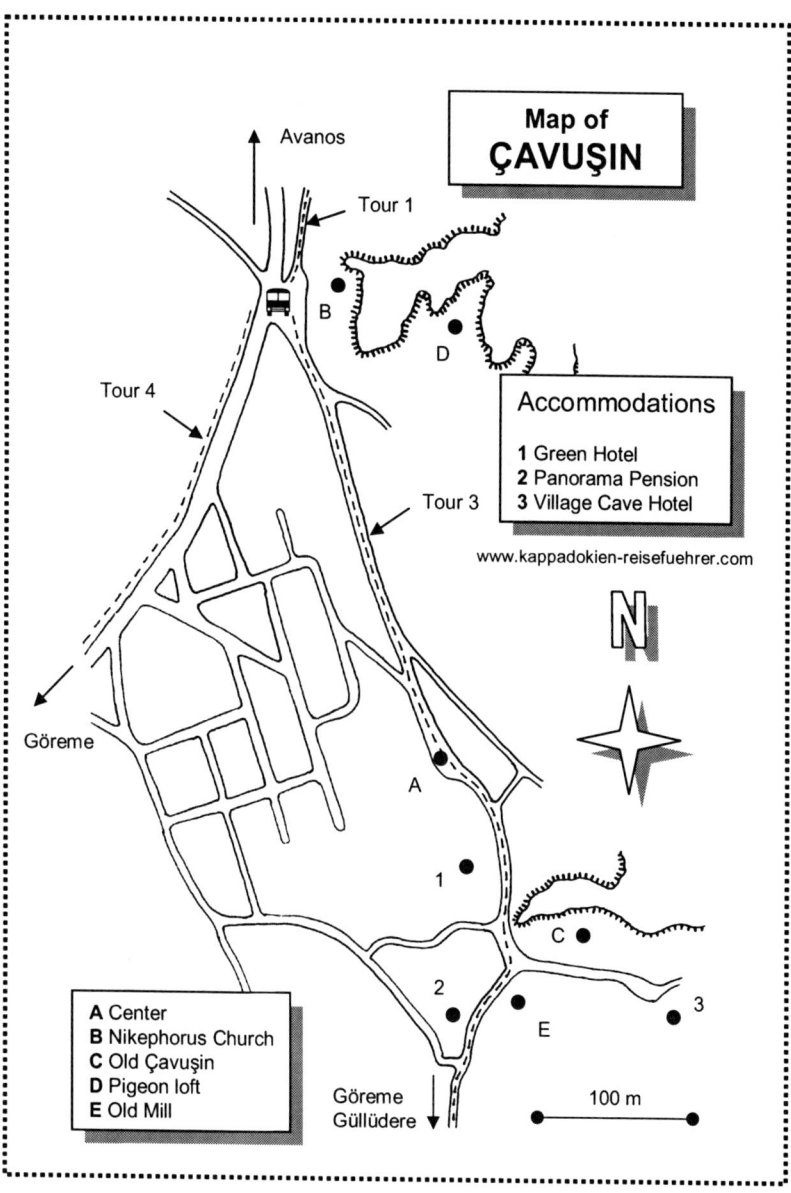

decay. The reason why this church was called 'Pigeon Church' can be seen on the front wall, where a large misshaped hole has been beaten through the rock and through the paintings to provide an entrance hole for pigeons. The complex is open daily from 8.00 a.m. to 5.00 p.m.

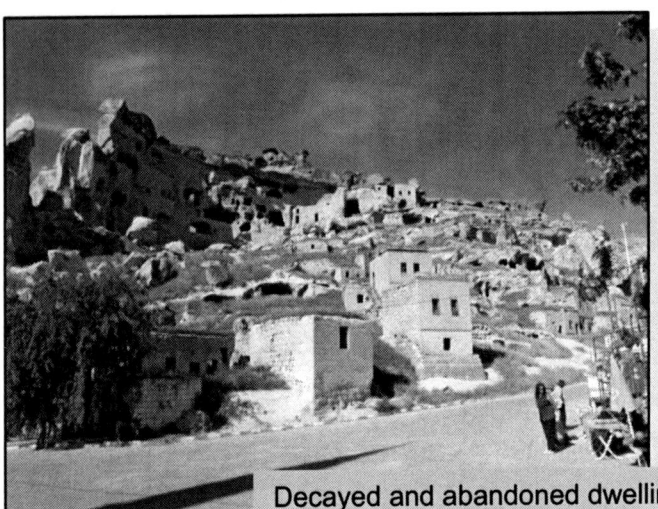

Decayed and abandoned dwellings on the slope of Çavuşin

Foto: Johann Munker

Accommodations in Çavuşin

➤ GREEN HOTEL

This hotel has existed for 20 years and was expanded gradually. It has a lovingly furnished lounge and a small cave restaurant where traditional food is served. The house is run by the whole family and it is very clean. Like all lodging houses in the village it is very quiet. A small camping ground is combined with it and can be used for 6 TL per person. Unfortunately, the trees that could provide some shade will still have to grow a little, and the maintenance of the grounds is not really a specialty of the house, although its name should be a motto for it.

1	40-50 TL	26	E – F – D	ⵟ 🍽	①⑤⑧

Phone: 0384 532 7050   www.motelgreen.com

➤ PANORAMA PENSION

An inexpensive and quiet alternative at the end of the village. The rooms are simple and quiet, partly with a marvellous view over historic Çavuşin. A cozily furnished cave room is available for cold evenings. Another one of those hostels which remind you of the boom era in Cappadocia when backpackers stumbled over each other here. At least the price-performance ratio is almost unsurpassable here. The proprietor is a flower enthusiast, and it would perhaps be a good idea if he tried to increase his income at the Green Hotel, for example.

2	30 TL	7	E – F	⟨Y⟩ ⟨🍽⟩	①⑤⑧

Phone : 0384 532 7002   Fax : 0384 5332 7115

➤ THE VILLAGE CAVE

Pure luxury and a successful combination of ancient Ottoman coziness and modern technology. The old cave complex was redesigned and transformed into a special hotel. Already the simple rock-carved passageway between the restaurant and the rooms evokes a feeling of walking through an underground city. The rooms are large and partly equipped with open chimneys. The position at the foot of the old town in a cul-de-sac promises very quiet nights, and any kind of hectic activity inside the house itself seems unlikely with only 6 rooms.

3	140-260 TL	6	E	⟨Y⟩ ⟨🍽⟩	①②③⑤⑧

Phone: 0384 532 7197   www.thevillagecave.com

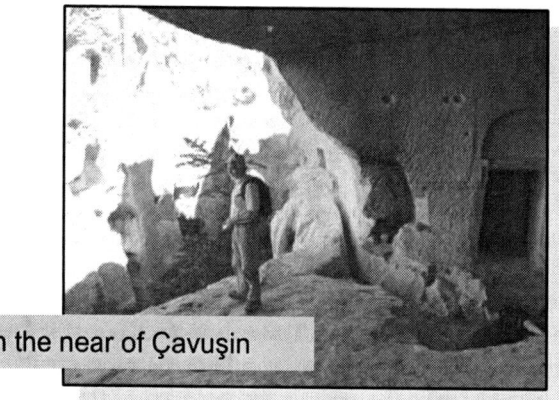

Hiking in the near of Çavuşin

Foto: Johann Munker

Paşabağı

This little valley, which is also called the "Valley of the Monks", is between Çavuşin and the museum village of Zelve and is famous for its many well-preserved fairy chimneys. By watching them, the erosive process typical of Cappadocia can be studied very well. The mountain in the background actually seems to be 'calving'. The individual layers of rock are clearly visible on the high rock towers. If you draw an imaginary line through one layer from one chimney to the others, the original stratification, as it is found with every mountain of the region, becomes easily discernible. It is especially the hard rock caps on the top which give the towers their bizarre appearance and which also protect them from deterioration. The collapse of such a cap would cause the tower to shrink to a little stump within a few decades.

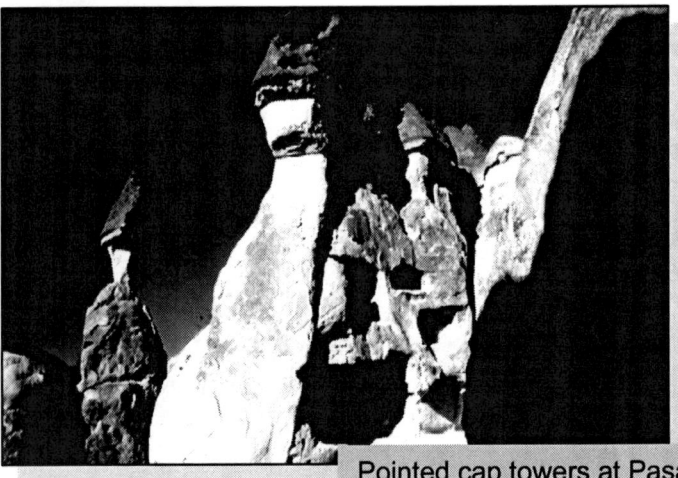
Pointed cap towers at Paşabağı

Here, too, man has used those structures as dwelling places from primeval times. In the south-eastern corner of the valley there is a large dwelling complex you can climb up to and where you will find a viewing window at a height of about 15 m. The Simeon's Tower is situated amost in the centre of the valley. In the lower part of the tower, a little chapel was built in which a statue of St. Simeon, the pillar saint, is supposed to be. The dwelling area in the upper part of the tower is more interesting than the inaccessible chapel. It can only be reached by a vertical shaft which is about 5 m high. Visitors who are good climbers will easily manage to put their hands into the indentations in the side walls and then climb up the shaft. Above there are two dwelling rooms, furnished with a bed and a seat, both carved out of the solid rock.

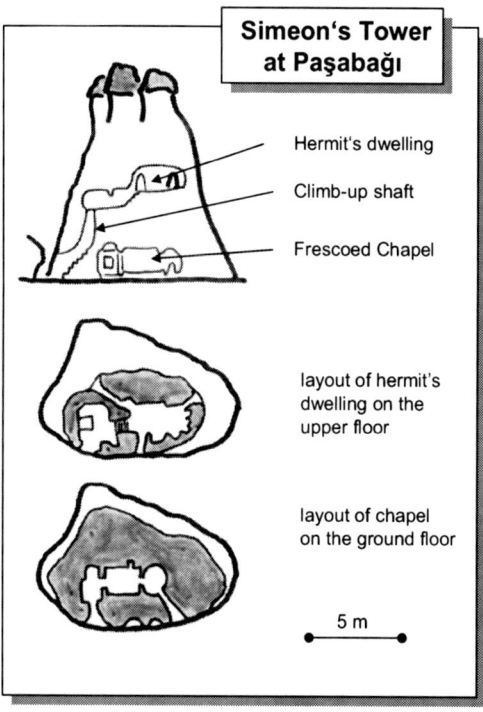

You can take excellent photos of the surrounding chimneys from here. Unfortunately, sales stands are spreading in a more and more uncontrolled manner along the valley. While 20 years ago there were only some simple canvas-covered stands, in the meantime a veritable shopping street has developed. And the stands are advancing further and further into the valley. If you watch the numbers of tourists in the morning and in the afternoon, you know why this happens. The best time for taking photos here is from late afternoon until sunset. The rush is not so great then anymore, and the towers start to shine and glow.

Zelve

The place was evacuated by the government in 1950 and the population was rehoused to a new village 1.5 km further to the north. Aktepe, which is the name of the new village, reveals at first sight why it has remained so small. In comparison with the inhabitants' original home, the place can be described properly as 'dusty' and 'desolate'. And therefore it is not surprising that so many former inhabitants moved on to other towns.

However, the huge boulders at the bottom of the valley to the right prove that the former evacuation did not take place without a reason. All those boulders have broken free from the sides of the mountain during the past 50 years and would most certainly have claimed many victims among the population. The thin wall of rock between the first valley on the right and the second one was also completely preserved until some decades ago. Today the front part of the valley on the right is even closed to tourists for safety reasons. Zelve was no small settlement, as is proven by the numerous rooms and dwelling units that had been carved into the rock on both sides of the valley. Up to 1923, the year of the great population exchange, Christians and Muslims had lived together in the village. Even in their wildest dreams the remaining Turkish inhabitants will probably not have been able to imagine that only 25 years later they, too, would have been forced to leave their habitat.

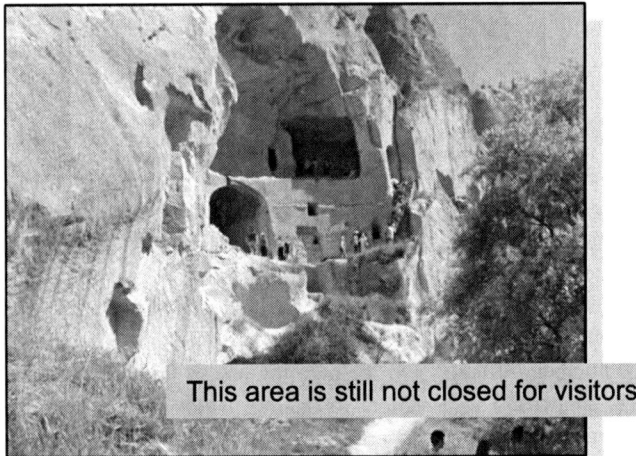

This area is still not closed for visitors

Foto: Johann Munker

Central Cappadocia 221

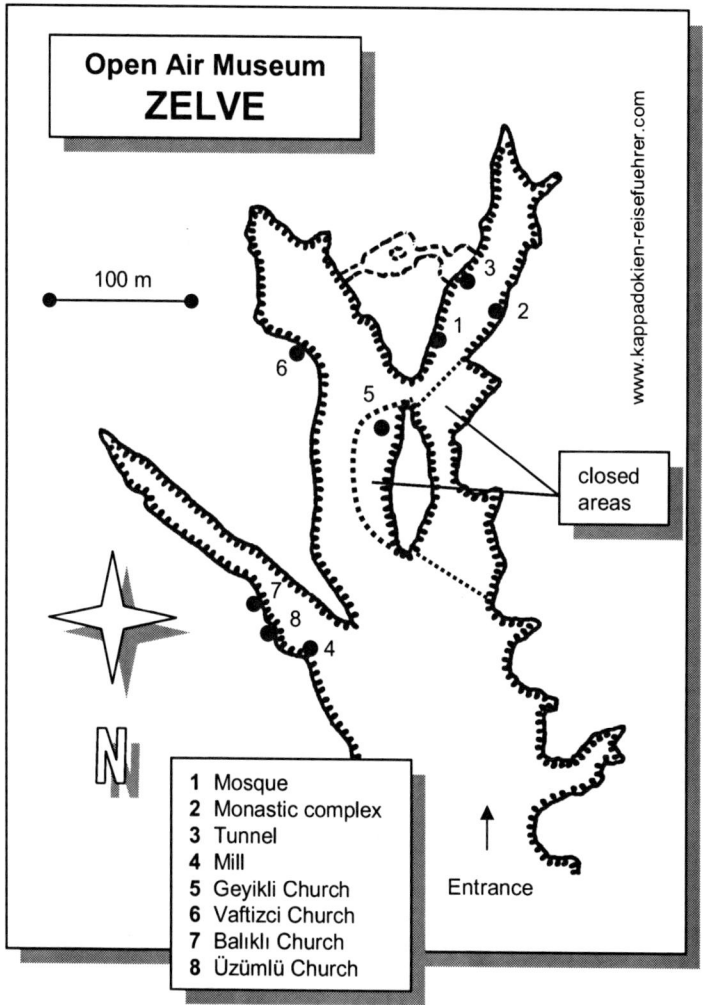

The place consists of three valleys, which have been cut into the mountain from the north. Two of these valleys protrude far into the mountain and have almost given it the shape of a 'U'. The third valley on the far left does not extend so far into the mountain and is often overlooked by visitors. However, there are several interesting rock-cut rooms right there. The old village mill with its large millwheel, which was kept in motion by a draft animal, has been preserved. Right next to it are two churches. However, their ornamental painting has hardly been preserved, and only some fragments of a painted decoration in form of vine branches indicate why one of them is called Üzümli Kilise (Grape Church). In general church decoration here in Zelve is very frugal, as the colourful decoration that was used after the iconoclastic period is not found here.The distinctive feature of Zelve is rather the fact that, apart from the little mosque in the valley on the right, there are no artificial buildings at all here. Up to the end the people remained faithful to their old cave dwellings. Today, this fact gives us a brief glimpse into the way that the Cappadocians must have lived in their villages centuries ago. Places like Avanos, Göreme or Ürgüp did not look much different then.

Another thing worth mentioning is the connection tunnel between valley number one and two. Today nobody knows when and for what reason it was first made. On the one hand it is of course a short cut between the two valleys, but perhaps also tactical, i.e. defense reasons were involved. In case of an attack the defenders could relocate their troops from one valley to the other promptly and effectively, just to wherever they were needed.

Today Zelve is a museum which can be visited between 8.30 a.m and 6.00 p.m. for 8 TL. For a walk through the tunnel you should wear sturdy shoes, have a torch with you and be free of claustrophobia.

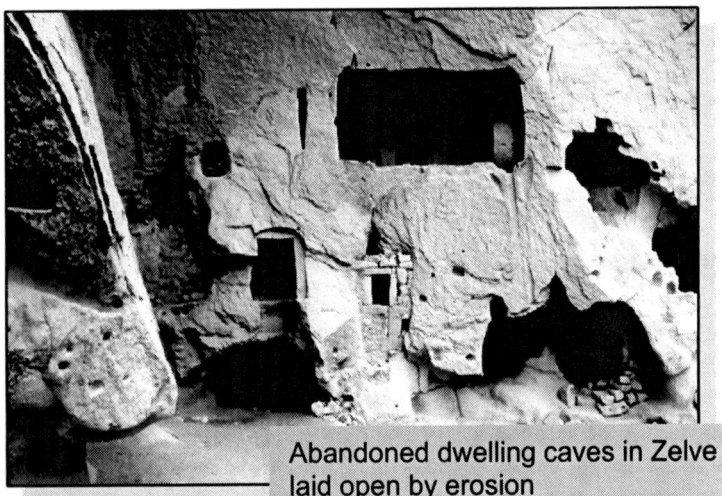
Abandoned dwelling caves in Zelve – laid open by erosion

The Devrent Valley

This valley is situated halfway between Ürgüp and Avanos, about 3 km from Aktepe. The characteristic features of this not very large valley are rather small tuff cones standing close to each other by the hundreds and making the horizon look ragged. If you try to get through between the individual cones, you will understand why the valley has never been inhabited. The narrowness and pathlessness among those rock formations did not leave any room for settlements. Photo fans should come here in the late afternoon when the small cones cast long shadows and glow in the sunset. Unfortunately, the valley is out of reach of the public bus service, and a walk across the shadeless plains towards the valley is not exactly a pleasure, either. But if you have rented a scooter, you should not miss this freak of nature and enjoy a romantic sunset here.

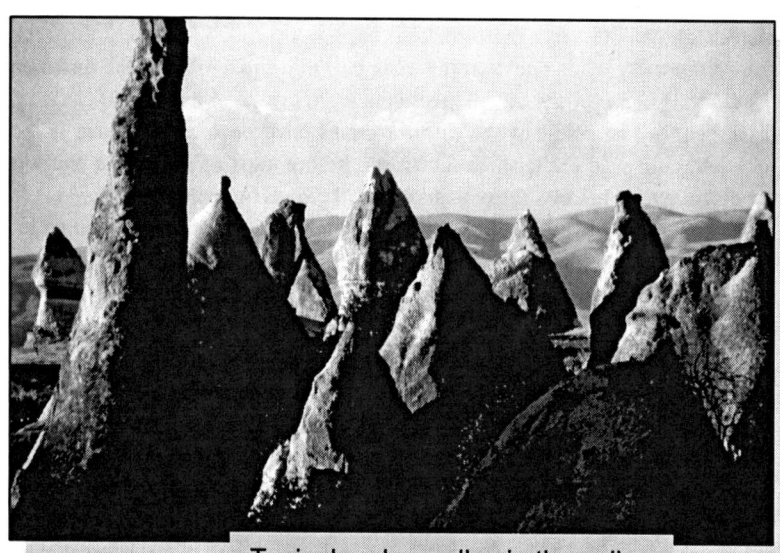
Typical rock needles in the valley

Ürgüp

This little district town represents a pleasant mixture of Göreme and Avanos. What is lacking in terms of tourism in Avanos and in normal life in Göreme, comes together here in a healthy manner. Today Ürgüp is spread out over a large space at the foot of three historically inhabited hills. They are not habitable any more, but they indicate how large the town must have been even in historic times. Its large size, which it was famous for already in the Seljuk era, remained the same until the population exchange in 1923. The tomb of the Seljuk Sultan Ruknettin Kilicarslan is proof of the extent of Ürgüp's fame in former times. He escaped to Ürgüp from his brother, who contested for the throne against him, in the 12th century. His tomb, however, was erected by the Ottoman Vecihi Pasa only in 1863. Thus the city was famous as a place of refuge for disgraced persons over many centuries. The numerous tunnels and secret passageways inside the three hills were ideal hiding places for refugees. The Seljuk Sultan's tomb was open for visitors high up on the first rock of the town until 2007. It is part of the new viewing plateau above the city, the Temenni Tepesi. In 2007, however, the rock gained notoriety when one morning a big part of it broke off and fell down on the central square of the city. Three lives were lost, as the rock had buried a discotheque. The result of the disaster could have been much worse if the rock had collapsed earlier than 5.00 a.m., before most of the guests had left the discotheque. In 2008 the plateau was still closed to visitors.

Like some other towns, Ürgüp possessed a large Greek community with a lot of Greek villas, some of which have been preserved. It is worth while leaving the town centre for a while to admire the architectural achievements of the former inhabitants.

The old vicarage with its large portico about 50 m to the left from the mosque at the central square is especially beautiful. The restoration, which had been due for a long time, was finally begun in 2008. The main square itself was spoiled some years ago by a true masterpiece of modern architecture, in which some restaurants and shops established themselves. Besides, there is everything that a tourist's heart desires in the centre of the town. Numerous travel agencies offer their tours of Cappadocia. Rug dealers are lying in wait for a big haul, and here there are also the offices of the big car rental agencies like Avis and Europ-Car, whose vehicles can be rented at their European branches already.

Central Cappadocia 225

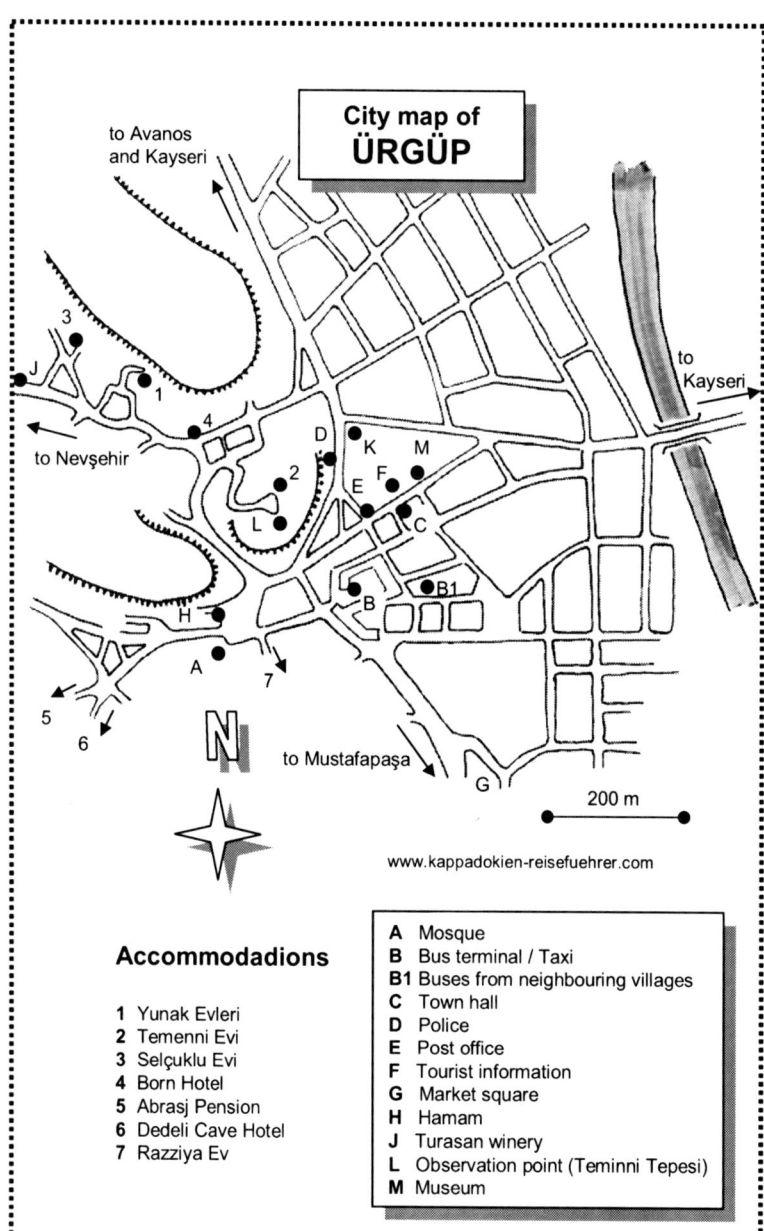

There is also an old hamam at the square, where you can spend a couple of hours of relaxation. The little museum can almost be called cute and displays historic finds from the vicinity. They are especially proud of the petrified mammoth tusks which were found near Mustafapasa. A bit further, on the road to Nevsehir, there is an attraction which is more interesting to local visitors: The 'Asma Konak', named after the Turkish soap opera of the same name, is located here. At certain times the fans of this successful TV serial step on each other's toes here. The success of this serial has led to the result that more films are shot in the town and that there are always camera teams present here. Still a bit further up the road you will find the Turasan winery, which has produced its wine in Ürgüp since 1943. If you are interested, you can indulge in a detailed wine tasting session here or take part in a guided tour of the factory.

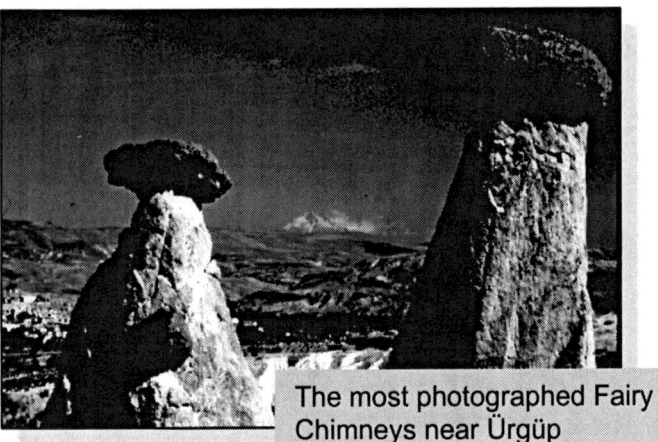

The most photographed Fairy Chimneys near Ürgüp

Accommodation in Ürgüp

Finding accommodation in the town is something special. Places to stay are not scarce; but compared to Göreme the price level is rather high. You pay 40 TL and more for a rather dated hostel. And after that, prices soon escalate very quickly. Many luxury hotels have established themselves, and by this we do not mean the large concrete hotels in the eastern part of the town. Lots of cute cave hotels have emerged in recent years on the north-western fringe of the ancient town hill, and their prices for a standard room are at least $100. Very nice hotels, no question, but just not affordable for everyone. But this price category seems to have motivated the owners of simple boarding houses to keep up with them in a way, only because they also offer a few cave rooms for rent. We have not included all these noble hotels because they are already mentioned in other travel books like "Turkey's Nicest Hotels" or "The World's 1000 Top Hotels". Due to the difficulties in finding an accommodation with a reasonable price-performance ratio in Ürgüp, our selection is rather modest, in spite of the almost 50 hotels and boarding houses in the town.

➢ YUNAK EVLERI

Let us start with a superlative. A wealthy businessman from Istanbul invested money in this seemingly crazy project and created a special class hotel. The complex itself is not directly seen as what it is, as the rock wall behind which it is hidden looks exactly like it has done for centuries. Here you live in a luxurious cave with a long view high up in the rock wall of Ürgüp and at the same time enjoy the amenities of a modern hotel. Of course, a private rock-carved balcony belongs to every suite.

| 1 | 180-300 TL | 30 | E | ⊤ ⦿| ①②③⑤⑥⑦⑧ |

Phone: 0384 341 6920   www.yunak.com

➢ TEMENNI EVI

Also one of the many noble hotels in the town. The hotel is located high up on the mountain, even a little higher than the public viewpoint which is directly next to it. The huge roof terrace equipped with plush corner seats is best for sipping one's cocktail under the town's starlit sky in the evening. All rooms have jacuzzi bathrooms, open fireplaces and are large and spacious in design. The cave rooms are supplied with daylight very skilfully by means of light shafts. The offered 'Romantic Dinner' is something very special. Through a tunnel of 30 m you go to a small cave with a balcony beneath the viewing platform high above the town. The hotel is well-known for its good cuisine and additionally offers cookery courses.

| 2 | 150-300 TL | 14 | E | ⊤ ⦿| ①②③⑤⑥⑦⑧ |

Phone: 0384 341 3341   www.temennievi.com

➢ SELÇUKLU EVI

The third and last of the noble lodginghouses included here. You should not let its outward appearance fool you. Only if you enter the inner courtyard, will you be able to discover its unique architectural charm. Here, too, good local cuisine is supplied. The owner, Mr Halil Elalan, is a veteran of the tourism business in Ürgüp. He has also been the owner of the 'Alan tourizm' travel agency for more than 25 years and will love to support his guests with advice and practical help.

3	160-500 TL	20	E – F -D	⊤ 🍽	①②③⑤⑥⑦⑧

Phone: 0384 341 7460   www.selcukluevi.com

➢ BORN HOTEL

A relatively inexpensive solution for Ürgüp. The old Ottoman house has been an inn for 21 years, and unfortunately it looks like it. The rooms are simply furnished, but the age-old doors, windows and wooden stairs still have a certain flair. The shady front garden which represents the outdoor hotel grounds, unfortunately is directly next to the road.

4	40 TL	10	E	🍽	①②⑧

Phone: 0384 341 4756

➢ ABRASJ PENSION

Very nice complex in an old house whose cave rooms have mostly been preserved authentically. The shady inner yard filled with small fruit trees and the very quiet location far from all noise make this inn an oasis of recreation. The Belgian operator promises a sumptuous breakfast and top local cuisine in case of full board. You should, however, arrange a pick-up service with the operator on your arrival, as the inn is situated relatively far away from the town centre and very hidden.

5	100 TL	6	E – F – NL - D	🍽	①②③⑦⑧

Phone: 0384 341 7032   www.abrasj.com

➢ DEDELI KONAK CAVE HOTEL

If you are standing in front of the narrow entrance door, you will hardly expect a hotel behind it. Here, situated in the middle of an ordinary and quiet residential neighbourhood, the whole complex gradually opens up to the guest from floor to floor, and distributed over several terraces. Here, too, lots of original pieces of the room furnishings have been preserved. On the roof terrace a comfortably funished barbecue area – entirely in Ottoman style – is available for the guests.

| 6 | 100-150 TL | 10 | E | ♉ ꧁ | ①②③⑤⑧ |

Phone: 0384 341 5840   www.dedelikonak.com

> **RAZZIYA EVI**

Finally the inn which we liked best here in the town. Beautiful, spacious and lovingly decorated rooms, which are partly furnished with an open fireplace, and a green and flowery garden have convinced us. With it there is promised a sumptuous breakfast adjusted to the home country of the visitor. An in-house hamam is a specialty devised by Romy Celik, the Swiss proprietress of the house. Other hotels with a similar ambience usually only start at triple-digit prices.

| 7 | 80 TL | 8 | E – F - D | ♉ ꧁ | ①②③⑤⑦⑧ |

Phone: 0384 341 5089   www.razziyaevi.com

The Karamanlı
Caviar Trade in Cappadocia

Very little is known about the origins of the Karamanlı nation. They are supposed to have originated from the present province of Karaman. According to some allegations, they were Greek people who had been turkmenized in the Seljuk period, but who had retained their Christian religion. Other historians maintain the thesis that they belonged to an ancient Turkmen tribe which had adopted the Christian belief in the Byzantine period. But in fact, no clear statement can be made on the origin of this nation. What makes clarifying their historic origin so difficult is their unique separation of language and writing. Although they spoke mostly Turkish, they used the Greek alphabet for writing. There is a similar situation in Iran, where the Persian language is recorded by using Arabic characters. In Cappadocia the Karamanlı mainly settled in Mustafapaşa, Ürgüp, Nevşehir and Kayseri. At the same time they established certain regional trade guilds.

In Kayseri they specialized in selling sausages and dried meat, and also today the city is famous for its sausages and smoked beef ham called Pastirma. In the other Cappadocian places they concentrated on trading in caviar and fish, which is rather strange considering the geographical position of the region in the centre of the Anatolian highland. But Cappadocia is in the middle of the trade route between the Caspian Sea, where the biggest sturgeons were caught, and the main market for those goods, Istanbul. Many Karamanlians had lived at the Bosporus since the conquest of Constantinople by the Ottomans under Mehmet the Conqueror. They were relocated by force then in order to rebuild the city after its destruction in 1453. They were also regarded as clever intermediaries between the new rulers and the local population. Most of Istanbul's new inhabitants came form Aksaray and some of them soon founded a new town quarter, which still bears the name of their home town up to the present day. But in 1923 the entire population of Karamanlıs had to leave what had been their home town for a thousand years. Because of their Christian religion, they fell under the Lausanne treaty and thus became part of the population exchange arranged between Greece and Turkey. This second forced resettlement was extremely hard for them, as they were deeply rooted in the Turkish traditions and did not understand the Greek language. Today their culture has disappeared completely, either lost in Turkish nationalism or fallen victim to assimilation in Greece. Only every now and then the name 'Karamanlis' in Greece reminds us of this ancient nation.

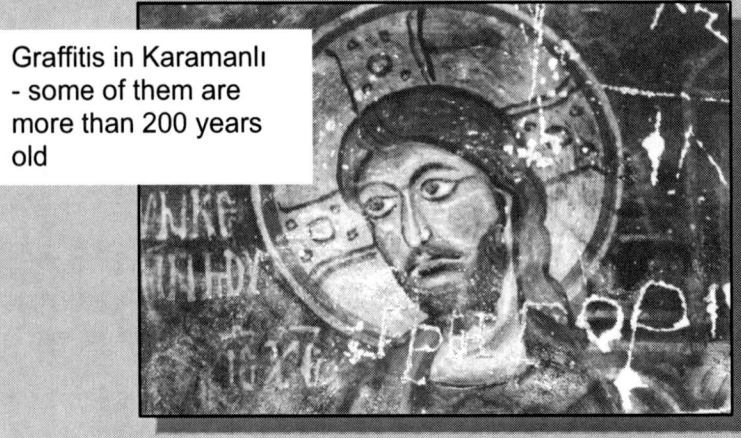

Graffitis in Karamanlı - some of them are more than 200 years old

Ortahisar

This is a small town situated south of the road between Nevşehir and Ürgüp. Although the place has only few tourist structures, it is full of life here. The whole town seems to be on its feet in the centre, and the teahouses and gardens round the central square seem to burst with men playing cards and palavering. Opposite the tourist information there lies, quiet and shady, the town's most beautiful teagarden at the foot of the 'Kale' mountain. Like Uçhisar, Ortahisar, too, has a huge perforated rock formation which is visible from afar. 'Ortahisar' means 'middle castle' and, contrary to its counterpart, Uçhisar, the impression of a castle can be seen more obviously here. The rock is actually somewhat smaller and the view is not so distant, as it is situated deeper, but climbing it is much more exciting. You will get a vivid impression of what it was like to live not only on and in the rock, but also with it. The ascent is only for people who are surefooted and you should also be free from giddiness here. Several metal ladders go upstairs through narrow openings, and now and again you walk along close to the precipice to the next ascent, where the rickety railings do not really convey a feeling of security. A magnificent view over the town and its neighbourhood finally rewards for much trembling of the knees. In 2007 the mayor of the town declared the rock closed to visitors. The commune complained about the insufficient safety installations with the Turkish Ministry of Tourism, as they feared accidents. The barriers have however been made rather half-heartedly. The fence is easy to get around and the entrance has been bricked up only half, so that only few tourists can be kept from climbing up the rock in spite of that.

Since a few years ago there has been a small privately installed ethnological museum which is situated opposite the mosque. In it, scenes from traditional Cappadocian life are shown by means of full-size figurative representations equipped with everyday objects from the pre-touristic time. These lovingly equipped dioramas are also explained in detail. The admission fee of 3 TL is well spent here. And do not be deterred by having to walk through a restaurant first, for both institutions are run by the same owner, for which reason the museum is closed from 12.00 noon to 5.00 p.m.

A visit to the numerous antiques shops at the foot of the Kale is also worthwhile. Though there is much competition here, you will not pick up a bargain. The second-hand dealers know their rates.

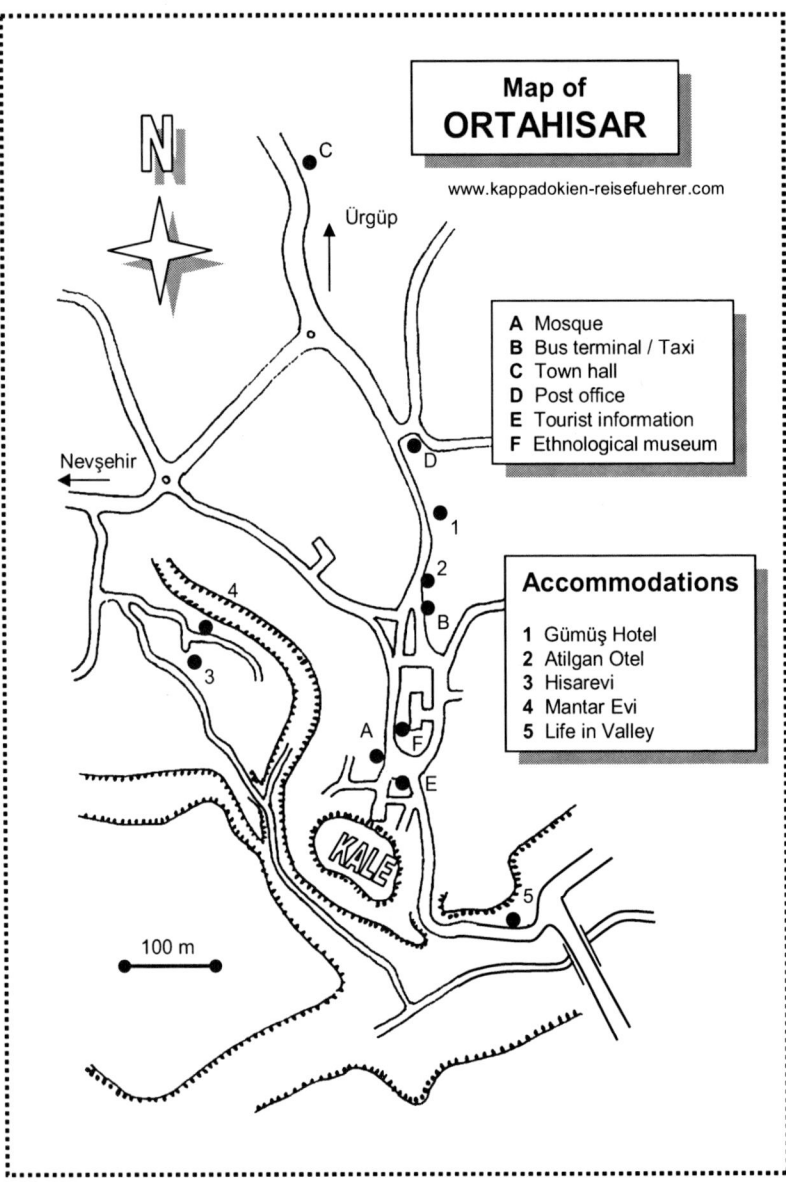

Accommodations in Ortahisar

➢ GÜMÜŞ HOTEL

Plain and simüple multi-storey house on the road to the main square. On the top floor there is the breakfast terrace with a view over the town. There are rooms in various sizes from single bed to six beds. Breakfast costs an extra 5TL.

1	50 TL	25	E	⌕ 🍽	⑤⑧

Phone: 0384 343 3127   www.gumushotel.com

➢ ATILGAN HOTEL

This is the foremer « Mersin Hotel » which got a new owner in 2007 and was completely renovated. The hotel is more oriented to Turkish tourists. It is a useful recommendation for travellers on a tight budget.

2	30 TL	35	E	⌕ 🍽	①⑤⑦⑧

Phone: 0384 343 2220   www.atilganotel.com

➢ HISAR EVI

The counterpart to the two hostels described before. The hotel is slightly away from the hustle and bustle in the old town centre, from here you have a magnificent view over the town, its neighbourhood and the Kale. All rooms are built in old caves, and the entire complex is romantically integrated into the surroundings. Lots of green, flowers and winding paths make your holiday dreams come true. Of course the price is also a bit different from the hotels metioned above.

3	200 TL	10	E - D	⌕ 🍽	①②③⑤⑦⑧

Phone: 0384 343 3005   Fax: 0384 343 23 28

➢ MANTAR EVI

Small family hostel with just 2 rooms on the first floor. The family lives on the ground floor, so you are right in the middle of Anatolian everyday life. Especially in the autumn, when large amounts of food are preserved for the winter, it is guaranteed that one never gets bored.

4	80 TL	2	E		②⑧

Phone: 0384 343 3687   zulfuyemantar@hotmail.com

➢ THE LIFE IN VALLEY

This small inn is situated out of the way and quiet above a gully on the edge of the town. Cozy cave rooms with private terraces, where you can excellently spend many a warm summer evening, and a family atmosphere are a guarantee for successful holidays.

| 5 | 40 TL | 6 | E | 🍽 | ②③⑧ |

Phone: 0348 343 3748   www.naziminyeri.com

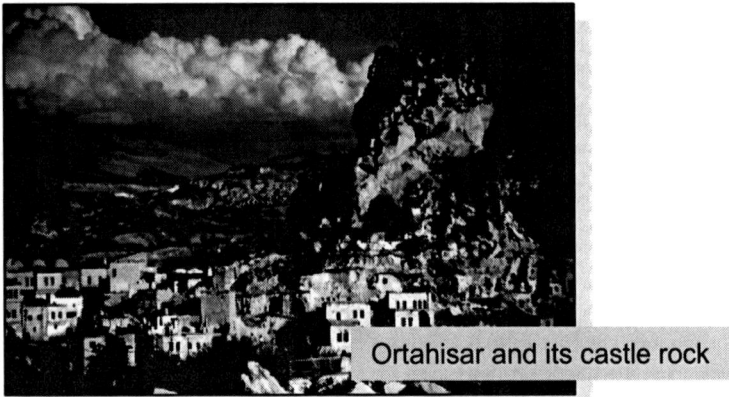

Ortahisar and its castle rock

Hospital Manastırı

This ancient rock monastery is located a little off the road between Ürgüp and Ortahisar, but there is a large sign which shows you the way. The clean and simple architectural lines are the special feature of this complex. The partly missing wall paintings underline the largeness of the prayer rooms, and you will get a certain idea of how many tons of rock had to be cleared away here. The church room on the left with its massive columns in the corners is especially interesting. On the left above the entrance door a statue in a peculiar pose has been left standing there when the rock was carved out. These rooms are from more peaceful times, as the facades were also smoothed and decorated with masonry. Taking a closer look at the painted decorations of the dovecote openings, which were carved out later, is also wortwhile.

Ibrahimpaşa

If you want to go on a little time travel into the past, you should by all means take a look at this place. It is only 5 km from the hustle and bustle of Göreme, but nevertheless those two places are whole worlds apart. No car noise, no spattering of scooters and no constant stream of music from the restaurants, but the warbling of birds, cock-crows and now and again the surreal braying of a donkey. Yes, there still are donkeys in Cappadocia. Here in Ibrahimpaşa they still belong to the daily life, also driving the cattle across the village to drink does. The two halves of the village just seem to be glued to the slope on both sides of the valley. Traditional village life is still practised here, untouched by tourism and seemingly unattainable for modern times.

The place is situated about 2 km south of the road from Uçhisar to Ortahisar, in the valley which connects Kavak and Ürgüp. Unfortunately, the dolmus service to it is very infrequent and irregular. The stone arch bridge, which connects the two parts of the place high above the valley and was built by the inhabitants in 1938 and 1939, is its highlight. There are no tourist accommodations in the village yet.

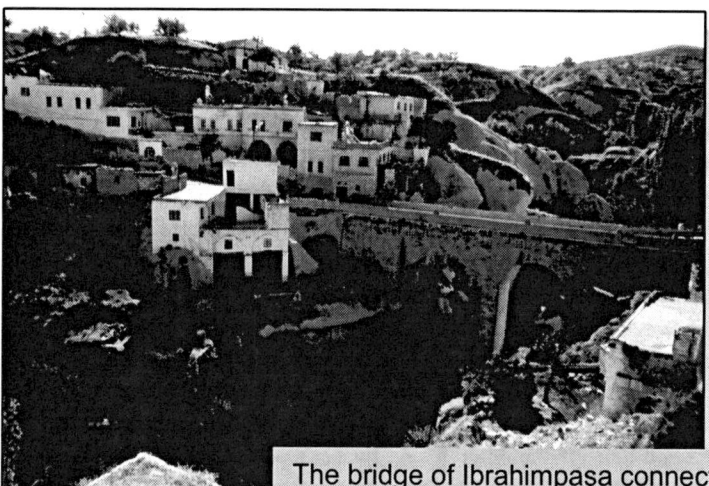

The bridge of Ibrahimpaşa connects the two halves of the village

Nevşehir

Economists would call it an expanding town, city planners are just throwing their hands up in horror. In the past 20 years the town has spread over the countryside like cancer. If you drive to Nevşehir you first drive through endless development areas and then you reach the traffic chaos of the inner city. Nevşehir has only had its own provincial administration since 1954, until then it had belonged to the district of Niğde. In tourism, the city has little to offer, although it once used to be the centre of Cappadocia. The most famous son of the city was named Ibrahim Paşa. On the career ladder he made it from simple kitchen helper to grand vizier at the Sultan's court. His marriage to Sultan Ahmet III's daughter turned out to be no disadvantage for him in that respect. In his role as grand vizier he presented the town of Muscara, as Nevşehir was called in those days, with a number of important buildings. Of these, only the Kurşunlu Cami (Leaden Mosque), the madrassa and the hamam have survived until today. After his death in 1730 the building activities came to an end, but the city remained an important trade centre up to the time of Atatürk's republic. Ibrahim Paşa also ordered the Seljuk fort high above the town to be enlarged and fortified more. The mosque is definitely worth visiting. Its large tree-lined inner yard and the wide arcades above the entrance exude an atmosphere of very special devotion and peace in the midst of this urban juggernaut. Next to the mosque is the ancient madrassa, which today contains a library, and below it, the hamam, which is still in operation today.

We will leave it undecided whether a visit to the fort is worthwhile, as the way up there is very tedious and hard to find. Besides the complex up there does not offer much to the visitor, providing it is open at all for a change. From a sociological and urbanistic point of view the steep way up is worthwhile. While the city is prospering with all kinds of modern buildings in every direction, the old town quarters on the slope offer a pathetic picture of decay. The city's poor people live here in dilapidated houses, some of which used to be real gems in former times. But the tedious way up is also worthwhile only because of the view over the city. Whoever has taken the trouble upon himself should go a step further still and venture further to the south. In this direction you can see a mosque on the next hill. Behind it a treasure of Christian religious architecture is hidden: built massively of hard rock, but unfortunately completely neglected and closed, rises the Panagias

Central Cappadocia 237

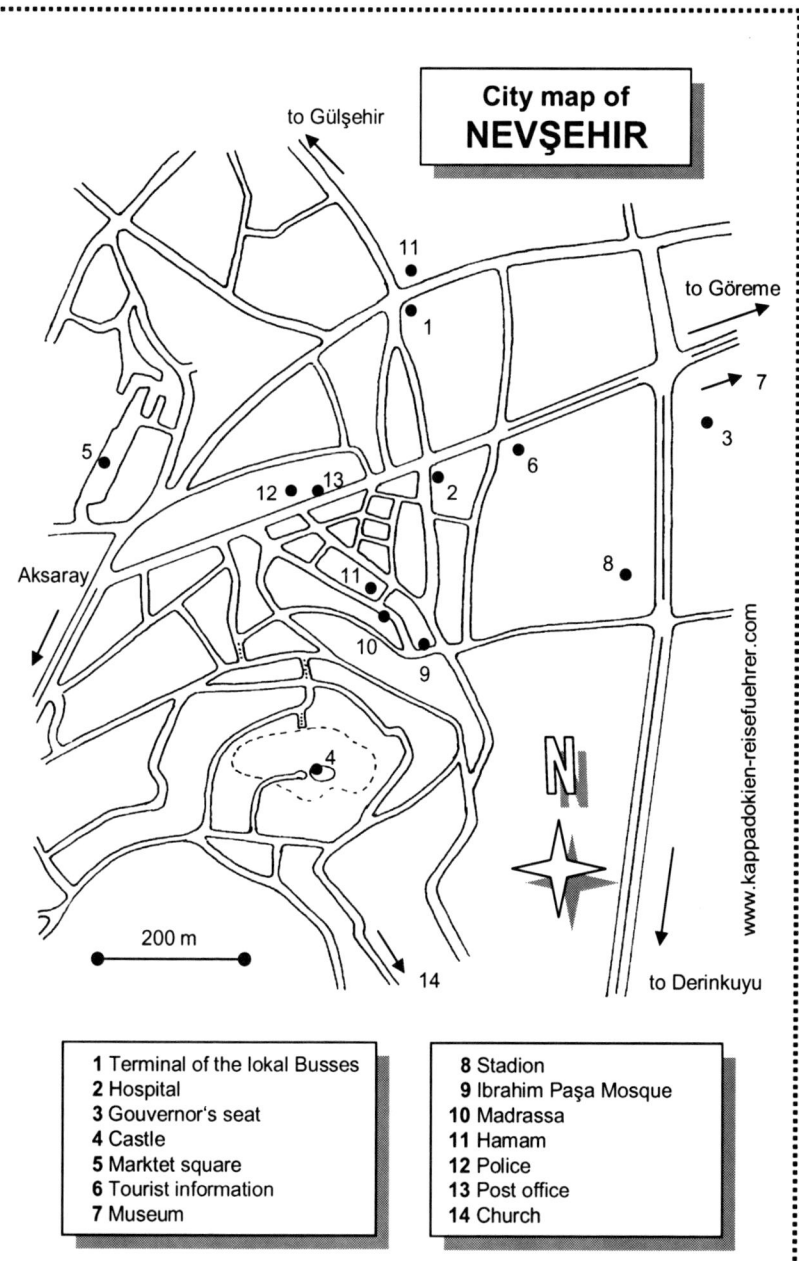

Church from 1849. Do not let yourself be deterred by the inhospitable environment and ignore the rubbish lying around. For decades nobody has cared for this sacred building, which seems to brave the wind and the weather. The columns at the end of the arcades are especially notable. They have no static function, but serve only for decoration and can be rotated. The different colouring of the pillar sides shows that they have not been moved for a long time. Try to memorize the environment as well as possible, and after this, visit the museum in Nevşehir. There, go to the top floor and turn directly left to the right corner of the room. There is an old view of the city on the wall. Upon closer inspection, you will at last find the church again, drawn a little darker and embedded in a huge town quarter. This is what the city looked like before 1924, before the Greek part of the population had to leave the country. Not a single one of the many buildings around the church is there anymore today.

The museum is tucked away behind the Ibrahim Paşa monument on the outward road towards the east. Exhibits from the Ottoman time are on the top floor. On the ground floor findings from the surrounding area and from earlier periods are on display chronologically and counter-clockwise. The earliest exhibits are from the time around 8000 B.C. and were found near Gülsehir. The museum is open from 8.00 a.m. to 5.00 p.m. and admission is 3 TL, provided they have not run out of tickets again. A longer stay or even overnight accommodation in Nevsehir is simply not worth it; therefore we have not mentioned any hotels or hostels here.

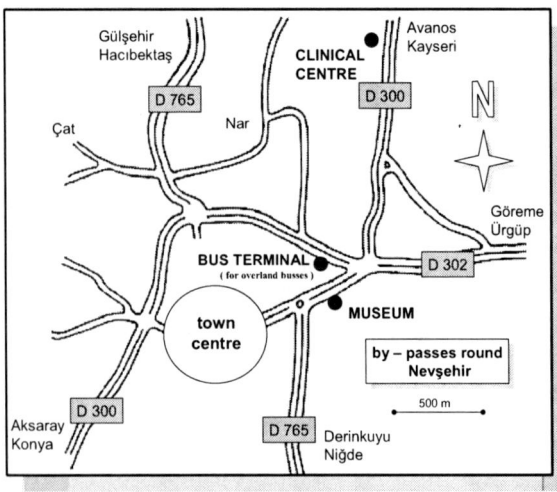

Avanos

This town is in the north, adjacent to the Göreme National Park, on both sides of the Kızılırmak. The river clearly divides two eras: in the north, on the slope, the old town; opposite, on the plain, the newer part, which was built in the sixties. The place has become famous for its century-old ceramic art. With clay sediments of several metres on its banks, the Red River supplies the basic material for it.

With its more than 10,000 inhabitants, Avanos is not a village any more, but a busy little district town with all the associated institutions, like a small infirmary, several schools and the obligatory administration offices. Just a typical Turkish small town which has been spared the onslaught of tourists; much to the chagrin of the local carpet dealers and hoteliers. At first glance the town does not have much to offer, apart from a pottery market in its centre. Thus, busloads of tourists are unloaded in front of the potteries, are given a demonstration of working with clay, often buy a souvenir, and just before the hour they continue to the next town. This is also the reason for the relatively limited supply of accommodations in spite of the size of the town. The few inns and hotels of the city centre make the offer very concise. The large hotels are all situated away from the centre and have dedicated themselves to the package bus tourism.

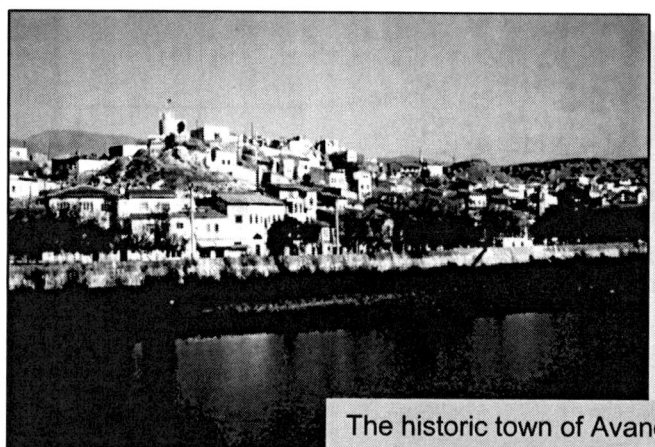

The historic town of Avanos – on the banks of the Red River

240 The North

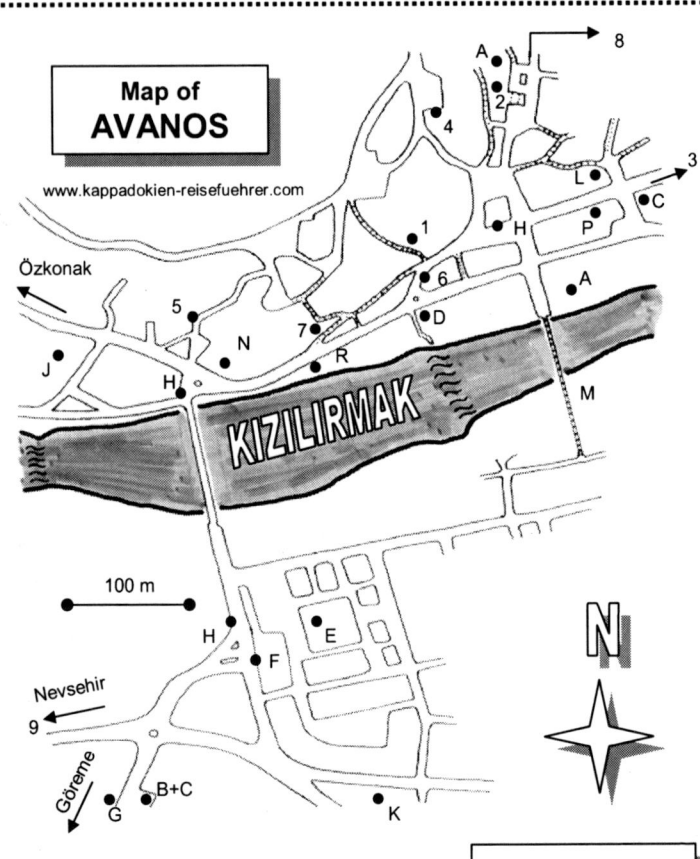

Map of **AVANOS**
www.kappadokien-reisefuehrer.com

A	Mosque	J Hamam
B	Bus terminal	K Health station
C	Taxi	L Potterys
D	Town hall	M Pedestrian bridge
E	Market spuare	N Evranos Restaurant
F	Petrol station	P Post office
G	Yandarma	R Tourist information
H	Bus stop	

Accommodations

1 Vanessa Pension
2 Tokmak Konuk Evi
3 Kavuncu Pension
4 Duru Motel
5 Sofa Hotel
6 Avanos Evi (Office)
7 Kirkit Pension
8 Günay Konukevi
9 Ada Camping

But Avanos can offer something which has become very rare in Cappadocia: ordinary Turkish life, almost unaffected by tourism. It is actually not easy to find a shop in Göreme which has not adjusted itself to visitors from around the world. But here in Avanos you get an insight into the daily lives of the Cappadocians. Here is a shop with household goods, there is one for paint and everything a workman needs. In between, a dark badly lit room where oil-stained hands repair bicycles, and not far away, perhaps a small glazier's workshop or one of those general stores which offer almost anything from cigarette lighters to dry biscuits. Pharmacies, butcher's shops, minimarkets and stationery shops supply the demands of the citizens of Avanos and of the surrounding villages.

Here, you are looking in vain for restaurants which have honed in exclusively on tourism. All of them have managed the balancing act between the needs of the locals and those of the foreign visitors. Even the smallest Lokanta with its traditional supply will be able to organize a small bottle of ketchup for the discriminating American palate.

If on the main square you do not turn towards the suspension bridge, but in the opposite direction, you will enter the old town. Tourists rarely happen to come here. If you have left the mosque behind on the left, you have also escaped the last pottery shop. The residential area of the old town begins here. Unfortunately it is partly in a bad state of decay. The owners and the town administration lack the funds to restore the buildings. But this offers an opportunity to observe the quiet daily life of the inhabitants. Stray cats, children playing ball games and women sitting in the shade of their doorways, chatting. Above it there is the smell of laundry tubs and steamy stews. Here in those sometimes narrow lanes, far away from the noisy traffic, birds warble in all keys and even the chirping of crickets strikes the ear of the beholder. It is also worthwhile making a walk across the pedestrian suspension bridge that traverses the river. Especially on Fridays, when it is market day and people from the surrounding villages populate the city, this is great fun. The construction squeals and shakes under the weight of the many feet, so that one is likely to be seasick. The market, which is situated near the main bridge, is an attraction in itself. It is an Eldorado for lovers of exotic fruits and spices; only here you can buy a supply of fresh fish. The cries of the many dealers who are loudly praising their wares echo under the roofing which covers the major part of the market. Strange smells waft through the construction, and the lightbeams from the roof windows make you dive into an almost forgotten world.

Pottery on the Red River

- a craft shapes a city

Since time immemorial, the Kızılırmak (the Red River) has flowed through Cappadocia and has made Avanos a centre of pottery. For here on its edges the river deposits its sediments which, having turned into clay, are formed into vessels, pots and bowls in the numberless pottery caves of the town. The clay contains much iron; and the iron gives the clay its red colour and the river its name. Iron in clay reduces the melting point in the firing process. Thus the formed vessels can be baked hard at only 900° C/ 1652° F in simple, straw-burning kilns built of tuff. The pots baked in one night can thus do their services for centuries – if they do not fall down. Glazing is not known by tradition in Avanos; the ceramic product is hardened by a very unusual method: the dried product is smoothed with a metal spoon so that its surface looks tight and shiny after baking. Glazed ceramic products were only produced with the high-temperature electric kilns.

Besides Kütaya in the west of Anatolia, Avanos is the largest ceramics centre of Turkey. Only 20 years ago there were about 200 potteries and almost all local families worked in this craft. But only the men learned how to work with the potter's wheel. The famous 'Güveç pots' were sold all over the country (see the chapter on "Food and Drink" p.134). Only few potteries have remained today. Some workshops have survived in the 'industrial area' of the town. The cave potteries, however, produce exclusively for tourists, which has led to a refinement of techniques. Today artistic considerations play a major role, the functionality of the vessels has moved to the background. Artists from all over Turkey have changed many a simple cave into a studio. Thus you find the country's largest supply of ceramic art handicraft in Avanos today, apart from the family workshops which still work in the traditional way. And it is of a qualtiy that can compete internationally. Valuable replicas of ancient pieces as well as elaborately decorated vases and plates can be found here. Only delicate hands can apply this delicate ceramic painting. This is why you sometimes see children sitting by the roadside in Avanos, holding a vase in their laps and drawing Hittite figures and ornaments on it with a fine pencil. But do not worry, this is no child labour, but the usual help in the household or with the home-work. This way, also young women get a chance to earn some money, though they are mercilessly underpaid.

If you watch a potter at work, as a layman you are amazed at the ease with which a beautiful vase is created from a lump of mud in his hands. But the craft looks easier than it is. An apprentice might need hundreds of hours of practice just to be able to 'centre' this lump of clay - as the expert says - on the wobbly potter's wheel; hours in which the lump slides off the wheelhead again and again and just does not run centrally. The potter learns this art - of forming an absolutely centrally moving lump of clay into a work of art - for a lifetime. There is always a higher level of difficulty. The Hittite beak-spouted jug is one of the most difficult vessels made on the potter's wheel: a fragile narrow foot, a widely drawn body which is drawn again to a long neck with a projecting spout after a sharp edge, and all this done with wafer-thin walls – this will always remain one of the greatest challenges for a potter, and you can watch the greatest experts in their craft at work in Avanos.

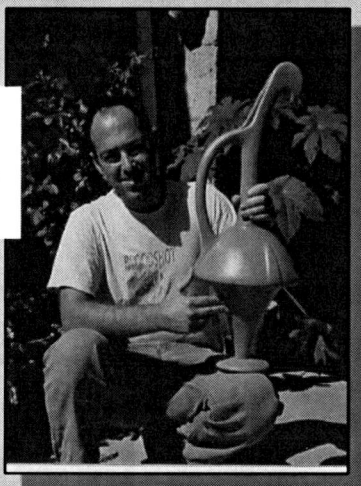

The Hittite beak-spouted jug – manufactured by the "Ikizler"

Hittite vases are objects of decoration which were formed here in Cappadocia already 3500 years ago. You will not find them in a Cappadocian household, but instead, there are huge storage vessels of up to 1,5 m. height, in which raisins, wine or pickled vegetables are stored up to the present day. The production of those vessels needs years of constant training at the potter's

> wheel, too – and Herculean strength is needed for centring more than 20 kg of clay.
> The wheel is kept in motion by one's feet on a wooden flywheel in the floor. On the wheel, separate ceramic tubes are mounted on top of each other, only fixed to each other by fresh clay. The construction is crowned by a wheelhead, often an ordinary flat stone, with a diameter of only 10 to 15 cm, on which the complete pot must find support. This wobbly structure, which threatens to collapse at every touch, represents yet another additional challenge.
> It is no matter of course that the pottery craft still exists here in Cappadocia today. Only some decades ago, the trade was threatened by destruction due to the advent of lots of brightly coloured plastic containers. It was tourism which finally aroused the old potteries to a new life again, in an unexpected artistic diversity.

If you are interested in pottery from Avanos, you definitely should visit the potteries off the main road. Often the same pottery is available here at a much lower price. You will find very creative and high quality pottery at the workshop called "The Twins" (Ikizler). It is somewhat away from the town centre. You turn in a western direction at the end of the stone bridge and follow the main road for about 250 m. up to a small grocer's shop on the right side. The two young men's studio is tucked away behind it.
www.katpatuka.org/izikler

Restaurant tip in Avanos: Evranos and Uranos

Two cave restaurants. The one is directly opposite the stone bridge, the other about 2 km away on the road to Gülschir. They are actually designed for tourist groups, but individual guests are no problem, either. For 35 TL you can eat and drink endlessly here – also alcoholic drinks – and you are offered a folklore program of more than 3 hours which ends with a belly dance. A pleasant change for all those who do not mind sitting together with about 300 guests in a huge cave room, taking part in the extravagances of tourist amusement. No joke, you must have gone through it. Reservations required.

Evranos – Phone: 0384 511 3750   Uranos - Phone: 0384 511 5636

Accommodations in Aavanos

➢ VANESSA PENSION
A cute little inn in a lane near the main square. The operator has a passion for everything antique. His collection of old Cappadocian photographs is especially pre-eminent, and all rooms are decorated with those treasures accordingly. Under the town houses which this hostel consists of there is a small underground town, through which the owner likes to organize tours for his guests.

1	60 TL	8	E		①②⑦⑧⑨

Phone: 0384 511 3840   www.katpatuka.org/venessa

➢ TOKMAK KONUK EVI
The inn consists of several historic and newly renovated town houses in the old town centre. The hostel is run by the family and is equipped with everything that makes the traveller' life easier, from an emergency lighting that starts into life when the electricity breaks down, to the hairdryers that are ready for use in the bathrooms. Some rooms are quite large, so that the room rates vary. It must be emphasized that one room for disabled persons and several specially equipped rooms for families are available.

2	50-170 TL	11	E – F - D		①③⑤⑥⑦⑧

Phone: 0834 511 4587   www.tokmakonukevi.com

➢ KAVUNCU PENSION
Small hostel which is situated about 200 m. off the main square on the road to Kayseri. The rooms are simply furnished and remind you of the old days of the backpackers. The friendly staff and a big lush garden make up for this, however.

3	50 TL	12	F		①⑤⑧

Phone: 0384 511 4244   www.kavuncupansiyon.com

➢ DURU HOTEL
High up above the town but still located centrally. Another new building from the eighties, to which some adjacent old houses have been added, however. Some family rooms with four beds are available here. The magnificent all-round view far over Avanos up to Uchisar on the far horizon

is a highlight. At the same time the hotel is situated very quietly and good parking space in front of the door is the reason why the complex was formerly called MOTEL .

| 4 | 65 TL | 17 | E – F | 🍽 | ⑤⑧ |

Phone: 0384 511 2404   www.hotelduru.com

➢ SOFA HOTEL

Nothing for people with a poor sense of direction, although the hotel is located directly at the end of the road bridge on the fringe of the old part of the town and cannot be missed. The owner gave up his career as a teacher in 1986, bought a small house and started his hostel with a few rooms only. In the course of time he added more and more old neighbouring houses to it, and this way a little romantic private village developed in the middle of the city. A good sense of direction is required inside the complex: narrow winding lanes, stairways, galleries, bridges, terraces and even little tunnels connect the tiny individual buildings. The whole thing is furnished with various antique things and densely leafy, cozy courtyards give rise to a relaxed atmosphere. Lounges in Ottoman style for all guests and a small coffee bar achieve the rest. Most of the rooms have their own little terrace area, which is open to the public, but where you can nevertheless be on your own outside the rooms. Even if you have another lodging, take a look at this little work of art; you will be thrilled.

| 5 | 100-150 TL | 30 | E – F | ☏ 🍽 | ①②③⑤⑥⑦⑧ |

Phone: 0384 511 5186   www.sofa-hotel.com

➢ AVANOS EVI

A real alternative for the travelling large family. It is a huge apartment high up on the mountainside. The view is magnificent and a large terrace is available. The two bedrooms and the lounge have been furnished with love, and the also spacey kitchen is fully equipped with everything you need for making the first omelettes. Additionally, the owner offers a full delivery and shopping service. The apartment is rented from two persons onwards, with the other room then being left unoccupied and not rented again, so that one remains undisturbed in the whole complex.

| 6 | 140-340 TL | | E | | ①②⑤⑥⑦⑧ |

Phone: 0384 511 2298   www.avanosevi.com

➤ KIRKIT PENSION

An archetype of Cappadocian tourism, which started its activities in 1981 in a small town house. Today the hostel consists of several houses bought step by step from the neighbours. This is why it is full of nooks and crannies, too, and the nicely furnished rooms are mostly accessible over several gangplanks and little stairways. The complex is owned by the Kirkit-Voyage Agency, which additionally organizes tours, has about 40 horses in its stable and rents a variety of vehicles or can provide them. Almost every day there is a short little folklore event in the inn, which can also be visited by non-resident guests.

| 7 | 50-80 TL | 17 | E – F - D | ▼ ⦿ | ①②⑤⑦⑧ |

Phone: 0384 511 3259   www.kirkit.com

➤ GÜNAY KONUKEVI

This little hotel first opened its doors in the spring of 2008. The owner renovated his parents' old house and created a little quiet oasis above the old town. From the terrace you have a magnificent view over the whole town and over parts of Cappadocia. The hotel is very family-run, and the guests are taken care of with love.

| 8 | 120-260 TL | 11 | E | ▼ ⦿ | ①②③④⑤⑥⑦⑧⑨ |

Phone: 0384 511 5255   www.gunaykonukevi.com

If you want a shave you are in the best of hands with Ömer Kubali. He understands some English and is always in the mood for a joke. Right next to him, there is the only Restaurant with draft beer, the 'Sancho Pansa'. Both are on the right side by the main square in the direction of the old town. Please make sure that Ömer is wearing his glasses while shaving you!

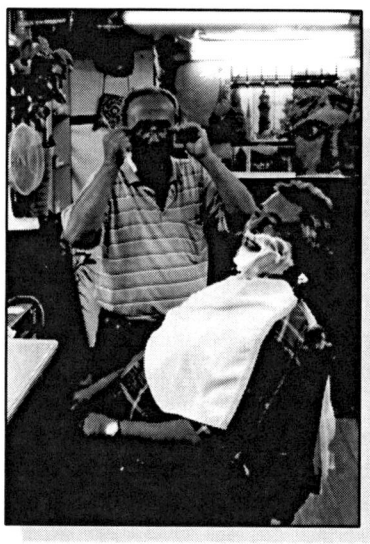

Özkonak

The town is north of Avanos, behind the mountain range, and is reached by a road distance of 14 km. Apart from a little underground town, it does not have much to offer. Perhaps you will be astonished at the many new and smartened up houses in the streets. Many of the inhabitants have worked in Germany, or their children and grandchildren are still living there. Those people invested their savings in new homes of their own and have thus changed the townscape a lot.

But let us return to the attraction of the town. If you have visited other underground cities, you will be astonished at the quietness here. There are no souvenir stalls here which you have to walk through before reaching the real historic location, and it can happen here that the ticket counter has to be unlocked for you first. If you are afraid of the long trip to Derinkuyu or Kaymaklı, you should proceed under the ground here. The complex is in fact considerably smaller, but as a conseqence the crowds of visitors are limited. The structure is basically the same as in the larger complexes. First you reach the stables with their feeding troughs carved into the walls. Then there are the storerooms and utility rooms, which can be identified by the slots in the floor in which formerly the large earthenware jars used to be put. One of those large jars is still standing in its hole, and you will ask yourself how this huge jar can have been transported down here. There are also two wine basins, where the grapes were squashed by the feet. The must flowed through an opening into a vessel on a lower level. In the rear part are the escape rooms with their big millstone doors for closing this section. Those millstones, which weigh up to 2 tons, could be rolled in front of the doors, and there are three of them closely after each other. The millstones of Özkonak are different in two aspects: first, in contrast to those from other underground settlements, they have no central holes and second, those millstones were carved from the rock down here. In all other settlements they were produced outside and are of a different, harder material. There is also no well below the big ventilation shaft, therefore the thermal ventilation effect does not work so well here. The somewhat bad air can be explained by the increased water level, which caused the lower rooms to become quite damp.

The underground town was actually discovered in 1972 by Latif Acar, the then muezzin of Özkonak, when he was working in his garden. One year after that the complex was opened to the public by the town administration, even though only very few tourists happened to come here. Latif Acar was in charge of the supervision and maintenance of his discovery until 1990.

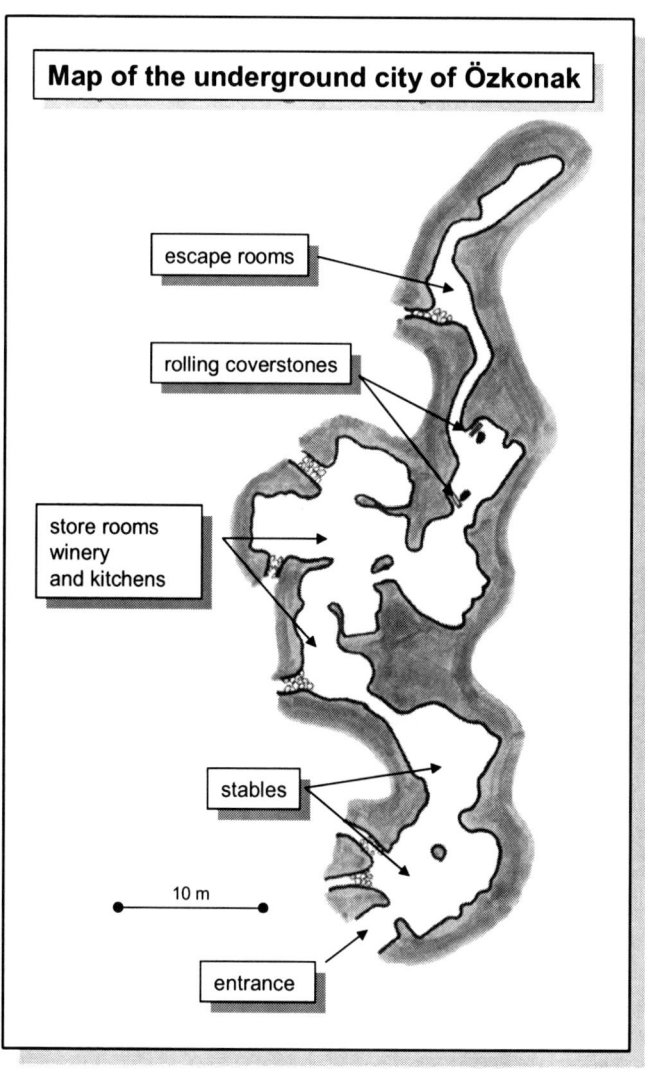

Bayramhacı

If there were no hot springs here, this town would be one of the many places which disappear in the wide plains of Anatolia. You have to drive through the village to reach the baths, which are a little away from the settlement. It is one of those places where you ask yourself whether the water is still pulled out of the well by hand. Foreign tourists do not come here. The health and recreation spa is located about 1,5 km south of the settlement and is well-known among the Turkish population in far more than the Kayseri area. You can rent a small room here for weeks and take your daily baths or enjoy your medical applications. Two large open air pools complete the institution, and you can rent the smaller Pool, which is protected from the eye by a brick wall, exclusively for small groups. The pleasure costs 10 TL per person – without any time limit, and open till 12.00 midnight. But there is another opportunity to take a bath in hot water.

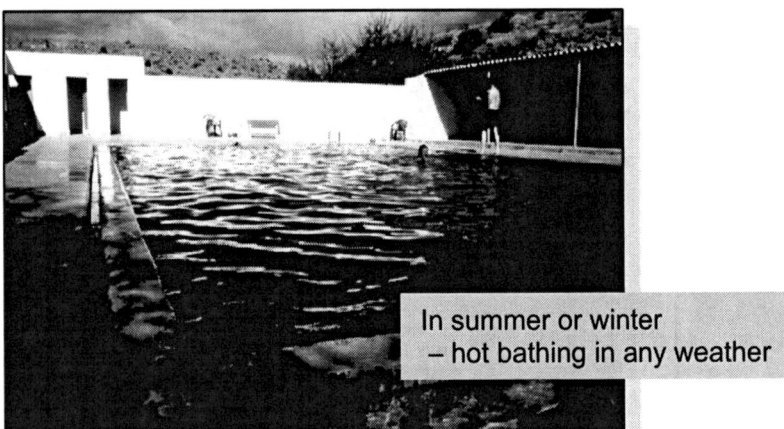

In summer or winter – hot bathing in any weather

At the end of the village there is a signpost to "Yale Camping". The complex has nothing to do with camping, it is rather like an open air swimmingpool. Here you can enjoy the ferrous and a little sulphurous water, which is always 35° C hot, for 5 TL (or, if the owner is in a bad mood, for 10 TL) a whole day long. There are some closable rooms with large masoned bathtubs next to it where you can soak and groom yourself properly. This is not for people with

poor circulation, however, as the narrow rooms quickly fill with hot steam. A teagarden with various beverages is connected with it and now and again the kitchen is also open, too. Campervans can stay for the night in the large parking area, too, if you ask the owner really politely. Nothing is more beautiful than a nocturnal bath under a wonderfully starlit Cappadocian sky. Unfortunately, a connection to the public transport network does not exist. From Avanos you drive in a northerly direction on the old Kayseri road down into the valley and then turn off to the right according to the signpost behind a little bridge across the river. After another 6 km you reach the village, which you drive through and then continue in a southern direction to the baths. From there, you follow the signpost to "Yale Camping".
In the village there also is the 'Bulut Hotel' with its own hot water pool; it can be contacted via the phone number 0352 399 7124.

Sarıhan

This old caravanserai is located about 4 miles south-east of Avanos, right on the new express highway to Kayseri. It is an impressive example of the great Seljuk architecture and proof of the fact that those times were anything but safe. If you have come to Cappadocia via Kayseri, you may perhaps have seen the many relics of those buildings along the route. 800 years ago, the Seljuks built such rest houses every 30 km, that is, at the distance of a day's journey. This shows how important this former trade route was, which connected Europe with the Middle East. Unfortunately, only a few of the many caravanserais have been preserved. One of them is on the Konya - Akserai road in the little town of Sultanhane, and another one – Sarihan - was built here in Cappadocia in 1249. In the mid nineties the decay of the building was stopped and it was completely renovated. For only 3 TL admission anyone can visit this historic rest house and can travel back to the time of the great caravans for a little while. The mystical music inside contributes to it. To secure the preservation of the complex, the Turkish monument preservation office has let the building to a contractor who stages the traditional dances of the dervishs from Konya every evening. The question what the whirling dervishes of the Mevlana Order have to do with Cappadocia can remain unanswered, but there could hardly be a more suitable place than this for their mystic dances and chants. The 45 minute show costs 50 TL admission. However, opinions diverge widely on this spectacle.

You enter the open courtyard by the large entrance gate. Above the gate is the Imam's pulpit from which he announced the prayer times five times each day. The quarters of the armed guards with stairs for quick access to the broad walkways are on the right. Next to them are rooms for a restaurant and various other service providers of the time. On the left there are arcades under which travelling salesmen used to put up their stalls. In the centre of the court, where there is a water basin today, the water used to be pulled up from a well in former times. Next you enter the main hall of the caravanserai by a second, richly ornamented portal. Here the animals were set free from their heavy burdens, and also the ordinary travelling people used to sleep here. One can well imagine the chaos that must have reigned here if by accident several caravans happened to arrive at the same time. The high and thick walls provided a constant and pleasant temperature inside, and the openings in the dome created the effect of a chimney which provided good ventilation. Even though it is out of reach of public transport, this ancient rest house is always worth a visit. You take the bus to Avanos and then change to a taxi for a few TL.

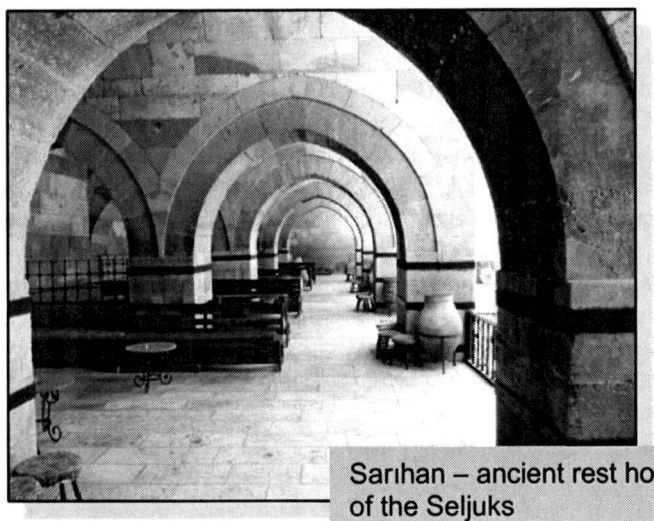

Sarıhan – ancient rest house of the Seljuks

Kayseri

Experience a city of a million in the middle of Anatolia - Kayseri is full of life. The whole city is a huge bazaar. And amidst the chaos of people and motor traffic rise the ancient buildings from Seljuk and early Ottoman times. The city is famous for its sausages and its Pastirma, that is, beef ham coated with paprika paste. And the sometime richest carpet dealers of the region live here. The people of Kayseri are famous and notorious all over the country as the cleverest tradesmen, and not without a reason do they call a clever dealer a 'Kayserili'. When you arrive on the outskirts of the city, you will probably ask yourself if the trip here will be worthwhile. Over the years, a huge industrial belt has grown all around the city, and people from Anatolia have followed the jobs. Kayseri has practically exploded in the past 30 years. While there were only about 170,000 inhabitants in 1973, the city is now heading for a million in giant strides. Correspondingly, it has grown in an uncontrolled and not always attractive way. But all this should not keep you from visiting the city centre and its sights.

The Cumhuriyet Meydani (Square of the Republic) (9) is the centre of the city, where the old citadel (1) from the 12th century rises. It has two entrances with narrow front yards and a third one from more recent times. All historic buildings have been built of the hard basalt which is typical for this region. The extremely hard material and the thickness of the walls have ensured that parts of these buildings have been preserved to this day. In the west of the old city centre there are only a few remnants of the old fortification wall which used to surround the city. The Fatih Mosque (5) inside the citadel was built much later by the Ottomans. Today there is a permanent market inside the walls of the citadel, which covers the whole area. Unfortunately, the round paths are not open to visitors, although there is a magnificent view over the inner city from them.

Opposite the citadel to the east there is the Mahperi Huant Hatun Külliyesi (12 and 13), a complex consisting of a mosque, a tomb, a madrassa and a hamam. This complex was endowed by the wife of the Seljuk Sultan Aladdin Keykubad in the year 1237 and was named after her. And she was also buried there, together with two of her daughters.

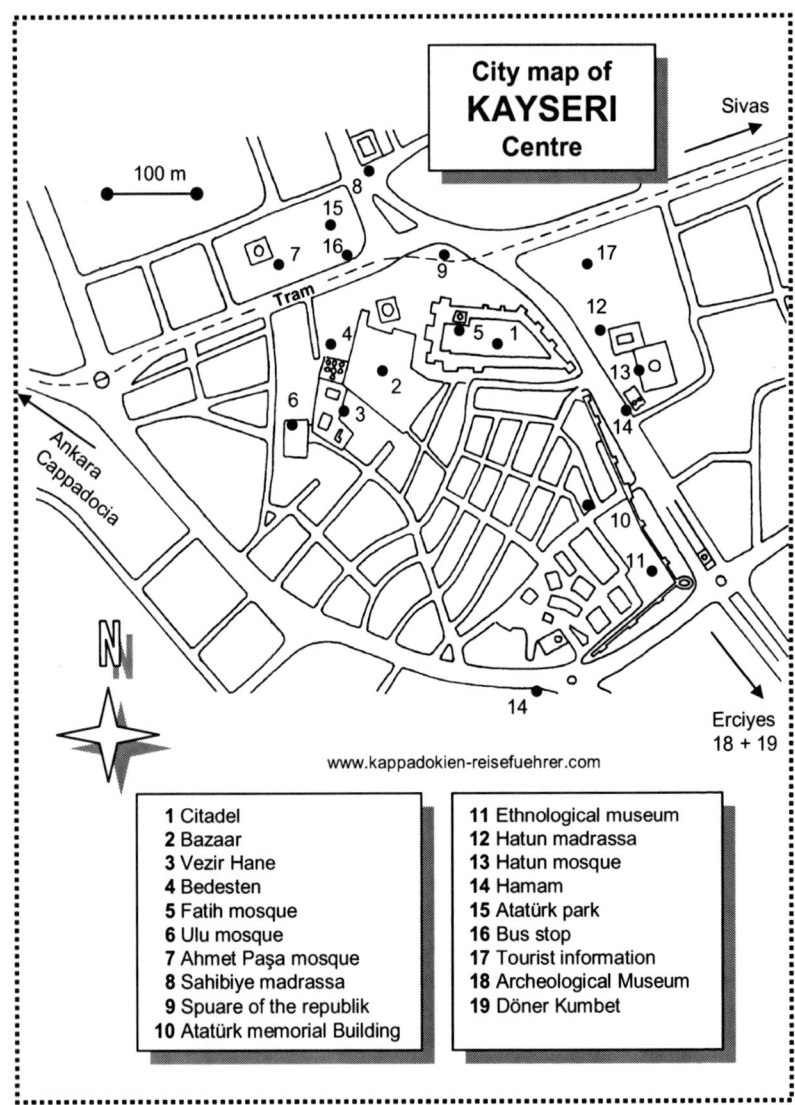

Today there is a shopping street with shops for various electrical appliances in the madrassa. It will remain a mystery to the visitor why the old museum had to move away from here, as one can hardly imagine a better location for such a museum.

A little further to the south, in the old city centre again, there is the Ethnological Museum (11), which is in a former manor house. The individual exhibits may not be that interesting, but the second section with its examples from the life in the Konak impressively represents the glamour of a lordly household in Ottoman times. It is definitely worth spending the 3 TL admission.
Two blocks further to the north is the Atatürk Memorial House (10). Atatürk temporarily commanded his troops in the defence operations against the Greek invaders from here. The working and private rooms of the founder of the Republic are on display. Those rooms illustrate the rapid change to a modern Western lifestyle, especially in comparison with the Ethnological Museum or the Ottoman Konak. Admission is free.

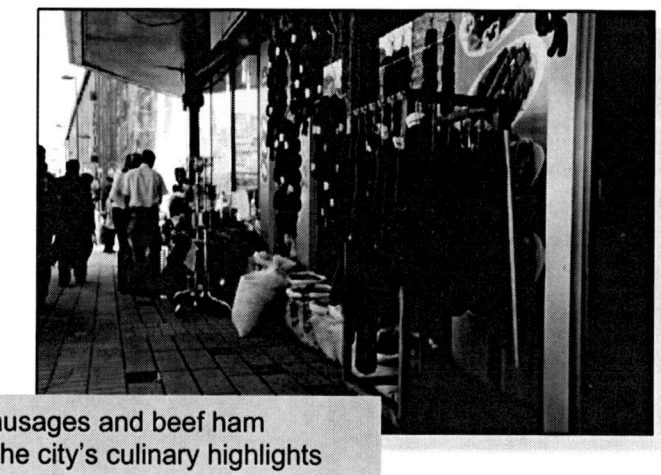

Sausages and beef ham – the city's culinary highlights

Kayseri also has a large indoor bazaar (Kapale Caryesı) (2), where the textile and jewelry dealers are. There are no products designed for tourists here. The local citizens have ever since been doing their shopping here and they bargain fiercely with the numerous dealers.
At the south-west end of the bazaar, an inconspicuous lane leads to the Vezir Hane (3), the city's oldest caravanserai. It makes a rather dilapidated impression, but you can still find the remnants of the ancient trades here. Hatters produce the traditional Turkish peaked caps here by hand, and you can still have a pair of shoes made to measure for yourself here, everything

produced with old machines or by much muscle power. Old carpets or kilims are repaired or mended meticulously here. Besides, the carpet dealers' zone begins here. While wool is sold on the ground floor, above it are the carpet dealers with the finished products, lying in wait for tourists who have lost their way. Right between the bazaar and the Vezir Hane there is the Bedesten (4), the old auction hall. The large building with its gloomy domes is firmly in the hands of the carpet dealers. You must remain very steadfast here not to leave the time-honoured building with a piece of textile floor covering after all. In any case you should not miss the Hane and the Bedesten, as both let you look back into another century - and we do not mean the 20th century by that.

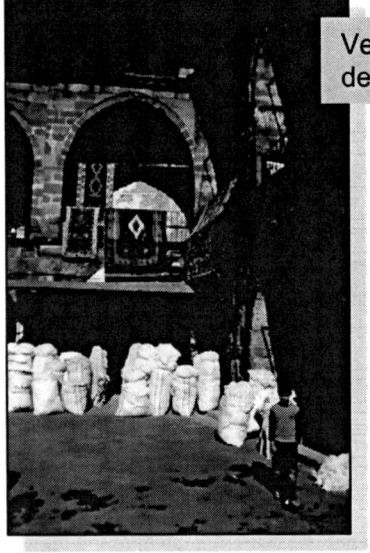

Vezir Hane – the carpet dealers are lying in wait here

Directly next to the Vezir Hane there is the Ulu Cami (6), a mosque whose construction was begun in 1135 and was finished by the Seljuks in 1205. It was built with 5 naves and with a small central dome, and the ancient Byzantine capitals of the pillars make one think of a church rather than a mosque. It is well possible that the building was planned or even begun in pre-Islamic times already.

Especially in the southern semicircle around the old city centre, the visitor will notice a rather low construction density for a large city like this, and if you look closer, you will find a host of old mosques, domed tombs (Kumbets) and other historic buildings there. The city is thought to have temporarily had up to 400,000 inhabitants already in the Seljuk period. Again and again you find ancient relics like wells or the remains of walls from that period among the modern new buildings.

About one mile north of the citadel there is the Döner Kumbet (Rotating Mausoleum) (19). It was bestowed by Shah Cihan Hatun in 1276 and is among the most impressive ones ever built. This building made of solid rock with its typical pointed roof is embellished with lavish ornamental decoration consisting of animals, pseudo arcades, and arabesques.

Nearby is the Archeological Museum (18) with finds from the Hittite and the Roman age. The presentation is not really spectacular, but the exhibits of Hittite pottery are definitely worth a visit. The typical ceramic jugs of that period can still drive many a contemporary potter to the brink of a nervous breakdown, as producing them requires an almost unattainable amount of skill and craftsmanship (see the chapter on 'pottery', page 242). It is open from Tuesday to Sunday and admission is 3 TL.

Mention should also be made of the Sahibiye Madarassa (8) from 1267, north of the city centre, in which presently some bookstores are located, and the Ahmet Pasa Mosque (7), which is also called Kursunlu Cami because of its rare leaden roofing.

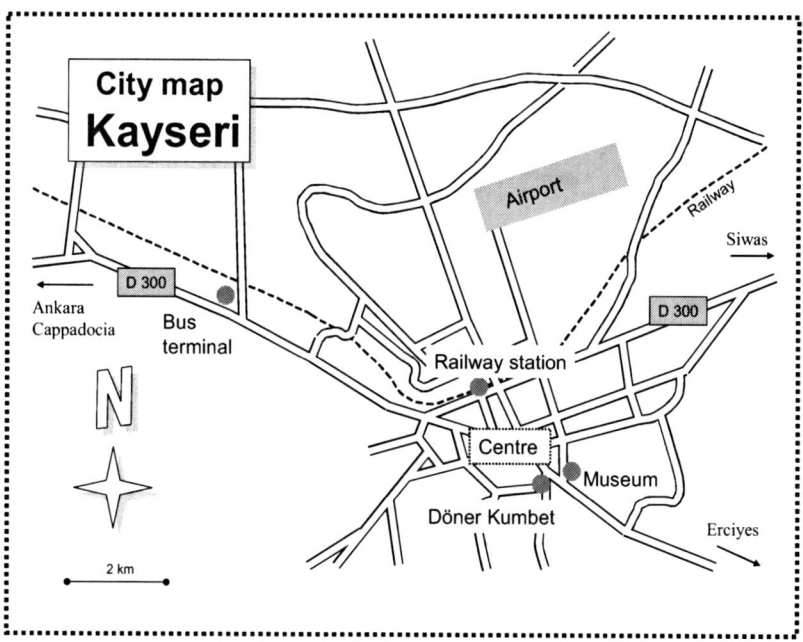

From Cappadocia you reach Kayseri by bus from Nevşehir, which also stops at Göreme and in Avanos (9 TL). Since the big ring road round Kayseri has been completed, heavy long distance coaches are not permitted in the inner city any more. A smaller shuttle bus takes you to the inner city from the bus terminal, which is quite far away from the old city. Returning to the bus terminal (Otogar or Terminal) is a little more complicated. The public service buses stop on the north-west side of the Cumhuriet Square (9) in the front bus stop section (16). The bus number and the destination are printed on a small metal sign behind the windscreen. Lines 142 and 131 go past the new bus terminal (Yeni Terminal) (1.5 TL). You must be patient, as almost all buses in this large city stop at that terminal at a 10 minutes interval, and they are usually overcrowded. You should expect a corresponding rush here.

The Erciyes

This mountain is about 30 km south of Kayseri. Located almost 4000 m above sea-level, its exposed position makes it seem particularly impressive, even though only the top 3000 m of the mountain are visible, as we already are at an altitude of 1000 m. Sometimes its two pointed peaks are covered under a white blanket of snow all year round. People like to tell a story from the old Ottoman days in which a salesman borrowed money from a money lender in the autumn and promised faithfully that he would repay the money when the snow on the peak of Erciyes would have melted in the spring. Both of them were unable to predict the arrival of a short interglacial period in the 17th century, and thus the borrowed money had to be repaid by the following generations.

In winter the slopes of the mountain are regarded as guaranteed to have snow to such an extent that a little skiing centre with tow lifts was able to be established in Hacılar. In summer the mountain can be climbed with a guide and with some alpine experience. Footpaths lead up to the volcano, which has been inactive for ages, either from Hacılar, which is 10 km south of Kayseri, but also from Kayakevı, which is on the road to Develi. The "Middle Earth Travel" agency in Göreme arranges two-day tours up to the twin peaks. But guides can also be hired in the two aforementioned villages. We, the authors, have not yet been able to decide to take part in an ascent of this majestic mountain. The view from up there must be simply gigantic, with the wide plains of the Sultan Marshes at your feet and, 150 km away, the snow-covered 4000 m high peaks of the Taurus Mountains.

Middle Earth Travel

This is a somewhat different hiking or tour agency. Mountain hiking tours through all the great mountains of Turkey are offered here: from the simple one-day tour through Cappadocia to an ascent on the 5000 m high Mount Ararat in the east on the Armenian border. This tour organizing company offers a wide range of variants for exploring the country on foot. On multi-day operations accommodation and food are included in the price. The organizer partly provides the equipment and there is also no extra charge for the transport from and to the airport. Tours of various levels of difficulty are presented in the program: anything is possible here from walking tours for Sunday strollers to high-altitude mountain climbs.

The ascent of Mount Erciyes is of interest in relation to Cappadocia. But this two-day mountain tour is only for experienced and strong mountain hikers. The tour is priced €175/ $245 including meals, accommodation and transfer. The also available ascent of Hassan-Dağı is somewhat cheaper, but also easier. The two-day tour costs €150/ $210, and beginners are also welcome again.

Cevizler Sok. 20
Göreme – Nevşehir
Phone: 0090 384 271 2528
Fax: 0090 384 271 2562
Email: info@middleearthtravel.com
Web :   www.middleearthtravel.com/de
(see also Göreme City Map, p.199, No. 16)

Round Trip:
Ürgüp – Theodore Church – Incesu – Ürgüp

We will not lead you directly to Ürgüp, but would like to propose this little round trip to you. Away from the tourist bustle, you can experience the diversity of the Anatolian countryside and the vastness of the unique country in the most impressive way on this route. A vehicle is required for it, though, as public transport services do not operate here, or only very sporadically.

Ürgüp is the starting and ending point of the little round trip is Ürgüp. There you take the eastern outward road, drive past numerous large hotel complexes and at the second traffic lights take the direction towards Dörtyol. A narrow asphalt road then runs through a valley to the south-east. After 5 km you reach the village of Karacaören. It is remarkable here that the old houses on the slope are mostly still inhabited. The valley is probably too narrow for new and modern development.

After 2 more km follow the signs to the Theodore Church. You turn right here onto a much narrower road, which leads to a valley which is very green for Anatolia. Next you drive through the villages of Karain and Karlik, which both have ancient rock dwellings above their houses, but they are very derelict. The road continues through a countryside which rather reminded us of the Greek heartland. Caution is required on this route, as the bus service operates to Yeşilös, and the drivers drive very powerfully on this route.

After some miles you reach the settlement, which is huddled in a corner of the valley. Follow the signs to the Theodore Church, which is on the right hand edge of the village.

Theodore Church

You enter the church in the classic manner through a large vestibule, before you proceed to the prayer room through a wide passageway on the left. Even though the frescoes – as in many other places – have largely been destroyed here, this church impresses the visitor by its sheer size, and it has a special feature in the form of a walk-in gallery at a dizzy height. The word 'walk-in' is only true for former times, however. The gallery is reached by a narrow tunnel which leads upstairs. However, we must warn against entering it, as it has been badly affected by water damage. When leaving the church, one should by all means pay attention to the lock mechanism in the passageway. Obviously the room of the church was rather firmly barricaded in the past, a sign of troubled times.

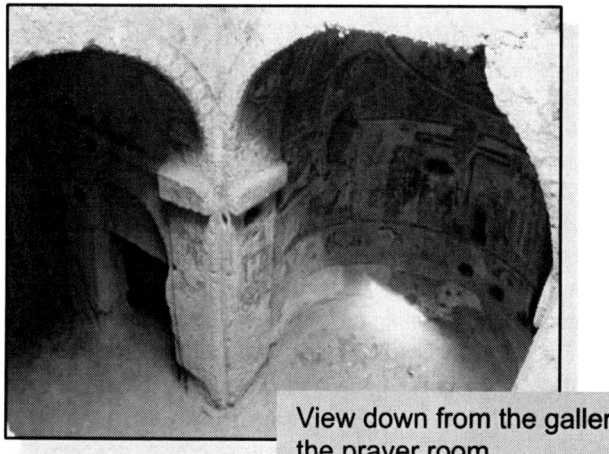

View down from the gallery into the prayer room

If you want to annoy your rental car company, you should drive up the very dusty track up the hill and turn down towards the village again shortly before reaching the top. Now at least you see why this valley is so green: everywhere in the village water rises on the mountain slope and irrigates the households and orchards.

But as you do not want to keep struggling with your car rental, you rather drive back to the main road on the direct route instead. The route climbs steeply shortly behind Yeşilös, and you reach the village of Ağcaören. At the village limit one gets the impression that nothing but threshing machines are sold here. At the end of the village you enter the plateau and have a wide view over the many grain fields, which has solved the mystery of the threshers.

In summer you often find a tent camp of the harvest hands along the small road; they come from far away regions of Turkey to earn their meager wages here. The term 'one-dollar job' is bitter reality here; if you depend on working as a harvest hand, you are among the poorest people ever.

The next place is called Başdere, and if you follow the winding road through the village, you will arrive on the main road between Ürgüp and Dörtyol again. Please keep to the right now and climb up the 1,535 m high Topuzdağı Pass. Shortly behind the pass, a gigantic view of the Mount Erciyes volcano and of the Sultan Marshes south of it opens up, bordering the foothills of the Taurus Mountains. On clear sight in autumn or in spring, even the snow-covered Four-thousanders of those mountains are visible, and one almost believes one can smell the sea.

The road now descends 400 m of altitude in the shortest distance and continues towards Dörtyol. Be careful at the level crossing! In 2009 it was out of order, the lights remained red and the gates did not open anymore or had been smashed by numerous trucks. Just do like the locals: make sure that no train is coming and cautiously cross the rails. And never fear, the top speed of the trains here on this dead straight route is just about 60 km/h.

It remains a mystery why Dörtyol appears as a town on many maps. A filling station, a hotel and an abandoned cement factory, that is it. We turn left towards Kayseri here at the traffic lights crossing and then drive through the monotony at the foot of Mount Erciyes for 20 km. Having arrived in Incesu, a sign points towards Ürgüp and leads us into the town centre.

Incesu

In the town centre of Incesu there is a cluster of important buildings from the Ottoman period. The town owes its origin to the builder of these complexes, Grand Vizier Kara Mustafa. It was the same grand vizier who stood before Vienna with his troops in 1683 and who, as is well known, lost the battle and, soon after, his head. In 1670 he ordered the large caravanserai, the mosque, the hamam, a madrassa and a bazaar in between to be built. Instead of the Cappadocian tuff, a darker and harder type of rock was used here. In 2007 the restoration of the carvanserai and the Turkish bath were completed. Unfortunately, the bazaar and the old madrassa are still in a pitiable condition. The bazaar would indeed make a good background for a period movie. The atmosphere becomes really rustic when on a weekend – the caravanserai being unfortunately closed then – you enter the complex through the bazaar or through the former guardroom. You have to walk though a tiny tearoom first, which spontaneously reminded us of the movie "A Season in

Hakkari" by Yilmas Güney. Such an archaic teahouse is probably not found within a radius of a thousand kilometers.
The inner yard of this ancient resthouse is huge. The many fireplaces and chimneys along the outer walls under the arcades are conspicuous.

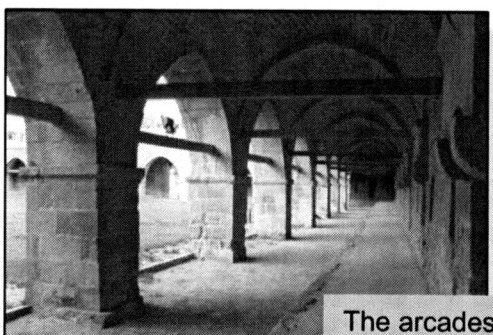

The arcades in the courtyard – In Ottoman times the travellers spent the night here

In summer, travellers used to spend the night here, while the goods and the animals stayed in the open yard. In winter, the same thing happened in the great hall of the caravanserai. On the edge of the surrounding platform the holes in the rock where the animals were tied for the night are still visible. Unfortunately, the community of Incesu does not really know how to use this gigantic hall. Only once a year, during the wine festival in autumn, the hall comes to life and is delivered from its existence as a storage depot. The newly renovated hamam is unfortunately not in operation, either.

Incesu is outside the administrative district of Nevşehir, in the Kayseri district, and is therefore difficult to reach by public transport. If you do not have a vehicle or do not want to do our round trip, you can take the Kayseri bus from Cappadocia and then try to intercept the public service bus at the junction of road 805 (Kayseri – Niğde). You should start on your trip very early in the day, as the bus ride takes some time and there is no accommodation for the night. Altogether, there is no tourist infrastructure at all in spite of the historic quality of this Ottoman complex.

After this you follow the signposts back to Ürgüp. The road rises slightly through green orchards which clarify the name Incesu (fine water) and you arrive at a little reservoir, which has become a fishing paradise for the local population. But, like the Damsa Reservoir, its banks are totally muddy and do not invite you to a swim. The road continues to rise and you arrive on the plateau again, on which far and wide no settlement can be seen, however. Agriculture is hardly possible here any more either, and you can well imagine the ice-cold Anatolian winds blowing across the plain here in winter. In the frenzy of speed on the dead straight route, do not forget to throw a last glance back on his majesty, Mount Erciyes-Dağı.

17 km behind Incesu you will reach the small town of Aksalur, which again, being located up on the mountainside, gives you a feeling of the horrors of the Anatolian winter. Steep roads and an early beginning of snowfalls at this altitude restrict the public life of the inhabitants considerably for several months of the year.

Shortly behind the town, which is ratherlong, you arrive at a pass of 1420 m altitude. No view over the whole region of Cappadocia can be more gigantic than this one. Even the big rock of Uçhisar seems tiny and small in the distance from here. Directly below your feet is Ürgüp again, where a narrow and extremely steep road will lead you back. Please be extremely careful on your way down, as the winding road has a downhill gradient of up to 20% in some parts. Do not shift higher than second gear, and frequently use the engine breaking effect. At the first set of traffic lights in the town you have reached your starting point, namely Ürgüp, again.

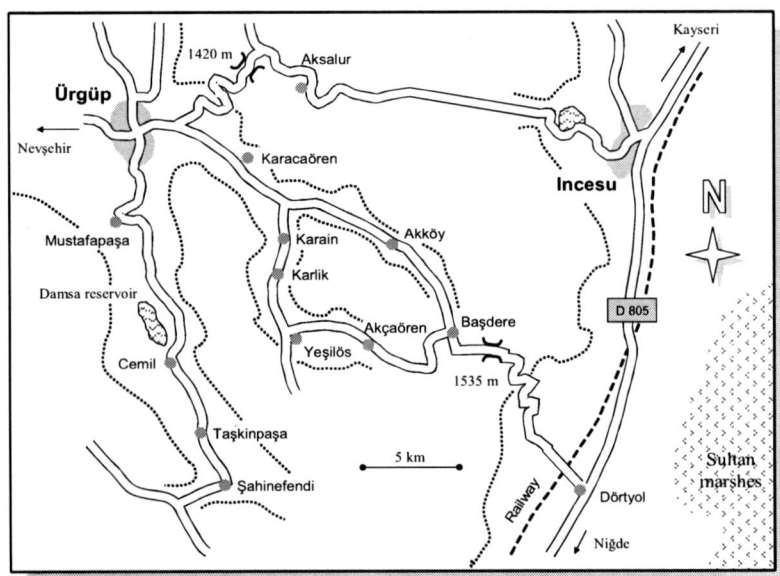

Kara Mustafa and the Gadzooks

- a Vizier has Great Projects

Grand Vizier Kara Mustafa is among the most ambivalent figures of Ottoman history. He reminds one a little of the vesier "Isnogood" from the popular comic book series of the same name. Arrogance, pomposity and greed for power are the attributes ascribed to him by the historians. Happily enough, also hubris and, along with it, an inability to command an army were among his other qualities. This was fortunate for the inhabitants of Vienna, in front of whose gates he was lying with a huge army in 1683, and probably also fortunate for the rest of Central Europe.

The Grand Vizier's career was very successful. After his father's death he was adopted into the famous Köprülü vizier's family, grew up together with their son, Ahmed, and later married the daughter of the house. He held the position of provincial governor for many years, became an admiral of the Turkish fleet, and finally inherited the office of grand vizier from Ahmet. As a clever tactician, managing Sultan Mehmet IV on the throne was plain sailing for him, as the sultan was regarded as idle and not much interested in government affairs.

During his career, Kara Mustafa always kept a watchful eye on the events on the western border towards the Habsburg Empire. State business was smooth under his leadership, taxes kept flowing abundantly, and the army was larger than ever before. In 1679 a message from Hungary arrived, in which Christian Magyars begged the Padisha of Istanbul for help against Austria. What had happened?

Well, Catholic Austria was more focused on harassing its Protestant subjects - among which was also the Hungarian nobility - than concentrating on the Turkish Peril. Thus it happened that many Magyars fled to regions under Turkish control, as they were allowed to practise their religion freely and without any repression there, and as the tax burden was also much lower. Nevertheless, the Hungarians kept on fighting against the Austrians in a kind of guerilla warfare from inside the Turkish territories. Those flying squads called themselves "Kuruzen", and this term later developed into the Austrian interjection "Kruzitürken" (a combination of 'crucifix' and 'Turks', used as an expression of annoyance). And it was those Cruci-turks who asked Kara Mustafa for support. Christians and Muslims were united in the fight against the last bulwark of the West. An idea which was meant to make the long-cherished plans of a power-greedy grand vizier come true at last. The march on Vienna could begin. On the way, the army grew to two hundred thousand men – the biggest army ever mobilized by the Ottomans – and on July 14th, 1683, over 300 cannons faced the walls of Vienna, the capital of the Habsburg Empire. But here the first chance had already been forfeited. The entourage of more than a thousand people that accompanied the vizier had slowed down the advance. If the army had arrived only a week earlier, they would have come upon a poorly secured city and could have captured Vienna in a surprise attack. After this, Central Europe would have been open to the Turks without protection. But Kara Mustafa made some more serious strategic mistakes. He allowed his elite troops, the Janissares, to become worn down in uncoordinated minor attacks and, out of avarice, he refused to release the city for plundering, which failed to motivate the army and, eventually, he forgot to secure the surrounding area. The latter was to give his troops the fatal blow. In spite of urgent warnings that a rescue army was on its way to Vienna, he did not give the signal for the assault of the city. On September 12th armies from Bavaria, Saxony and Poland assembled above Vienna without a single Turk having confronted them. The surprise effect was so much that the greatly outnumbered Turkish auxiliary squad was thoroughly defeated. They left behind over 40,000 dead Turks and 300 cannons which the Ottomans had forgotten in their precipitous retreat. Kara Mustafa was to survive this disaster for only three months. On the 25th of December he was executed in Belgrade by order of the Sultan. One of the most arrogant and greedy grand viziers that the Ottoman Empire had ever seen died with the hangman's noose around his neck.

According to official Turkish history, however, Kara Mustafa is said to have been captured - and executed soon after - by his enemies.

Sarıca Kilise

This church is not far behind Ürgüp, about 2 km off the Soğanlı road. Actually nothing special, if one has seen enough of the old cave churches. The complex consists of a monastery and two churches in the valley. But here you see that something has been done for the 3 TL admission. In the monastery you do not walk over dusty floors strewn with cigarette butts, but you see an excellent example of successful renovation and for once also feel something like the sacred atmosphere appropriate to the dignity of those temples. Not for nothing did the costly renovation of the complex receive an architectural prize in 2004.

Mustafapaşa

A small village located 5 km south of Ürgüp. Only small groups of visitors from foreign countries are seen here, and very occasionally you see a family speaking a totally foreign language walking round houses of the place. Those are visitors from Greece who have come here in order to walk in the footsteps of their ancestors. Mustafapaşa is exemplary for the misery of the eviction of the Greek-orthodox population from Cappadocia. The Muslims and the Christians lived side by side, but also together with each other in harmony. The population exchange of 1923/24 after the end of the war between Greece and Turkey made the village community break up, that is, be destroyed for political reasons. The Muslim inhabitants were not enthusiastic about this officially prescribed measure, either. Apart from the insecurity about how the new Turks from Greece would integrate into the village society, numerous business relations, friendships and perhaps also family bonds between the two religious communities had developed. Dramatic scenes are said to have happened in those weeks, which were told of long after by the older people. The fact that the town uses its old name, Sinasos, in tourism advertising again today shows that the relations have not been cut off completely.

So, once a year it gets hectic in the village. Even the Patriarch of the Orthodox Church, who actually still resides in Istanbul, comes to the little village then and reads Mass in the old church at the village square. Some of the expatriates even come from the USA to preserve the memory of their

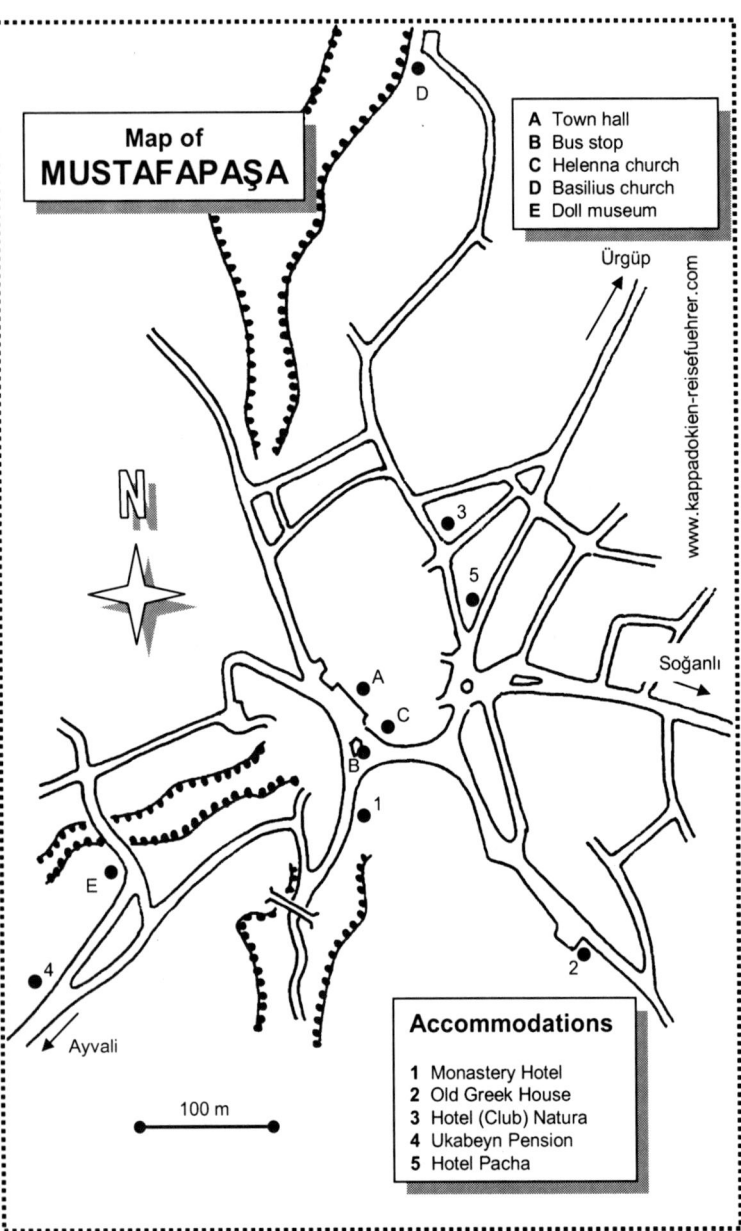

ancestors. All this is supported by the present population and especially by the town administration, which seems to have fully understood the importance of Mustafapaşa's history.

Apart from this, the place is very quiet, but not without life. If it is not Ramasan, the majority of the male population will assemble in the village square to play tavla and drink tea, aways ready for a little chat. There is no main road that would cut through the village, and the many little valleys which subdivide the settlement seem to increase the inhabitants' desire for communication.

If you walk through the village with open eyes, you will discover some differences from the usual architecture in Cappadocia. Pointed gables and religious ornamentation bear witness to the past. Greek inscriptions can be discovered above the entrance doors of many houses, and sometimes a building that reminds you of a church is just a normal dwelling house in reality.

Sibel Radiye Gül, born a Caucasian, has installed her doll's museum in one of those houses. Besides a small collection of dolls from all over the world, the exhibition is focused on the presentation of everyday scenes from the Ottoman time. Everything is there, from the pompous procession of the Sultan with his entourage to the rural teahouse scenery. All those many hundreds of dolls have been handmade by Mrs Gül. The little museum can be visited for 4.5 TL admission.

Another worthwhile side-trip is a visit to the St. Vasilios Church (D), which is located about 2 km off the village centre high up on the edge of a valley. It is controversial among the experts as to exactly when this cave church was built, but the paintings and reliefs were affixed not before 1901. The complete room has not been frescoed, but the few excellent paintings are strongly accentuated by the mostly whitewashed walls.

Mustafapaşa is an ideal starting point for multi-day hikes. You will mostly see only local people who are working in their fields or gardens – and rarely other tourists.

The Population Exchange

- a tragedy of two nations

In 1920, Sultan Mohammed VI sealed the official end of the Ottoman Empire by signing the Treaty of Sèvres. The rest of the empire was to be divided among the British, the French and the Italians and to be governed in a colonial style. Strengthened by this restrictive policy, the Greeks felt tempted to make their dream of a 'Great Greece' and of the repatriation of the ancient Greek settlement areas in Anatolia come true. Probably, also vindictive feelings for the more than 400 years of Ottoman occupation of their country played an important role. In 1919 they began to occupy the west of Turkey and declared it Greek homeland. But after little less than 3 years of boody war, this dream was to burst like a soap bubble. The former Ottoman military followers under Mustafa Kemal Atatürk had reassembled in the east part of the country and formed the new nationalist Republican Army. Under the leadership of the future founder of the state, this army succeeded in driving the Greeks back and reconquering Izmir, the last Greek stronghold, in 1922. The worn out armies of the European victorious powers could only look on as the new Turkish power thwarted their plans.

In 1923, the representatives of newly strengthened Turkey met with the Europeans in Lausanne and saw to it that the major components of the old treaty of 1920 were nullified. From that moment on the country was given full souvereignty and the Turks were given permission to found their republic. The Greek attack was to have painful consequences. As the new government in Ankara regarded the country's two million orthodox Greek inhabitants as a security risk, a population exchange between the two counties became part of the Lausanne treaty. To the Turkish rulers, nothing was of greater importance than the national unity within the remaining Turkish rump state. After all, Atatürk had realized that basically the burgeoning nationalism of the preceding century had been an important reason for the decay of the Ottoman Empire. Turkey could not afford a further fragmentation of the country into ethnic groups or religious minorities. A policy which, incidentally, has not changed until today, as can be seen from the treatment of minorities like the Kurds.

On May 1st, 1923, the agreement on the exchange of the Turkish and Greek minorities in both countries was published. A shock went through the ranks of the people affected – on both sides. Within a few months they had to pack their belongings and ship them or even sell them. They were to leave their homes, which had also been their great-grandfathers' homes, they were to give up their holy places and leave the graves of their ancestors to an uncertain fate. In Cappadocia, the villages of Mustafapaşa, Ürgüp, Güzelyurt and Nevşehir were the ones affected most by this rule. Often more than half the population of a village had to leave the country, so that those places were hardly able to survive. The remaining Turkish inhabitants were divided over the new government's actions. Both population groups had depended on each other during centuries of coexistence, and sometimes their attachments were more that just business relations. But of course there were also beneficiaries of the situation. There were many who took advantage of the Greek people who had to sell their houses and farms quickly, and thus gained possession of real estate and land for a ridiculous price. According to the Lausanne Treaty the emigrants were allowed to take all their possessions with them to their new home country. But here, too, clever transport businessmen took advantage of the chance for a profitable bargain. The Greeks from Cappadocia were taken to Mersin on the coast in order to be shipped to Greece from there. But they had to leave the remaining part of their belongings behind in the harbour. They were actually promised that everything would be sent after them later, but corrupt officials and numberless thieves looted the crammed storehouses, so that after a few months only a fraction of the goods or even nothing at all arrived at their new home. But on the other side, in Greece, it often proceeded in much the same way. Many expatriated Greeks were placed in the north of the island of Evia, near the town of Estia. Today a little museum commemorates the former expulsion. The Turks in West Thrace and the Greeks in Istanbul were exempt from the forced eviction. In Greek Thrace, the minarets of the mosques of the local Turkish minorities still rise today. But in spite of the exemption agreement, only a few of the once many thousand Greek people still live in Istanbul today. Disputes with the Turkish state caused many of them to leave Istanbul in the following decades. Most of the new Turkish citizens came from the border region near today's Macedonia. They were eyed with suspicion by the locals, as they had brought their very own culture and habits with them.

Today the old houses of the Greek people are the only testimony that reminds us of them in Cappadocia. But these silent witnesses are in danger, too. Only a few families can afford the maintenance of those buildings, which are sometimes very large. They have been scheduled as monuments, but cannot be renovated due to shortage of communal funds and are thus exposed to dilapidation. The expatriates have never broken their contact to their former home countries. Again and again, Greek people can be seen in the villages and towns of Cappadocia, who with great sadness are visiting the land of their forebears – a land which was their people's home country for centuries.

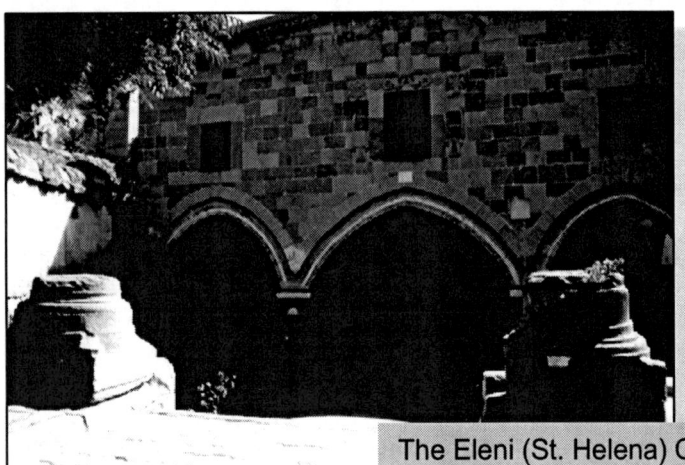

The Eleni (St. Helena) Church in the village centre

Accommodation in Mustafapaşa

➢ MONASTERY HOTEL

Close to the central square but nevertheless quiet, like all hostels in the village. This hotel is thought to have been opened in 1968 as the first inn in Cappadocia. It was given its name as the rooms of an old monastery were partly integrated into it. Meanwhile, the hotel is run by the third generation, by the grandson, who also gladly offers hiking tours through the region. In general, this family hotel is very helpful with solving problems, and in the shady courtyard there is always an open ear for the guests' questions.

| 1 | 50-70 TL | 132 | E – F - D | ␣ ␣ | ①②③⑦⑧ |

Phone: 0384 353 5005   www.monasteryhotel.com

➤ OLD GREEK HOUSE

Again one of those hotels you do not dare to dream of. But unlike the hotels which have been newly built or renovated beyond recognition, everything is genuine here. Virtually nothing of this 250-year-old building has been changed. The only concession to modern tourism is the sanitary facilities that had to be integrated. The vast salons, whose old wooden ceilings remind you of the glamour of the padishas, are decorated with wall paintings from 1886. And the ground floor, which almost entirely consists of a courtyard vaulted by an enormous arch, reminds you of a caravanserai rather than of an ordinary dwelling house.

2	140 TL	16	E	🍴	①②⑤⑦⑧

Phone: 0384 353 5306   www.oldgreekhouse.com

➤ HOTEL NATURA

Another ancient Greek house that has been preserved in its original form. The rooms and salons are decorated with 17th century wall paintings and elaborate ornamentation. A large sunny courtyard and the orchard behind the house make staying outside a pleasure, too.

3	120 TL	9	E - D	🍴	②⑤⑦⑧

Phone: 0384 353 5030   www.clubnatura.com

➤ UKABEYN KONUK EVI

Small inn full of nooks and crannies at a quiet location at the edge of the village. Modern ambience with several interlocking terraces. Open fireplaces keep the beautifully furnished rooms warm in autumn and spring, and a pool in the lowest terrace provides coolness in summer.

4	120 TL	7	E		①②④⑤⑦⑧

Phone: 0384 353 5533   www.cappadociapensiyon.com

➤ HOTEL PACHA

The hotel is unfortunately on the main road through the village. But that does not mean a lot in Mustafapasa. At least it has the best view over the countryside around the village. The little family business is run with much vigour, and in the large cozy lounge with its panoramic view you will inevitably take part in the family life. One-day or multi-day hiking trips are available.

5	50-60 TL	12	E - F - D	☕🍴	①②⑦⑧

Phone: 0384 353 5331   www.pachahotel.com

Cemil

The small village is about one kilometre behind the southern end of the Damsa reservoir, and at first glance does not have much to offer. Nothing but a sign at the entrance points to the special attraction of the settlement. Once Cemil must have had a large Greek community; the reason why such a large church was built in such a small village cannot be explained otherwise. Drivers should park their vehicles on the small central square, as the narrow cobblestone lanes are only something for hard-boiled drivers. It is a walk of less than 5 minutes to the church, which is on the other side of the hill. Large and powerful, it dominates the village. Unfortunately here, too, a picture of neglect presents itself. The furniture and most of the paintings have been destroyed, and only its massive construction has saved the 19th century building from total dilapidation. Even today the place still reminds one of a Greek mountain village. Perhaps the reason is that here the old trees are still standing at the crossroads, while elsewhere they have become victims of the cold Anatolian winters.

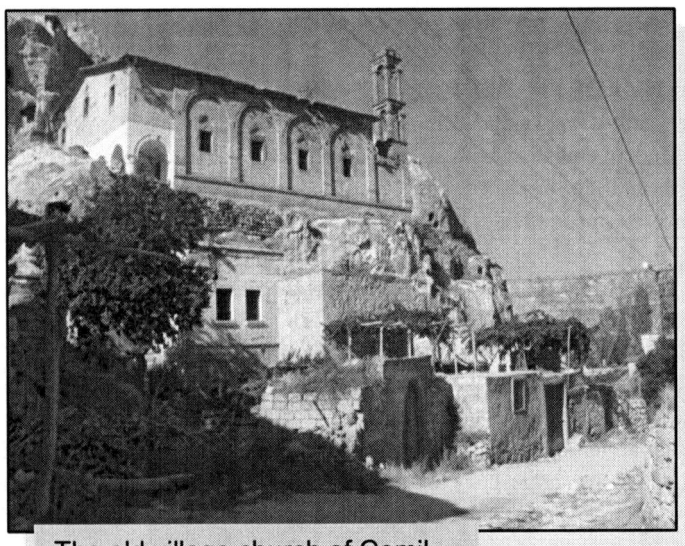
The old village church of Cemil

Keşlik Manastırı

This very large monastic complex is 12 kms from Ürgüp on the Soğanlı road. It must have been in operation for very long time, as it shows architectural features from different periods. There are partly the old defense facilities again, but other rooms have been also been designed open. The refectory, which has been carved into the rock up to 25 m deep and with two naves, already shows that a large monastic community must have lived here. Up to 200 people could have dined here, sitting closely to each other. On the whole, a number of winding corridors, climb-down shafts and rooms can be discovered here again. It takes some time to examine everything, as numerous store rooms, kitchens and stables have been built on several floors here in order to feed many people. The religious paintings were unfortunately destroyed by fire or blackened. Greek graffiti, the oldest from 1755, show that this must have happened already a long time ago. The new masonry which can be found in this complex is not a restoration, but mainly for the protection of the church rooms or for stabilizing the rock cones. In another rock cone there is a large prayer room, whose floor has collapsed, Here, the cave-masons have probably been careless again. Up above in the ceiling, at a dizzy height, there is another pigeonhole again, which was beaten through afterwards. Lovers of narrow cave tunnels will find a lot of pleasure and many things to explore here for 3 TL from April to October.

Taşkınpaşa

About 9 km behind Mustafapaşa you reach this village with a 600 year old Ottoman house at its entrance. Its erector, who has also given the village its name, is said to have been buried here, too. The building was recently renovated and a library was opened in it. Already the main entrance door, still in Seljuk style, and the three feet thick outer walls are worth seeing. Do not have any inhibitions about going inside, as readers are rarely present and the librarian has got used to foreign visitors meanwhile.

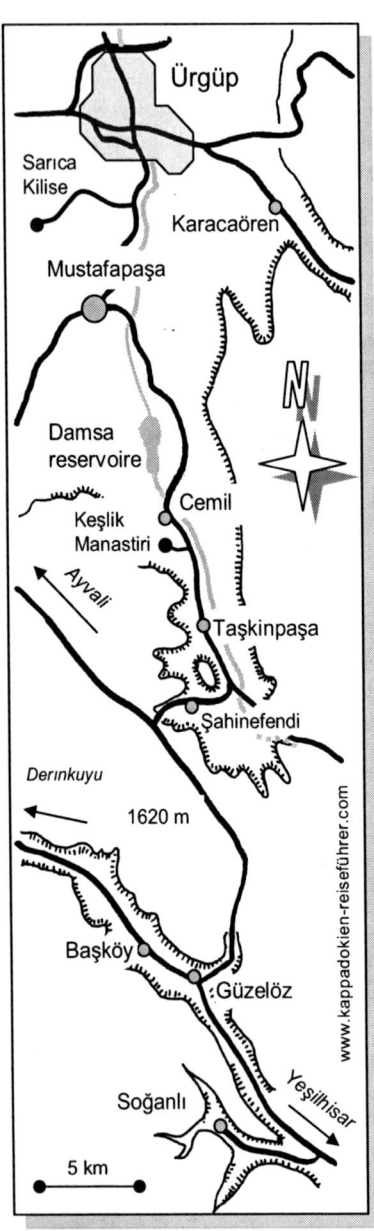

Soğanlı

Already on the way to the Soğanlı valley, the changes of the countryside cannot be missed. Deeply cut valleys are situated between the mighty table mountains which have been accompanying you for a while already. They are not mountains, however, but the sharp edges of valleys which have been cut into the Anatolian plateau for millions of years. The village of Soğanlı lies hidden in such a hollow. A village like many others in Anatolia: cubic houses with their typical flat roofs, that seem to be crouching down into the hillside and are overshadowed by biblical silence. If 1400 years ago Christian communities had not begun hollowing out numberless churches and monastic buildings into the rock here, too, Soganli would most probably have fallen into oblivion. There are said to have been more than 150 churches and chapels in the vicinity. But most of them have decayed, been filled up, or have simply disappeared off the face of the earth by erosion. Today only ten of those temples are open to the public, and even some of these are difficult to reach. However, some of those churches have a special feature which cannot be found anywhere else in Cappadocia: Here the churches were not only decorated on the inside, but the rock was also sculpted and ornamented on the outside. We would like to visit four of those churches on a little walking tour. Behind the pay kiosk (1) we keep to the right along the asphalt road and after 300 or 400 m reach the **Karabaş Kilise** (Black Head Church)(4). It consists of several prayer rooms, the front rooms dating back to the 6th century, that is, to the Roman and Byzantine periods. The other rooms were added in later centuries. Here, in the oldest part of the church, painted decorations from the different eras can be seen and distinguished easily. You see paintings from the time before the iconoclastic period, painted directly on the rock with earth colours. During the dispute, a layer of plaster was spread over them and the church room was decorated with simple ornaments.These ornaments have not been preserved, however, as after the end of the controversy new colourful figurative motifs were painted over them. Next to the church are several large cave rooms, which were used as utility rooms for a long time. (At least the many fire pits in the floor suggest this.)

After about 300 m, also on the right side of the road, there is the **Yilanli Church** (5) (Snake Church). There are graves in the side areas, and it was also redecorated with new paintings in the 14th century. Some people might criticize the bad condition of the frescoes and blame it on the distinterest of the Muslim population. But if you look closer you will discover that the majority of the scratched graffitti already disfigured the paintings in the 18th century, as they are almost entirely in Greek. Again, there are also side rooms next to this church arranged round a courtyard. A refectory and openings in the floor for supply vessels suggest a monastic community must have come together here, and at the end of the middle section there is a tunnel with an escape room and a millstone door.

We turn left now, cross a little creek that runs through the valley, and proceed back towards the village on the opposite side of the valley. After another 300 m we reach the **Kubbeli Church** (6), which had already been clearly visible from the other side of the valley. The rock cone ensemble stands out markedly from the hillside.

The dome of the topmost rock cone is worth remarking, as the inside and outside have been carved out of the rock most artfully. This building technique is only found here in the Soğanlı valley. Besides, the location of the upper church room has been precisely coordinated with that of the lower room. If the opening between the floors had not been closed, there would be a magnificent view from the columns of the lower floor up to the concave upper dome. The columns in the lower church room bear witness to the great skill in working the rock material and also of the playful design of the former master builders. Further down in the rock are cave rooms with graves in the floors, which, as the Turkish travel guide informs us, are "unoccupied at the moment".

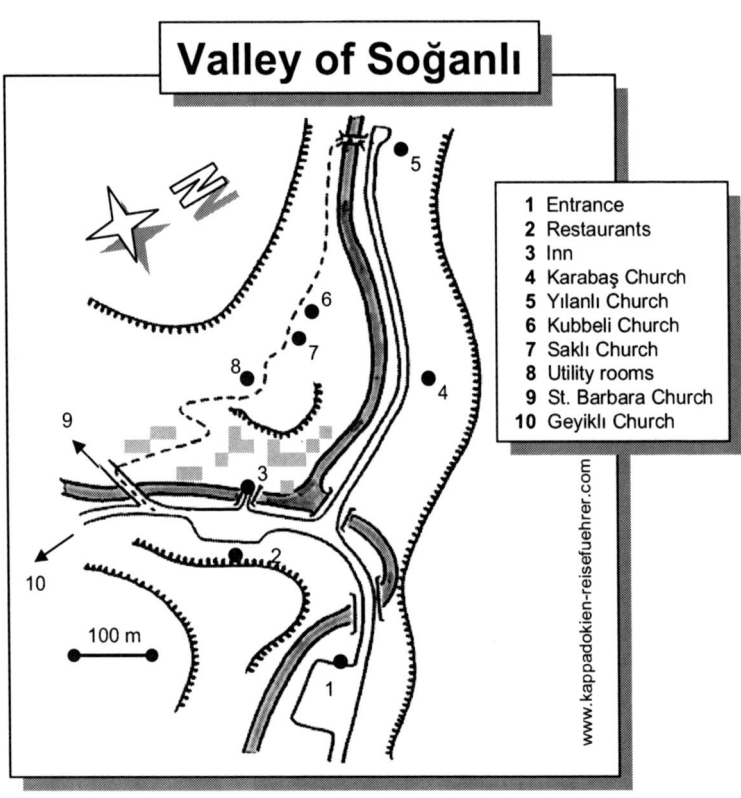

are difficult to reach. However, some of those churches have a special feature which cannot be found anywhere else in Cappadocia: Here the churches were not only decorated on the inside, but the rock was also sculpted and ornamented on the outside. We would like to visit four of those churches on a little walking tour. Behind the pay kiosk (1) we keep to the right along the asphalt road and after 300 or 400 m reach the **Karabaş Kilise** (Black Head Church)(4). It consists of several prayer rooms, the front rooms dating back to the 6th century, that is, to the Roman and Byzantine periods. The other rooms were added in later centuries. Here, in the oldest part of the church, painted decorations from the different eras can be seen and distinguished easily. You see paintings from the time before the iconoclastic period, painted directly on the rock with earth colours. During the dispute, a layer of plaster was spread over them and the church room was decorated with simple ornaments. These ornaments have not been preserved, however, as after the end of the controversy new colourful figurative motifs were painted over them. Next to the church are several large cave rooms, which were used as utility rooms for a long time. (At least the many fire pits in the floor suggest this.)

After about 300 m, also on the right side of the road, there is the **Yilanli Church** (5) (Snake Church). There are graves in the side areas, and it was also redecorated with new paintings in the 14th century. Some people might criticize the bad condition of the frescoes and blame it on the distinterest of the Muslim population. But if you look closer you will discover that the majority of the scratched graffitti already disfigured the paintings in the 18th century, as they are almost entirely in Greek. Again, there are also side rooms next to this church arranged round a courtyard. A refectory and openings in the floor for supply vessels suggest a monastic community must have come together here, and at the end of the middle section there is a tunnel with an escape room and a millstone door.

We turn left now, cross a little creek that runs through the valley, and proceed back towards the village on the opposite side of the valley. After another 300 m we reach the **Kubbeli Church** (6), which had already been clearly visible from the other side of the valley. The rock cone ensemble stands out markedly from the hillside.

The dome of the topmost rock cone is worth remarking, as the inside and outside have been carved out of the rock most artfully. This building technique is only found here in the Soğanlı valley. Besides, the location of the upper church room has been precisely coordinated with that of the lower room. If the opening between the floors had not been closed, there would be a magnificent view from the columns of the lower floor up to the concave upper dome. The columns in the lower church room bear witness to the great skill in working the rock material and also of the playful design of the former master builders. Further down in the rock are cave rooms with graves in the floors, which, as the Turkish travel guide informs us, are "unoccupied at the moment".

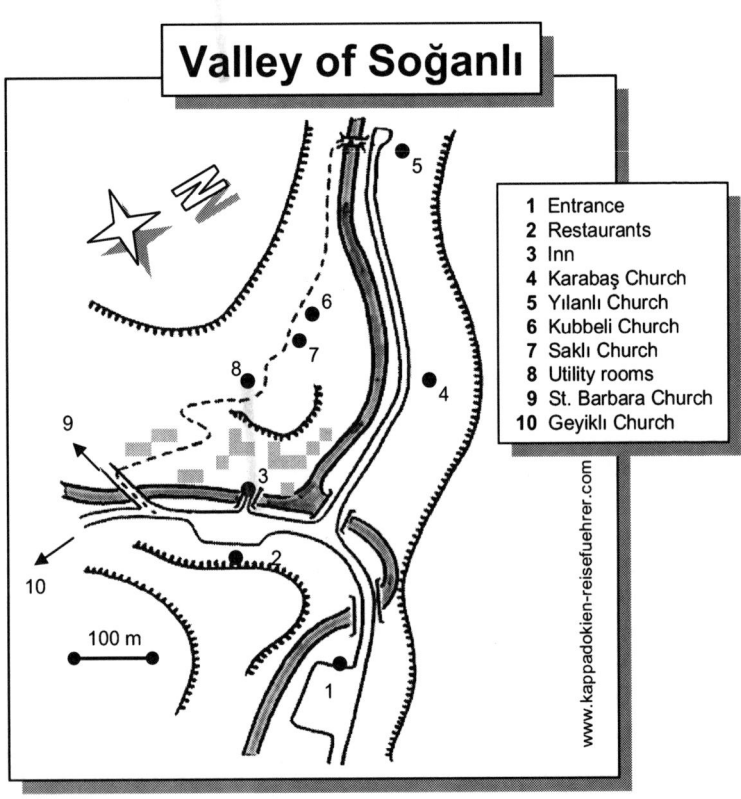

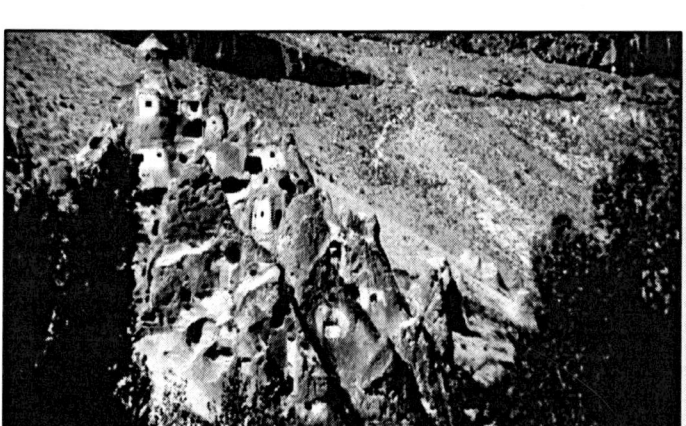
The rock complex of the Kubbeli Church

Only a few metres away from it is the **Saklı Church** (Hidden Church) (7), which looks very small and inconspicuous from the outside. Unfortunately its dome collapsed a long time ago. Apparently the cave masons had been a little too ambitious here. But oddly enough, entire groups of visitors disappear in it for a long time and you wonder where they may have gone. The secret lies hidden on the other side, behind an unconspicuous entrance door, where a lower – and larger – prayer room extends into the hillside, followed by a utility room further inside the mountain. Hidden still further in the mountain is an escape room with a millstone door. The difference to the tuff in Göreme can be recognized very well in this church. While the latter is very homogenous, rather soft and with few inclusions, the tuff here appears almost like concrete. The colour of the rock and the many gravel inclusions make the inexperienced visitor start wondering whether George Lucas might not have left another movie background behind here. 200 m up the path, there are several large open cave rooms on the right side. The eyes protruding from the ceilings and the rows of holes in the walls show that they were used as utility rooms.

The path now surmounts the hilltop and winds down through the village to the village square, where some restaurants have been established. Diagonally across from it, and only accessible over a little wooden bridge, there is the only hostel in this village (3). Those who want to see still more churches in this valley will find accommodation in the classic Anatolian style here. Breakfast, a traditional evening meal and free tea or coffee all day are included. If you are still not yet fed up with Cappadocian cave churches, you will also find lots of them in Güzelöz, which is about 10 km before Soğanlı.

Unfortunately the place is not accessible by public transportation, so that you will have to book a day trip to it via an agency or rent a scooter for a day. Soganli is about 50 km from Ürgüp and can be reached by the road to Mustafapaşa. In Mustafapaşa you keep left in the roundabout and follow the road through the villages of Cemil, Taşkınpaşa and Şahinefendi. Behind the latter, the road rises steeply and forks at its highest point. There, at km 26, you turn left again across the highland until reaching an altitude of 1600 m until the road winds down into the Güzelös valley. From there it is about 10 km to the fork to Soganli and 4 more km to the village.

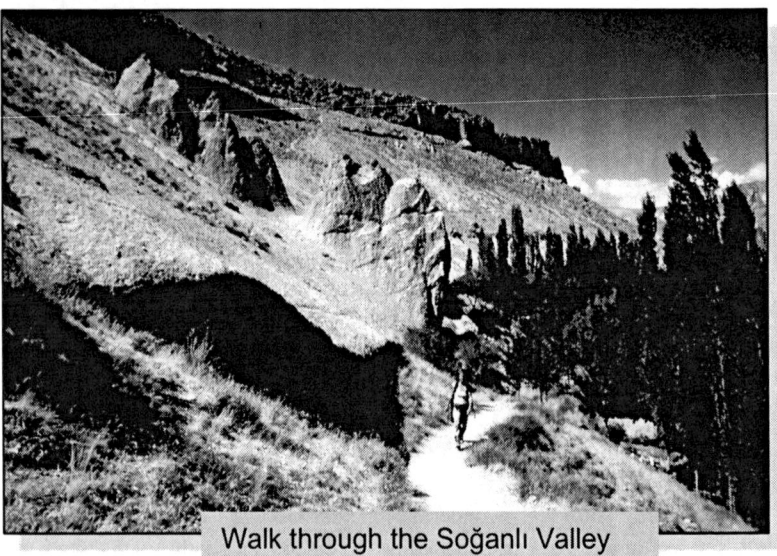
Walk through the Soğanlı Valley

Foto: Uwe Schmitz

Kaymaklı

The town is about 20 km south of Nevşehir on the Niğde road. Hardly any visitor would take notice of it if there was not this brown sign with the inscription "Yeralte Şehri" on it in white. Surrounded by spacious potato fields, the small town makes a rather sleepy impression. Only in the centre, exactly where its attraction is pointed out by the sign, is there some more life. An assemblage of souvenir stands shows visitors the way to one of the most frequented sights of Cappadocia: an underground town. Located right below the central hill of the settlement, it has been able to be visited since 1964. Initially the inhabitants themselves guided the visitors through the maze of corridors and tunnels with torches. Today however, this tourist magnet has been fully electrified and can also be visited without a guide.
As with all underground settlements in Cappadocia, the whole complex is not accessible here either.

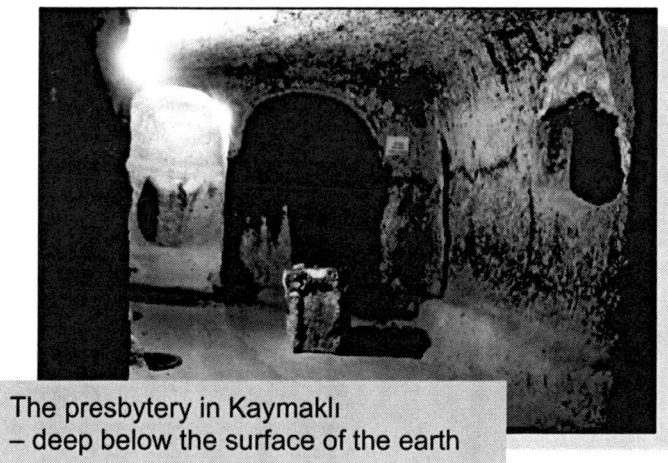

The presbytery in Kaymaklı
– deep below the surface of the earth

On the one hand there are parts which are in danger of collapse; on the other hand, large parts have not been fully opened and explored. Nothing is known about the origin of this settlement, as is also the case with all other underground settlements scattered over the region. Two factors make precise dating impossible: first, there is no written or pictorial evidence at all inside the caves; second, the uninterrupted use of the complexes until well into the 8th century destroyed all traces of the original builders. While above-ground dwelling complexes were always built on the debris of the older cultures, the remains of the former residents had to be removed or cleared out first before expanding an underground settlement. This meant that the archeologists could not find a single shard from a former settlement period any more. It is estimated, however, that already more than 4000 years ago humans had begun to carve small underground rooms into the rock. These dwelling caves were the best protection from the icy cold Anatolian winters for man and animal, and they could also be carved out with very simple tools.

The rock material of the different floors was submitted to a stability test by scientists, which showed that the rock of the top floors was a lot harder than that of the lower floors. As tuff hardens more and more under contact with air in the course of the years and as this process is very lengthy, it can be concluded that the first floor was used at a very early period. Finally, later generations and populations paved the way to deeper and deeper levels. Contrary to the lower rooms, there are also no tool marks found on the walls on the higher entrance levels, which is another evidence of their great age. The first written evidence of underground settlements is from a Greek document of the 4th century BC.

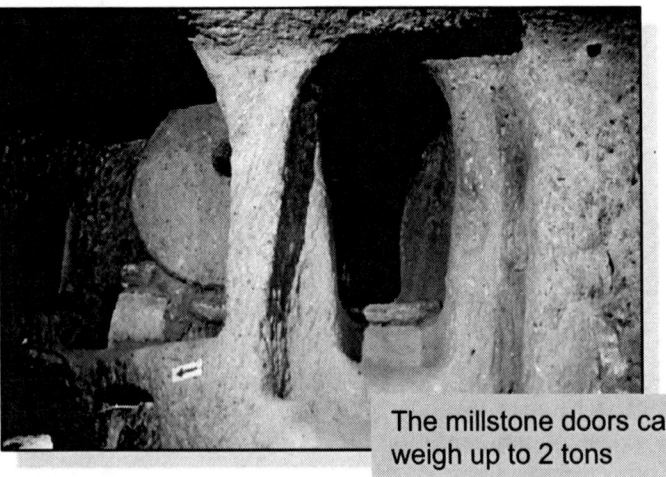

The millstone doors can weigh up to 2 tons

Kaymaklı's underground settlement is full of nooks and crannies, and some tunnels can only be crossed in a 'duck walk'. Also, the common rooms are not very large here. But basically the complex has been designed in much the same way as the underground settlements of other communes here in Cappadocia. The top floors housed stables, store and work rooms which were also used in times of peace. These rooms often had several larger entranceways to the surface for transporting goods and livestock in and out. Only from the third floor downwards the visitor has to squeeze himself through narrow tunnels, which could be closed by a heavy millstone. This is where the part of the settlement begins which served as a refuge from enemies to the inhabitants. Due to its extreme narrowness, the complex at Kaymaklı is an eerily good example how closely the people were crammed together in times of danger. Thousands of them are believed to have survived months of besiegement this way. Toilets, however, have not yet been discovered in them.

Kaymaklı can be reached by a minibus which operates between the settlement and Nevsehir every 15 minutes. 15 TL admission fee per visitor will be collected at the pay booth.

Derinkuyu

If the underground town at Kaymaklı should be too narrow for you, we can recommend a visit to Derinkuyu. The rooms there are much larger and one can walk upright in almost all the corridors. The functions of the various rooms can be recognized better here, too. There is a church with an almost cruciform layout almost at the deepest point of the town, and way down there you can easily watch how the excellent air conditioning system works. Still somewhat further down there is a well at the lower end of a shaft. It is more than 50 metres to the surface from here. Even though smoking is forbidden in underground settlements, smokers should nevertheless light a cigarette near a shaft just in order to show their fellow travellers how well those historic ventilation systems are still working. The huge chimney sucks the smoke in from below and thus provides continuous fresh air in the corridors.

In Derinkuyu, too, only a fraction of the existing tunnels has been made accessible to the public. The complex is believed to spread out below the whole town and to have various entrance doors, many of which are inside private houses, though. Some of the current inhabitants are still using the top floors as storage rooms or stables, and many of them obtain the water for their animals from the old air shafts, hoisting it from a draw well as in historical times. Those wells guaranteed the town's water supply up to 1967, but in spite of that, nobody suspected for centuries the big Swiss cheese that was lying hidden under their feet.

The underground town of Derinkuyu spreads over 5 levels and is up to 60 m deep. Perhaps in 1924 some of the inhabitants did guess what was hidden below their feet when they renamed the place "Deep Hole". About 400 to 600 additional rooms are believed to exist in the closed part of the complex, many of which have not even been documented. Also, in the underground town of Derinkuyu the usual layout can be found. On the top levels are the stables and utility rooms, further down the lockable escape rooms. Actually, all the millstones in the underground complexes, except Özkonak, are not from the caves themselves, but were made of much harder granite elsewhere and were built in later.

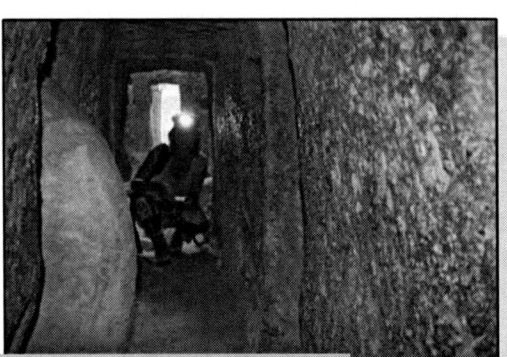
You can only continue crawling here   Foto: Uwe Schmitz

The monastic school on the second floor is somewhat unusual for such a complex. There is a large refectory combined with several study rooms there. It can be supposed that the school was used also in times of peace. For down here it was simply easier to maintain a cool head while studying the Holy Bible.

Derinkuyu is about 30 km south of Nevsehir on the Nigde road and is served by bus from the provincial capital every 30 minutes. The admission fee to the underground city is 15 TL.

Çat Valley

Walking tours through the Çat Valley have been offered by the local travel agencies for a few years only. This is due to the fact that this valley is somewhat away from the main tourist activities. The valley and the settlement of the same name are halfway between Nevşehir and Gülşehir, about 3 km west of the D 765 main road. If you book a walking tour there, the advantage is that you do not depend on the rather sporadic means of local transport. If you dare going on your own despite everything, you have to go to Nevşehir first and then take the minibus to Çat. The bus company has a little office near the terminal of all bus lines in Nevşehir. At the end of the 8,5 km walk, near Acik Saray, you finally intercept the Gülşehir – Nevşehir bus, which will take you back to Nevşehir. You should schedule at least one whole day for transportation and the rather long walk through the valley.

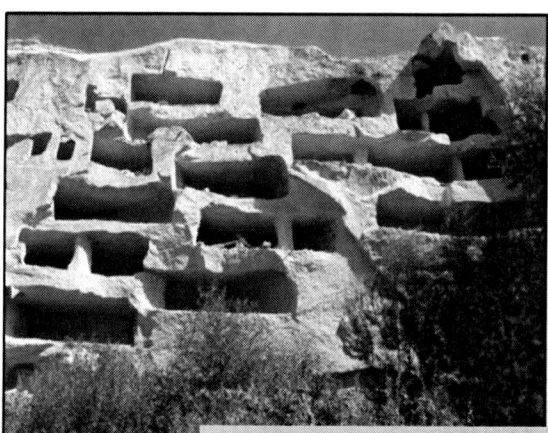
Dove highrises in the Cat valley

The village of Çat, where the walking tour begins, has 2700 inhabitants, at least 5 large mosques and is dominated by agriculture. From the town centre, which consists of the town hall, a shop, two teahouses and a large fountain in the middle, you follow the narrow road out of the village, past the town hall on the right side. Still in the village, you go slightly to the right, following the signs. The first km is not spectacular, because the road leads along the side of the mountain. You simply follow the little driveway paved with natural stones to its end. There, stairs lead down to the actual valley. You walk through it for the next 3,5 km, always accompanied by a small brook. At the outset there is a shaky steel staircase on the left side. Spare yourself the acrobatic feat of climbing up this unstable construction, because in the caves behind it there is only stinking rubbish.

Something else is to be found down here in the Çat Valley, something that is very untypical of Cappadocia and is not missed by anybody: stinging nettles. Over the following miles you will find millions of dovecote openings in the steep walls on both sides – the Çat Valley is the actual "Pigeon Valley". After about 2 km you will reach a place where the rock wall has slipped down on the right side and where you can have an excellent view of the inner labyrinth of dovehouses inside the rock. You cannot lose your way in this first part of the walk, as you need only follow the little stream between the sheer rock walls.

Halfway through, the rocks on both sides become smaller and smaller and the valley widens out into a plain. The brook, which you had to cross several times until now, has also disappeared. From here you always follow the dry river bed north, straight on through farm land, past hidden farms and lightly forested areas. Do not let the driveways which appear now confuse you. At the end of the route you reach an area of typical Cappadocian rock formations again, and now you have reached 'Açik Saray'.

Açik Saray

The experts are not unanimous on what this complex, the size of about one square kilometre, could once have been. Some speak of a caravanserai, others of a monastic centre, and still others of a historic military base. But according to its size it seems to have been an agglomeration of clerical institutions. Even an offshoot of the Bektaşı Order is said to have settled here, whereupon the Christian inhabitants provided – or had to provide – a church for their disposal as a mosque. One can imagine life in this spacious valley, which is still very green, only too well: the dwelling places up on the sides of the low hills, the large orchards and the plantations down on the flat valley bottom – an ideal place for a larger settlement. Perhaps Acik Saray also was the predecessor of the town of Gülşehir, which begins a quarter of a mile north of it. The complex has almost nothing to do with an "open palace", which is the English translation of its name. Perhaps it has been called that in the vernacular because the front walls of many of the large church rooms had collapsed.

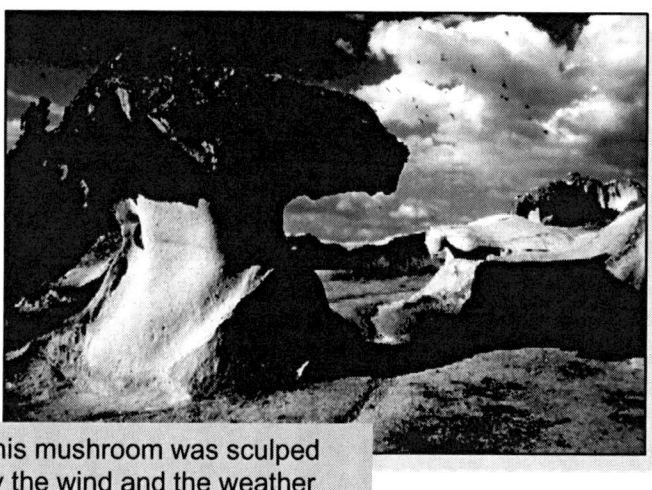

This mushroom was sculped by the wind and the weather

As soon as the wanderer is among the rock formations of Açik Saray again, he turns to the right on a narrow driveway towards the first rocks. Here again, several church buildings lie hidden in the rocks, and here rises also the famous "Mantar Kayası" (mushroom rock), unique in Cappadocia, which a freak of nature caused to erode to a monumental rock mushroom.

Having returned to the main route, one reaches the second part of the complex after about 300 m. Here, too, numerous clerical complexes are situated next to, and on top of, each other. You can traverse the complex walking through these rooms and will reach the exit, that is, the road to Nevşehir after 100 metres.

If you do not want to walk through the complex from Çat, you reach this open air museum by bus from Nevşehir. There is no bus stop here, but the driver will stop in front of the entrance gate on special request. Admission is free.

Hacıbektaş

This settlement, which bears its founder's name, is known far beyond the borders of the country. The Bektaşı Order has supporters all over the world today, many of whom come together here for a big feast on August 16th. Its centre is the old monastic school, where also the tomb of the founder of this religious sect is found. Although Haçı Bektaş Veli spread his teachings already in the time of the Seljuks, the present building was erected by Paşa Orhan Gazi later in the Ottoman period. In spite of that the buildings were designed in the ancient Seljuk style. Since 1964 it has been a museum which is open to everybody, that is, also to tourists. One should however bear in mind that this place is a sanctury and a place of contemplation to many religious persons. One should rather not enter the burial chamber of Hacı Bektaş, as one would only disturb those devoutly praying here.

The area consists of two large yards, the first of which is entered through a large doorway. On the right side there is the Üçer well, which was built in 1902 and which, remarkably, is decorated with a Star of David. Through another door you reach the middle yard with a water basin. Here again there is a well on the right side. This one has been giving water since 1554, but it got its name, Aslanlı Çeşme (lion's well), only in 1853 when the lion statue, a present from Egypt, was put up. The right wing houses the kitchen, and its eight large fireplaces with their big cauldrons show how large the brotherhood must once have been. The mosque behind it was built only in the 19th century, by Sultan Mahmud II. It is remarkable that there is a mosque at all on the site, as the religious community of the Alevi, the supporters of the founder of the order, meet for prayers in so-called Cem houses (see next chapter). The guest house is on the left side, with the oldest date of the building, 1367, above the entrance door. Next to it are the assembly rooms and the study rooms of the complex, which have been furnished with big seating platforms in order to make large discussion forums possible. In the third yard are the tombs of the great scholars. Straight on is the Pir Ev, in which the tomb of the holy Bektaş is. Also some objects from the daily life of the order are on display here, among others, an alleged original manuscript of Ali, the son-in-law of Mohamed and the founder of the Shiite religion.

Some other sarcophagi of later leaders of the order are on display beside it in the room. Further right in the yard is Sultan Balim's tomb, who built up the order with his great organizational talent and finally helped it to achieve real

Monastic complex of the Hacı Bektaş Order

1 First courtyard

2 Well

3 Second courtyard

4 Kitchen and diningrooms

5 Mosque

6 Reception und instruktionrooms

7 Third courtyard

8 Seprulchral building of Pascha Balim

9 Wishing tree

10 Tomb camber of founder Hacı Bektaş Veli

11 Exposition of islamic Relics

12 Tombs of other leader of the order

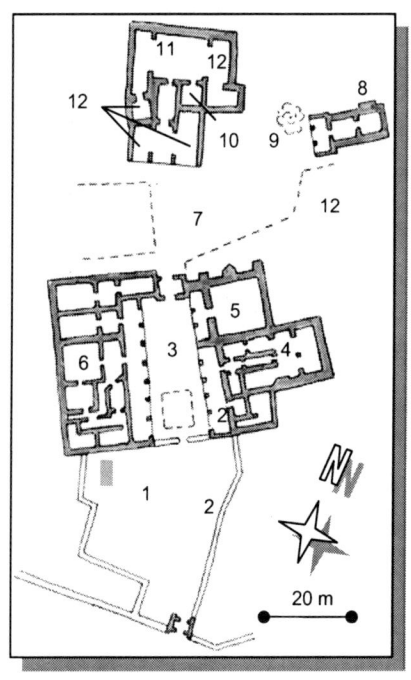

greatness. He is regarded as the second saint and leader of the order, and his tomb was erected in 1519. You will not find him on the list of the Ottoman sultans, however, for now and again also the leaders of the dervish order were allowed to bear this title. An old supported mulberry tree grows in front of the entrance door, which some years ago was still wrapped in numberless ribbons in different colours. It is a wishing tree for the Bektaşı, under which you say a prayer, express your wish and then wind a colourful ribbon around one of the branches. The tree was probably in danger of withering under all those wreaths, and thus all ribbons were ordered to be taken away by the museum administration. The town itself mainly lives on agriculture, apart from which it has not much to offer, and it is completely set to the needs of the pilgrims. The goods in the many souvenir stands around the monastic complex are completely adapted to the religious visitors, and the local hostels are not prepared to receive foreign holidaymakers, either.

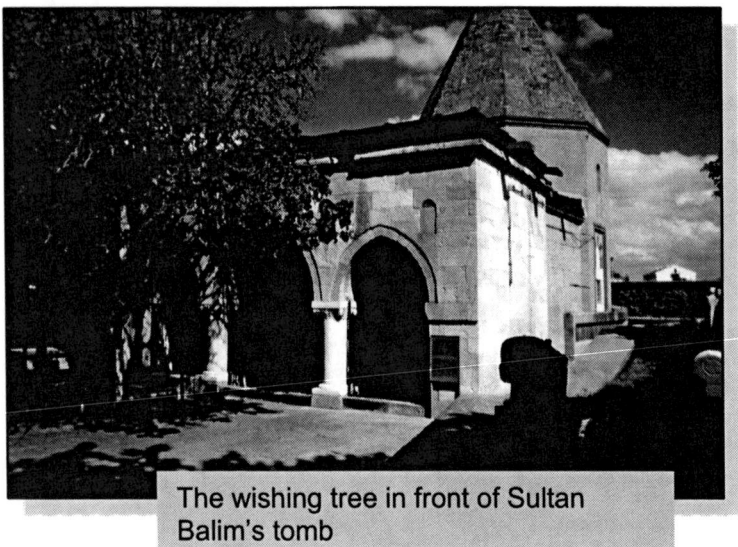

The wishing tree in front of Sultan Balim's tomb

If you nevertheless end up here for the night, there are two hostels at your disposal in the town centre: firstly, the HÜNKAR OTEL for 25 TL per person and per night and then also the YAGMUR PENSION for 10TL per person for a night in a quadruple room.

On a hill above the town there is another Bektaşı sanctuary, the Çillerhane. The hill is impossible to miss, as a huge Turkish flag is waving on the top. The founder of the order is said to have often climbed up here to receive inspiration. Many monuments of Alevi artists commemorate their work and their commitment to this religious community on the site, and the people assemble up here on the festival days in August to celebrate together. The complex is also open to visitors of other religions.

Haçı Bektaş Veli

and Anatolian Humanism

The founder of the Order, whose tomb can be visited in the town of the same name today, is said to have come from the east Persian region of Khorasan. He was not the only person who had to flee from there from the approaching Mongolian tribes in the 13th century. To the Anatolian nomads the term "Khorasan erleri" (soldier from K.) was another word for the wise men who came from there. However, it is doubted that Hacı Bektaş was really active here in Cappadocia. He is believed to have lived in Amasya instead, which is about 200 km north-east from here. Some historians also do not believe that he was buried here in the chief monastery of the Order. On the whole, very little is known about his life, and the legends circulating about him are quite contradictory. In some of those stories he appears as a wise and gentle philosopher, whereas in others he blesses the swords of Turkmen warriors to slay disbelievers with them. The policies and the philosophies of his followers and successors, who led the Order to undreamt-of greatness after his death, were as contradictory as those legends. To the simple population, they preached tolerance and charity. At the Sultan's court in Istanbul, however, the Bektaşi practised a realistic policy of power by exerting massive influence on the Janissaries, the Padisha's elite troops, thus taking part in deciding the fate of the Ottoman Empire.

Many mystics of that period then formulated the theories of what today is called Anatolian Humanism. They turned their backs on the so-called 'pure' religious doctrine and with the help of philosophical approaches and mysticism they tried to build up a tolerant and liberal popular religion. Mevlana Celaleddin-I-Rumi, the founder of the Dervish Order in Konya and a contemporary of Haçı Bektaş, was temporarily the most famous of these men. But in contrast to him the Bektaşi did not preach in the then official Persian language, but propagated their teachings in plain Turkmen language, which was understood by the population. This was to become one of the most important factors in the propagation of the Order and its principles. But the Order's tolerant attitude and its many adaptations from Christianity caused the conservative Muslims to take a hostile attitude towards the sectarian Dervishes. In their eyes, they were traitors to the pure doctrine of Allah and had to be fought against. The current Turkish word "tekke" with its two meanings shows how far this discrimination of the Bektashi could go: On the one hand it means "Dervish monastery", on the other hand it denotes an "opium den". Also the fact that they had brought their Shiite religion with them to Anatolia did not make them any more appealing to the Sunni leaders in the country.

But the Bektaşı Order could not be controlled so easily. While the Mevlana dervishes at Konya had a positive relation to the Seljuk sultans, the Bektaşı formed their alliances at the Ottoman court in Istanbul. Orhan, the son of Osman, the first Ottoman sultan, was the one who created the first elite corps of the Janissaries. In order to build up this army he claimed a 'boy's tribute' from the Christian population. Every Christian family had to hand over one of their sons to the Sultan at the age of 8 to 12 in order to make him a fighter in the Padisha's bodyguard. The boys had to convert to Islam and underwent harsh training to become fighters. But they were also trained in mathematics, reading and writing and in the Islamic religion. For this purpose the Sultan had appointed the Bektaşı, as they were most skilled in bridging the contradicitions between the old Christian education and the new religion forced upon them. Those dervishes believed in a trinity of Allah, Mohamad and Kalif Ali, his successor. They disobeyed the Prophet's ban on alcohol by introducing a kind of Holy Communion, they practised auricular confession of their sins, and quite a number of them advocated celibacy. This way the Dervish Order was to maintain its influence at the Sultan's court for centuries, and not infrequently it was those monks who stirred up one or another Janissary revolt in order to force through their political aims. In 1925, Mustafa Kemal Atatürk banned the Dervish Order in the country, as he was aware of their alliances in the old power system. Many dervishes emigrated to Albania then, where the Order had already gained great influence on the Nomad tribes in the 16th century. The largest community of active Bektaşı lives there today, and they form the majority of the Muslim population in Albania.

But the Dervish Order was to leave a much larger legacy to Turkey: 20 per cent of the Turkish population are so-called Alevi who trace back their religious belief to the teachings of Hacı Bektaş. They, too, are eyed with distrust by the conservative religious Imams. To the Alevi, only the confession of faith is of importance. Attending the mosque, the pilgrimage to Mecca and religious fasting during the month of Ramasan do not make any sense to them. Often, wicked rumours about their secret meetings circulate among the rest of the population. Hardly surprising, as they always hold their meetings - closed to the public - in their Cem-houses. You cannot join the religious denomination, either. You are born an Alevi and you also marry a partner of the same religion. They do not pray in the direction to Mecca, but sit together in a circle when praying, without any segregation of the sexes. And dancing means a form of prayer to them. Thus it is inevitable that the rest of the population suspects wild orgies behind such secret meetings. But in recent years the Alevi community has taken the offensive, as they feel more and more put under pressure by their Sunni opponents. Meanwhile there is an Alevi radio station and an Alevi cultural centre in Istanbul. Both are meant to help reducing the misunderstandings and prejudices against this religious community.

**The grate does not glow by itself, but from the fire.
Reason dwells in the head, not in the crown.
And what you are searching for, you will find it inside yourself,
Neither in Jerusalem nor in Mecca.**

Hacı Bektaş Veli

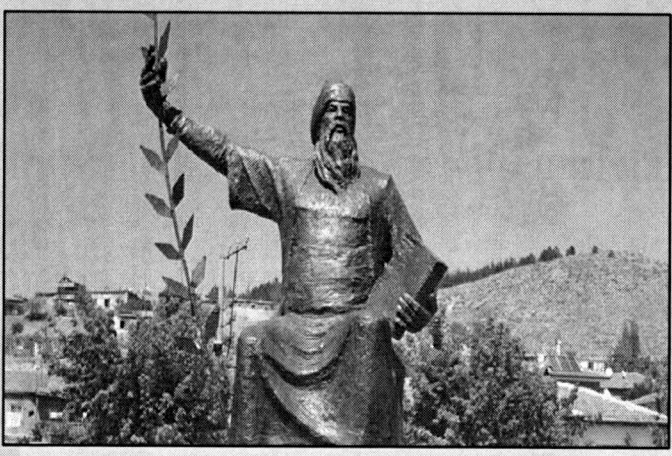

Nargöl

If, coming from Derinkuyu, you want to visit the Ihlara Valley or Güzelyurt, you definitely ought to make a short detour to the Nargöl. This is the last maar (volcanic crater lake) filled with water in the region. The little road to it leads up left into the mountains shortly after the provincial border of Aksaray. Unfortunately, the signs leading there promise too much. No geothermal installations whatsoever will be seen far and wide. After about 1,5 km you will be standing at the edge of a crater, looking down at the lake, which is surrounded by a steep crater rib. At a height of 1350 m and 60 to 70 m deep, one expects a cold mountain lake here. But now, a geothermal factor comes into play: the water temperature is pleasantly mild, as underwater springs of volcanic origin supply the lake with hot water. A little road goes round the lake, and on it you reach the beach on the opposite side. Here you can administer your own volcanic mud packs to yourself. But inside the water you will sink equally deep into the sludgy soil. So, take a run and then dive into the slightly sulfurous water. Great care is required on the crater ring road, as an extreme risk of falling rocks has to be expected.

A little tip for a short interruption of the Ihlara trip: about 4 miles in front of the exit to the crater lake a road leads off left to the village of Kayırlı. To your right on the opposite side you will see a mountain with two artificial mounds on the top. Such man-made hilltops are frequently found in the region, but nobody knows any precise details about their origin or their purpose. They are assumed to date way back to pre-Hittite times.

Gaziemir

Approximately 8 km after the turnoff to the Nargöl you reach the small town of Gaziemir. There, an underground caravanserai was made available to the traveller in 2007. Anyone who has not yet visited an underground city, regardless of whether he is claustrophobic or dislikes crawling through narrow passages, or cannot do this due to a physical impairment, should be sure not to miss this place. The facility is well accessible and does not lead straight into the deep. The large rooms just run into the rock and can be visited easily. As in other underground cities, one finds kitchens, stables, store rooms and of course the obligatory cave church in it. The great wine press and the many caves for wine storage in the floor of the complex are striking. One might think that all this could have been an antique wine wholesalers.

Residues of grains which were found in amphorae here, were subjected to a C14 analysis. The age of these grains could be backdated to the time of the Hittites. Also, some remains of walls in the courtyard of the complex were built in the typical Hittite construction.

The local guard unfortunately speaks no foreign language, but with the help of a leaflet and with the existing signs, the visitor should get along well in the complex. Admission is 3TL.

Güzelyurt

The name of the settlement means "beautiful homeland" in English, and this could not be more appropriate. At least the old village centre, which is located deep down in the valley, has the qualtites of an intact ideal world. Lots of green and the steep rock walls at the back of the valley convey a feeling of security from the harsh world outside. As in a paradise, the people have been living here for centuries in a kind of oasis in the middle of the Anatolian highlands. The crowing of roosters, the country air and the perennial necessity to walk around animal excrement make the world still seem alright here. But this is deceptive. Only a few families live inside their own four walls here and their houses are in danger, too. Not by erosion, as in many other places, but the Turkish museum board and its plans jeopardize the existence of the last few inhabitants of the valley. As in Göreme, it is intended to open a large open-air museum here. And in this case, another eviction would take place here for the second time in a short historic interval. Already in 1924 the Greek inhabitants had to leave the village in connection with the former population exchange. Numerous Greek-style houses and the many overground churches inside and around the settlement show that the old village, which was called Kalveri or Karbala, was mainly inhabited by Christian people until the most recent times.

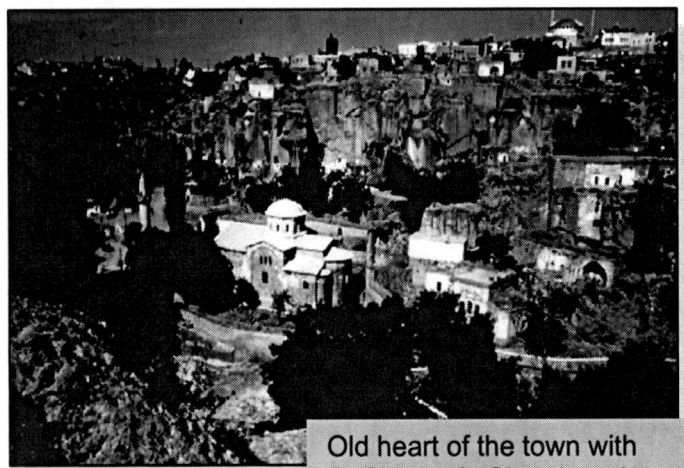

Old heart of the town with St.Gregory's Church at the centre

In the middle of the valley there is the Church of St. Gregorius from 1886, which was turned into a mosque in 1924. Unfortunately the frescoes were painted over with whitewash then, but in a very few places it is peeling off, making little fragments become visible again. The only preserved clerical evidence inside it is the wooden pulpit which is decorated with numerous carvings. The minaret shows the speed of its transformation: it was built with unplastered bricks and above the entrance door, which is an uncommon type of construction in this region. The relics of St. Gregorius, who was born here, were transported to Greece in 1924. He had been one of the great supporters of the orthodox doctrine in the great Council of 381 A.D at Constantinople and climbed fast on the career ladder, all the way to the position of Archbishop. The grounds of the St.Gregorius Church were renovated in 2008. The old rectory was rebuilt and the whole complex was cleared out. In a few years it will be impossible to distinguish the new parts from the old ones, because the work has been done so exactly.

Several more ecclesiastic buildings are scattered over the valley. The Sivisli Kilise from 1887, whose one half was carved out of the rock, is situated opposite the new village centre and a little way above the valley. Its few frescoes show Jesus surrounded by his 12 disciples, once in the apse and once in the dome, too. The notches in its walls at floor height are a specialty and indicate that the church once must have had a wooden floor. Some kilometres away from the village towards Niğde there is the very dilapidated "Red Church" and towards Aksaray, on a rock above the reservoir, is the "Yüksek Kilise" (High Church). Especially from the latter there is an excellent view over the whole region, all the way to the Hasan Dağı. On the way to this church you should not miss noticing the stacked rocks. Evil tongues say that the commune has piled them up with an excavator, but this is of course not true.

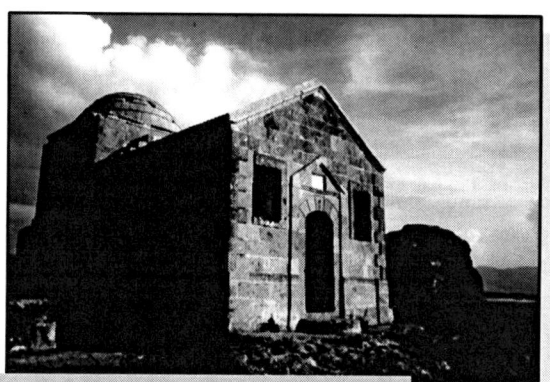

The Yüksek Kilise just outside Güzelyurt

There are two small underground settlements within the limits of the old town centre, but they can only be visited by good climbers, as the different floors are connected by steep climbing shafts. A 4 km long valley, the Monastery Valley, leads away from the village and through a fairytale-like landscape, past many more old dwelling-caves and chapels. As the more interesting section of the valley is about 1 km away from the town centre, driving visitors should feel free to drive into the valley. A small shady parking lot is accessible on a half paved road. From here you can explore this wild and romantic valley really well. It is like a mixture of the valleys of Göreme and of Ihlara.
The new town centre is situated above the steep slope of the valley. But there, too, you can admire the traditional Greek architecture with its multi-aisle way of construction. Not far above the new town centre there is a former Christian-Orthodox theological school, which was renovated in 1998 and

which now houses a hotel. The building is a good source of revenue for the small town, as it is rented out again every five years to the highest bidder.

And also feel free to enter the tourist information on the main square. You will be surprised at the foreign language competence, the high standard of knowledge and the plethora of information the young ladies there will provide you with. This is found seldom enough in Cappadocian municipalities.

The town can be reached by public transport via Aksaray, from where there is a dolmus every hour. A day trip from Göreme is only worthwhile in your own car, or if you book a trip there at one of the many local agencies. The easiest route there is through Nevşehir and Derinkuyu to Güzelyurt. You should take into consideration, however, that the town is about 90 km away from the centre of Cappadocia. There are several shorter routes there, but they are mostly poorly marked and you can easily lose your way.

Another thing about the admission money: the Ihlara Gulch, the church and dwelling complex of Selime and the Monastery Valley near Güzelyurt are all under the administration of the little district capital of Güzelyurt. You pay 5 TL for a one day ticket and you can visit all three sights with it. A ticket system which could be followed as an example by the cultural administration of Nevsehir; it is visitor-friendly and simple!

Accommodation in Güzelyurt

> ### HOTEL KARBALLA

This hotel has rented the former theological school built in 1856, which is situated a little above the main square. Its architecture corresponds to this. All common rooms of the hotel complex are huge, and above all the vaulted dining room goes beyond all dimensions. But the bedrooms are not small either. A shady front garden with big trees completes the sacred atmosphere of this hostel. The price is not for low budget travellers, but the price is in accord with the performance.

110-130 TL	20	E – F - D	¥ 🍽	②④⑥⑦⑧

Phone: 0382 451 2103   www.kirkit.com

> **HALIL PENSION**

This rather new hostel is situatued about 500 m from the town centre. The rooms look like at the first occupation; they are spic and span decorated with a lot of knick-knacks in the typical Turkish manner. Unfortunately, the courtyard exudes the charm of a never-ending building site.

60 TL	7	E		①⑦⑧

Phone: 0382 451 2702   www.halilpension.com

> **HOTEL KARVALLI**

It is situated far outside the town, but it offers a magnificent view over the wide countryside and of the Hassan Dağı. This somewhat larger hotel is run by a German emigrant, who had it built 8 years ago. The furnishings are accordingly Middle-European and include a large well-assorted bar and a billard table. Under the roof there is a large open terrace, an ideal place for a long drink at sunset. A conference room for seminars and congresses has also been made available recently.

80 TL	26	E - D	⛄🍽	⑥⑦⑧

Phone : 0382 451 2736   www.karvalli.com

The Ihlara Canyon

This canyon is one of the most popular excursion destinations in Cappadocia and every local travel agency offers a visit to it. It would be 8 km long if the Melendiz River had not carved so many serpentines into the Anatolian Plateau in thousands of years. Thus you have to walk almost twice as far from its beginning near Ihlara to its end near Selime. A hiking tour through the valley is so popular because it offers the visitor a totally different picture than in the valleys near Göreme. Gone are the gentle rounded rock formations, here the rocks are considerably harder and therefore rougher and sharper-edged. The steep walls of the valley are not shaped elegantly by wind and water, but huge boulders are splintered off by frost fissures and splittings and leave a sharp and jagged edge behind in the sky. In the sky - this is at least what it seems like - because the canyon is often very high and narrow. The rock walls rise up to 150 m and form the edge of the plateau up there. The river in this valley is also unique. In contrast to the other rivers of the region, which dry up in the summer, the Melendiz River carries water throughout the year and thus creates a lush vegetation on the bottom of this valley. Dense birch forests which rustle in the wind, waving grass and sometimes muddy footpaths are very rarely found elsewhere in Cappadocia, especially at the height of summer. And the ever-murmuring brook gives the valley a very special atmosphere. The little river manages to make it to far behind Aksaray, where it trickles away into the soil of the swampy plains of the great Salt Lake.

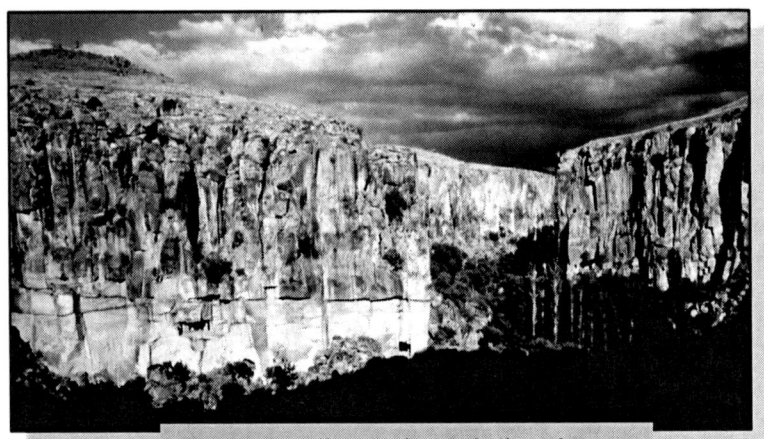

Rugged walls cut through the plateau

Here in the Ihlara Valley ancient dwelling complexes, caves and sacred buildings can again be discovered in the rocks. The deep and easily defensible gorge virtually offered itself as a refuge area to numerous Christian separatists. The upper part near Ihlara was inhabited by Christian people already at a very early period. Those church rooms from the 6th century show strong Persian and Syrian influences. The artistic representations of the Three Wise Men and of the Flight to Egypt show a reference to Oriental models. Further down in the valley, you find Byzantine church frescoes again, which are typical of Cappadocia. Even after the Seljuk conquest of the region, sacred buildings like the St. Gregorius church continued to be erected. All Christian building activity finally came to an end in the 14th century.

If you have booked a hike through the valley, including transfers from and back to Göreme, you are often shown only a small section. You are driven to

The West

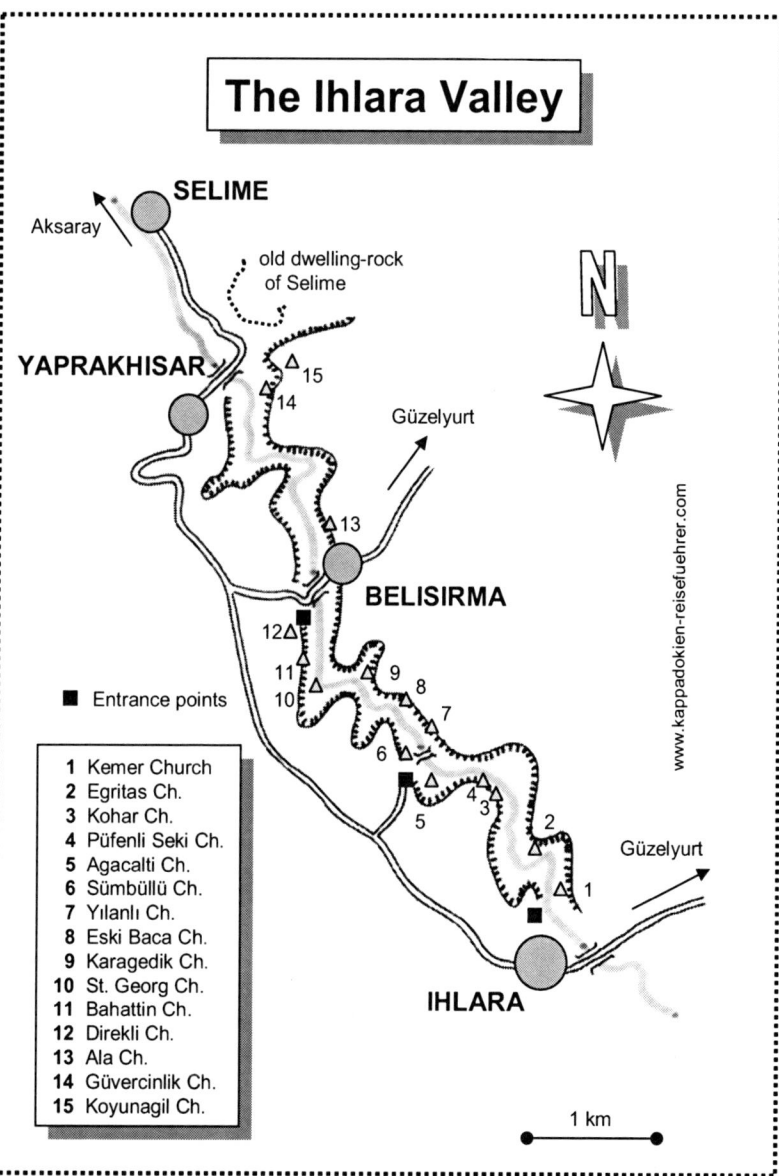

the entry point of the valley, which is some km behind the town of Ihlara. However, the view over the valley is really impressive from here. A stairway of several hundred steps goes down to the valley bottom here. After a two or three hour walk you arrive at Belisirma, which is situated halfway between Ihlara and Selime, and stop by in one of the cozy local restaurants by the river. If you want to head out on your own and with your own vehicle, you have two ways to explore the valley: as the first option, you drive to the entry point mentioned above and walk through the valley on the opposite side of the river. Having arrived at Belisirma, you change sides, refresh yourself in one of the little restaurants and walk back on the western river bank. The second option should be begun early in the morning. It goes through the complete valley to Selime and one must expect a walking time of at least 6 hours.

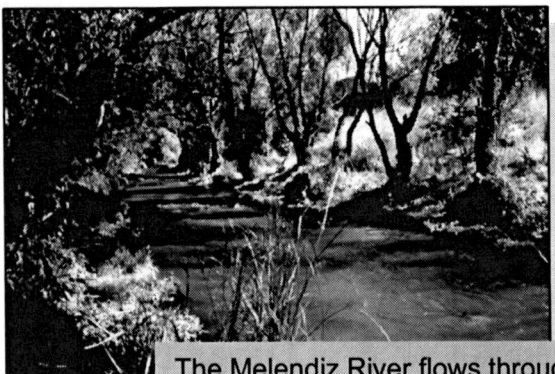

The Melendiz River flows throughout the year at the bottom of the Canyon

If you want to do this long walking tour, you can book a room in advance at the Çatlak Inn in Selime. The useful thing about it is that the Çatlak Restaurant is situated at the end of the hiking trail, on the opposite side of the road near the bridge which connects Selime and Yaprakhisar. You can stop by there for dinner and afterwards be chauffeured to your sleeping quarters by the young tourist entrepreneur Beytulla. Your tour should be planned in a way that you can take the bus to the end or to the beginning of the valley in the morning, as the last bus already leaves at 7.00 or 5.00 in the afternoon, according to season, and is mostly totally crowded. During the day and in the week, the Aksaray-Ihlara bus leaves every hour.

Selime

The town itself cannot exactly be called really beautiful. But it has a large dwelling rock with an interesting church complex high up above the valley. You reach the platform with the old cave churches over hazardous footpaths and through a system of tunnels and you have a magnificent view from here. On the opposite side you see the counterpart of this dwelling rock, which belongs to the commune of Yaprakhisar. But this complex has not been made open to the public yet. Below the old Selime dwelling complex there is the tomb of a Seljuk sultan. Perhaps he was not very popular among the people; at any rate, many bricks were used for building it. Other monumental tombs from that time were always built of massive stone and are therefore often preserved better.

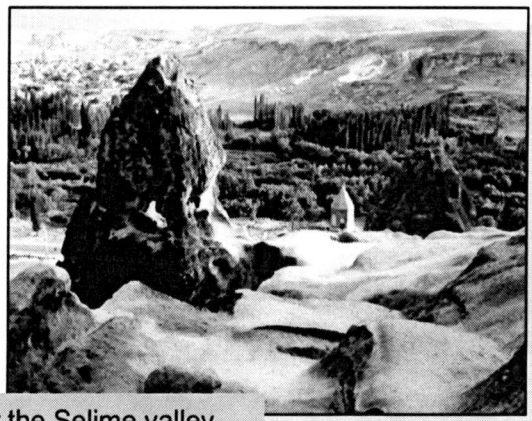

View over the Selime valley

The Çatlak Inn is the only acceptable accommodation in Selime. The 18 double rooms are very plush according to Turkish custom, but they are large and clean. It is 60 TL for two persons, with breakfast, hot beverages all day and free internet access.

For campers, there is an area behind the Çatlak Restaurant near the bridge between Selime and Yaprakhisar available. It is 10 TL a night, with free electricity and hot drinks all day.

For information see: www.catlakturizm.com.tr

Places for your own notices........

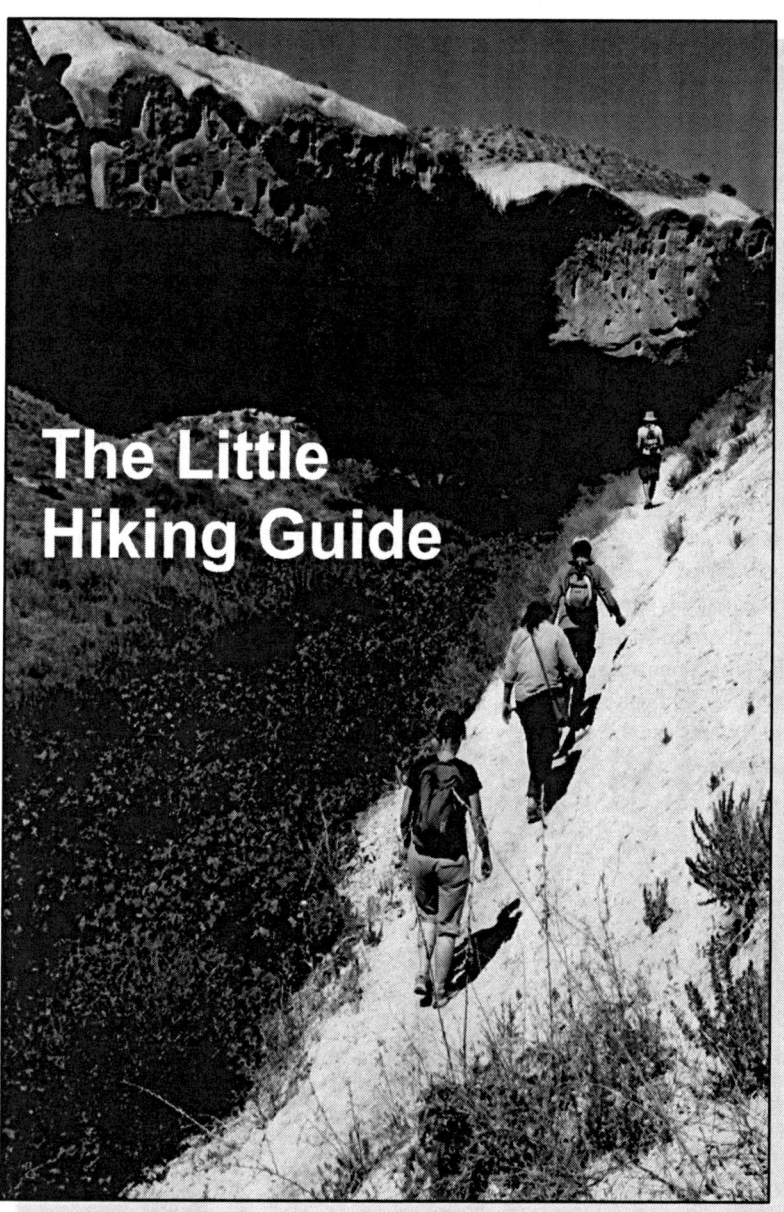

Foto: Uwe Schmitz

Some Words in Advance

Here in the 4th part of this travel guide you will now find some hiking routes which we have explored for you.

As we have already described in the chapter on "walking", we want to point out to you again that the roads and footpaths that wind through the valleys are often very narrow. You should abstain from doing the hiking tours described here if you do not feel steady on your feet, as there is no mountain rescue service in Cappadocia. Unfortunately, the National Park administration still has not managed to mark the hiking routes. The few colour spray markings are often quite contradictory or have been destroyed by erosion and originate from the commitment of the local tourism companies. However, wooden signs have meanwhile been put up at the start and the end points of the hiking routes.

We advise special caution on the narrow paths after heavy rain. The tuff grit on the paths will then change into a slippery mass on which you will find only little support. After rainy days you should change your plans and do the hikes uphill, though this makes orientation more difficult. All hiking routes – except route 3A – are described in a downhill direction.

Finally, a remark on the times given for the various routes. Of course the time needed for one of the walks can vary considerably individually. Our statements can therefore only serve as indications and should not be taken too literally.

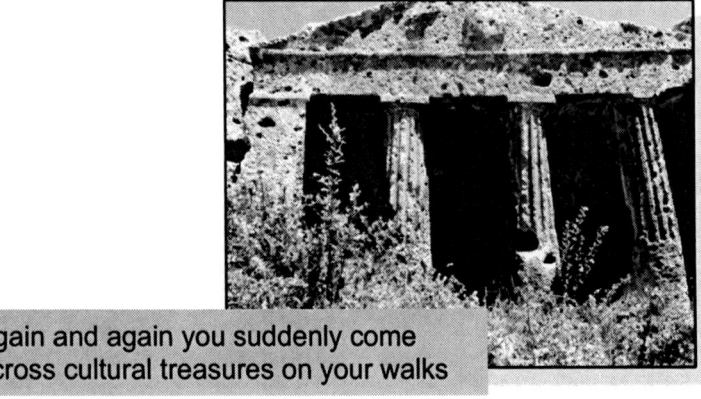

Again and again you suddenly come across cultural treasures on your walks

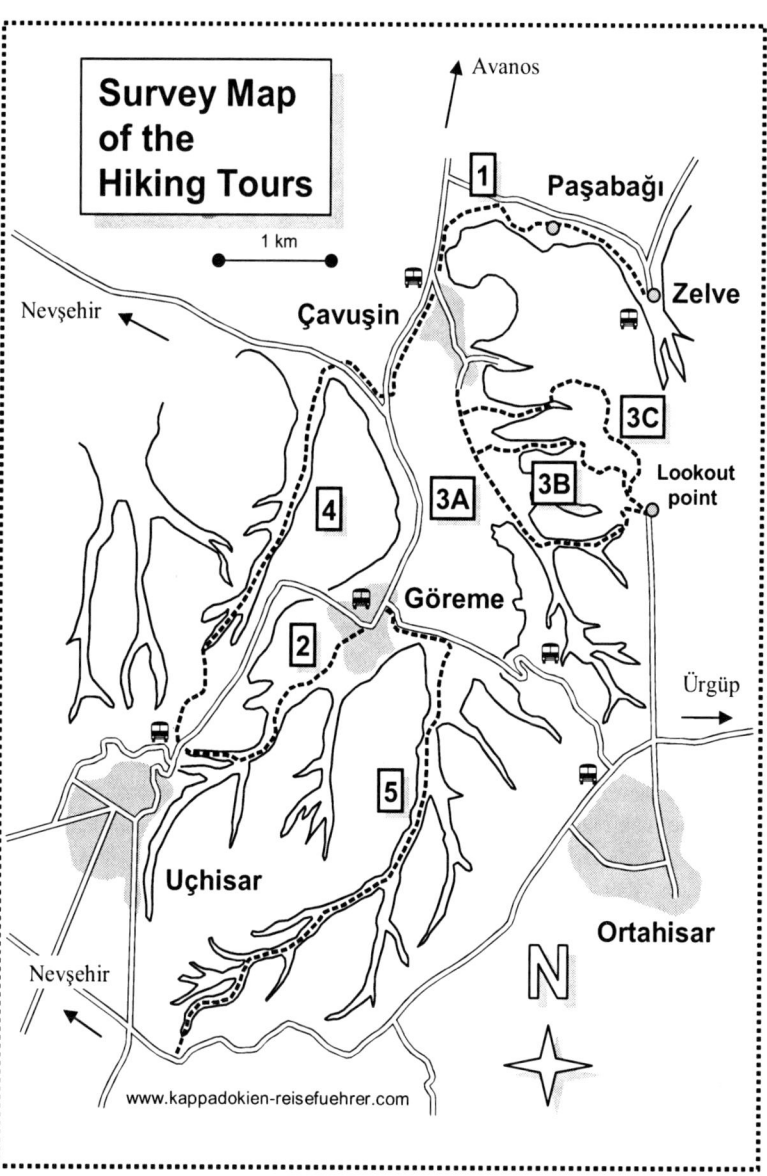

Tour 1:

Çavuşin – Paşabağı – Zelve

This 1 to 1,5 hours tour is meant to accustom the inexperienced hiker to the paths and beaten tracks that are typical of Cappadocia. You find all levels of difficulty here which are also found in the large valleys. If this walk is too difficult for anybody, he will always be able to return to the road which accompanies the path at a varying distance. Even though orientation is a little more difficult than in the valleys, nobody can lose his way here. On your right are the steep walls of the table mountain, which cannot be surmounted by hikers, and on your left there is the road leading from Çavuşin via Paşabağı to Zelve. A small hint: begin your walk rather early in the day, as there are only a few shady places on this route.

The route begins in front of the church at the town limit of Çavuşin and first runs almost parallel, as a wide sand track, to the road leading north to Avanos and then slowly turns to the east in a wide arc. This first section is not particularly challenging, as far as the walking capacity and the countryside are concerned. After about 10 to 15 minutes, and about 100 m before you reach the Zelve road, a driveway forks off to the south on the right side. It winds towards the south and towards the east for a while, gradually getting closer to a mountain in the south, or rather, a rock promontory of this mountain. But before you reach this rock wall, you arrive at a large level space. From there, a beaten path forks off left again towards the east and runs round some rock chimneys and up a small hill. On the top you walk across a small ruined wall, a little down the hill, and then left again along the small valley in a northern direction. You walk along among fairy chimneys, and in front of one that looks as if it has been turned into a spiral, a path leads off on the right and then up the white tuff wall. This path requires some climbing on the crumbly rock. The route is a little longer, but easier instead, if you ignore the fork and keep to the narrow driveway north for about 150 m, and only then turn into a little path on the right side. Doing this, you walk round the chain of hills running from north to south, then get closer to the road again after about 50 m, then cross a broad farm track and reach the hill above Paşabağı. Here we meet the climbers again. Now you cross the Paşabağı valley from west to east on a paved road, walking past the Simeon's Tower,

Hiking Guide 309

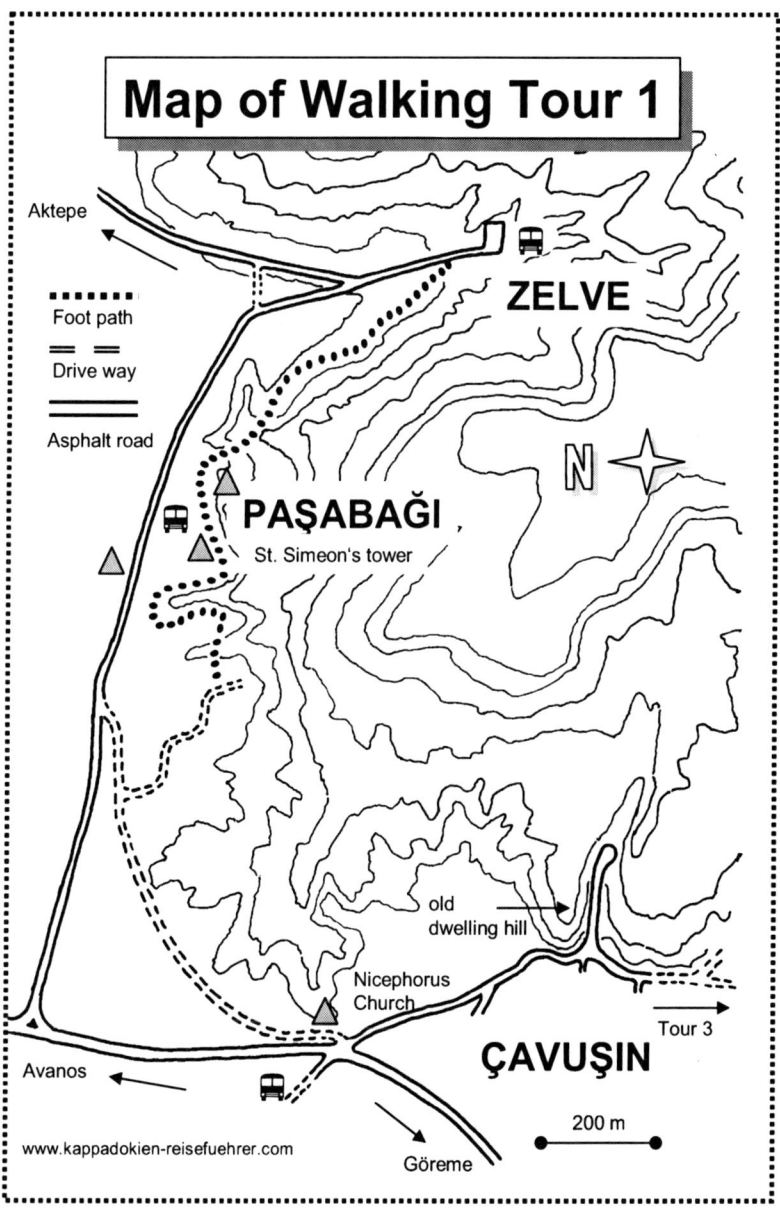

which can be identified by the many souvenir stalls around it. East of Paşabağı, right above the road, a little path runs up a hill again and then towards the south-east, across a wide plain of large soft tuff slabs. Here the path peters out a little, but its further course can be seen in the distance. It crosses a driveway and you walk past the ruins of an old quarry on your left. The flat stone slabs were beaten out of the ground here, and it also can be seen that grooves were carved around the slabs first in order to split the slabs off with wedges afterwards.

The road disappears from your view again, the path turning south, following the shape of the mountain. Walking through vineyards and past fairy chimneys, you arrive at the museum village of Zelve soon after, including the offshoots of its touristic infrastructure.

If this tour is too short for you, you can easily turn it into a day trip. Coming from Göreme or Avanos, you go to Çavuşin by bus and visit its decaying old town, then walk to Paşabağı, where you should take your time to walk around among the fairy chimneys. Then you continue to Zelve on the described route, and if you still have not had your fill there, you rummage through the local old museum village. Finally, you return towards Göreme or Avanos by dolmush again. - The descriptions of the towns of Çavuşin, Paşabağı and Zelve are in the chapters of the same name, and the bus departures are on page 110.

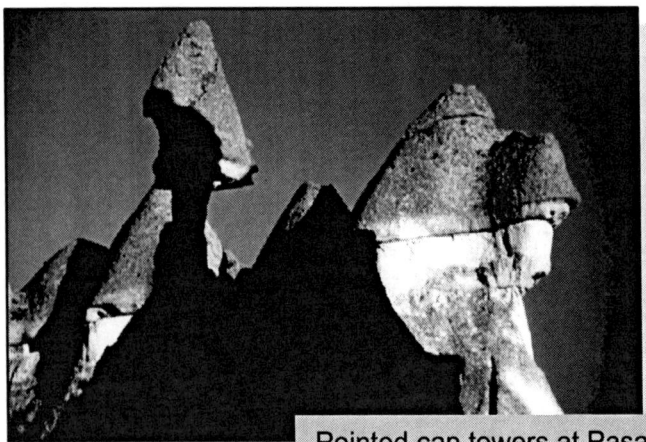
Pointed cap towers at Paşabağı

Tour 2:

Uçhisar – Pigeon Valley – Göreme

The hiking route through the lower part of the Pigeon Valley consists of the traditional old footpath between the two villages of Uçhisar and Göreme. Orientation is very easy, as the path is well-beaten and it follows the valley downwards. The red signs, which were once put up, are only rarely seen here, however.

The tour begins at the Özel Center Artisanal at the asphalt road from Göreme to Uçhisar, where the bus stops on demand. From there you walk down the little cobblestone road leading up to Uçhisar for about 150 m, until a paved walkway forks off it in front of the first fairy chimney on the left. This walkway now leads down into a valley and after about 50 m narrows to a footpath. Shortly after, it runs towards a dune-like rock wall on the left. You are alright here, although the path now seems to be somewhat overgrown with bushes and small trees, and you only have to follow the well-beaten path. A little spring with a reservoir for refreshment is situated on the right side (but please do not drink the water).

Soon after, the path descends along the rock wall on the right, down a steep slope. The path forks after 15 minutes of walking. On the left it runs into a tunnel, which soon ends, though. These are the remains of an old irrigation canal, which was cut through the rocks more than 1000 years ago. If one continues towards the right side, the path goes more and more downhill, and the course of the former canal is now clearly visible in the rock wall on the left. Meanwhile the valley widens and after 20 minutes you reach the bottom of the Pigeon Valley, which extends in an east-western direction. Be so kind as to look out for tourists who are looking for a way down from the top of the steep rock face on the right. Please warn those people, for there is no such path. There is only a steep wall of about 20 m here, which has already claimed several victims in the past.

From now on there are two options for continuing your walk. Either you follow the valley down to the bottom, or you turn to the left earlier and walk along the rock wall a little above the valley floor level. Both routes meet again after about 10 minutes. If you choose option 1, the path goes down to the bottom of the Pigeon Valley across a small rock – and here the seat of your trousers might have to be used for the first time. The path forks again

Hiking Guide

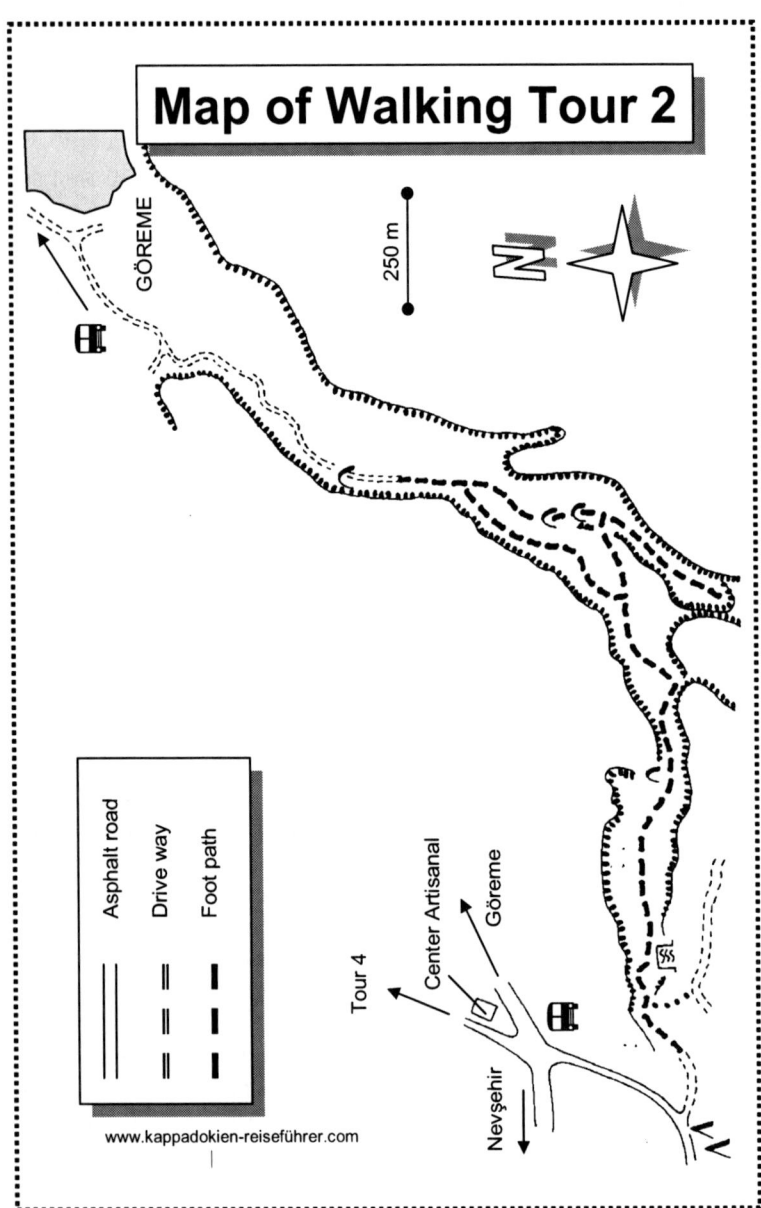

now. On the right, you walk up the Pigeon Valley through old canal tunnels, until after about 10 minutes the path ends in front of a waterfall, which is about 30 m high. But it is only really spectacular in spring or in autumn. On the right, the path runs towards Göreme through several tunnels, then merges with option 2 and soon widens to driveway size. After a few more minutes, another larger valley comes from the right. Next there follows a broad tunnel which has been enlarged for tractors, and after a 30-minute walk the valley becomes very wide. Five minutes later you reach the edge of Göreme near the "Gümüş Kave Hotel". Walking along the broad canal on the left, you reach the town centre of Göreme after another 5 to 10 minutes, where the bus picks the weary hiker up again.

As this tour is very short, it is well-suited for visiting the towns of Uçhisar and Göreme on the same day. If you are coming from Uçhisar, you just follow the little cobblestone road down the eastern slope of the settlement and turn off into the footpath described above at the last fairy chimney in front of the asphalt road. This tour can also be done up the valley without any problems, as you will hardly lose your way here.

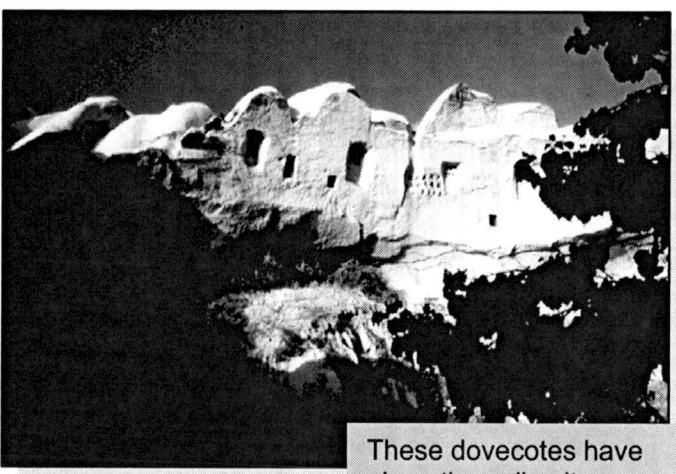

These dovecotes have given the valley its name

Tour 3 A:

Çavuşin - Lookout point

This tour already takes a little longer and belongs to the ones most frequently done in the region. This means that you will occasionally meet larger groups as well. They are transported by coach to the lookout point, the highest point of this route, and are picked up again at Çavuşin. Some kiosks for drinks or even picnic gardens by the wayside are evidence of an increased amount of tourists. But this should not keep you from making this tour.
It is a peculiarity of this tour that, in contrast to all the other tour descriptions in this book, it goes uphill. Thus you are able to return to your starting point either on route 3B or 3C - which means, you are able to make a round trip.
The start is at the bus stop in Çavuşin. You cross the village and go slightly to the right at the foot of the ruined old town. At the end of the village a dusty cart track leads through the graveyard and runs south-east towards the mouth of a wide valley. After about 350 m you turn slightly left, continue in the same direction and ignore the following junctions with the signs indicating the ways to Güllüdere (Rose Valley). The first third of the tour is not very spectacular or demanding, as you always walk straight along the dusty driveway. After a while you reach the first short tunnel. The valley forks 50 m behind it, and you turn left. After 50 more metres a little footpath forks off towards a rather large cave complex. This short detour is definitely worthwhile, as the caves are distributed over several floors and there is a magnificent view over the valley from the top floor. In one of the back rooms is an old shaft of a well, which extends deep down into the rock. On the first floor is an old water channel which runs along the external wall of the rock and which, like all rooms that can be recognized from outside, was previously hidden from the gaze of strangers in the rock. Daring hikers reach the crest of the hill, which is high above the valley, over a steep staircase. Back on the walkway, you reach another tunnel after 100 m, and you walk through it. Here you find the remains of old route signs in the form or red arrows painted on the rock. The path narrows and begins to become overgrown here. The wall rises steeply on the left and you walk through a third tunnel. After this the valley divides and and you keep fully to the left, where you have to cross another tunnel. Only a few yards behind it you reach a tea garden, which you can use for a short break, or not, as unfortunately it is

Hiking Guide 315

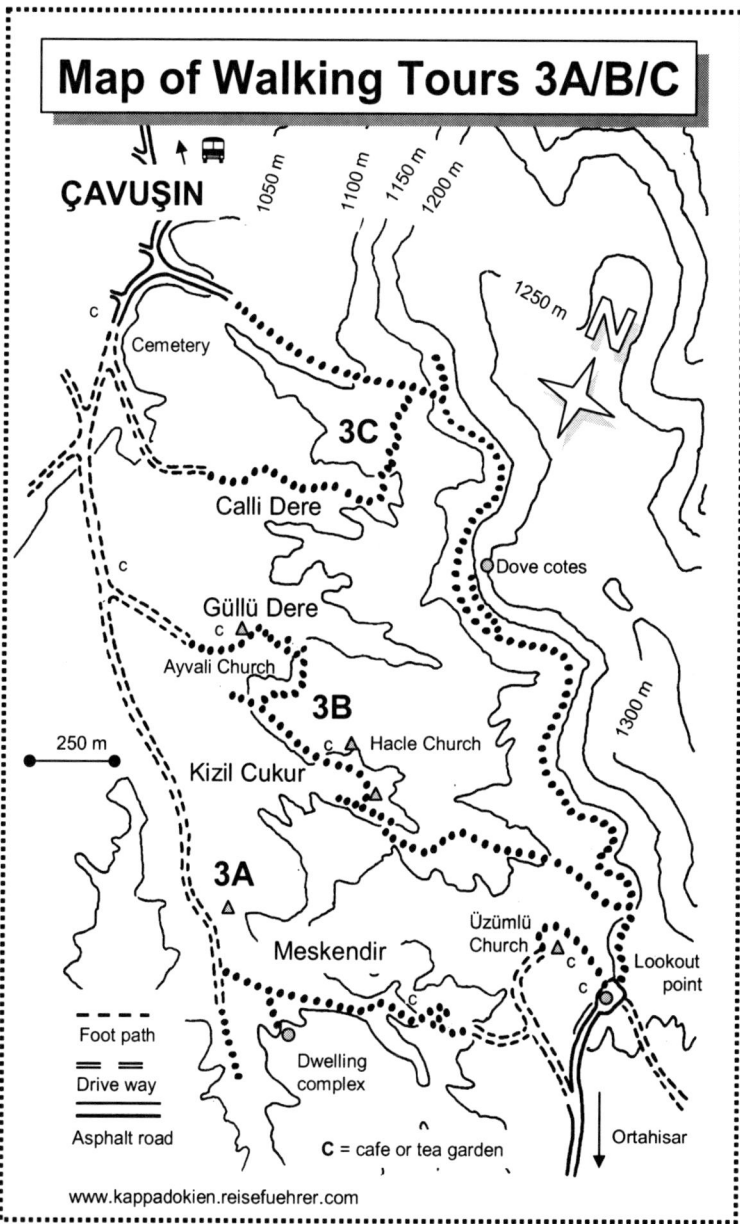

seldom open. Now the path runs past a fruit orchard and steeply up the hill in serpentines and onto a first plateau. The high safety fences along the way are not really integrated harmoniously into the landscape, but they are really helpful for people who suffer from vertigo. Up above here, we best turn our gaze east-southeast first and discover the lookout point at a distance of about 300 m. Now we follow the walkway, which has meanwhile broadened to driveway size, and turn off into another wide driveway. A sign indicates the Üzümlü Kilise (Grape Church), where we arrive after only 100 m. Beside this church, which is closed with an iron grille, there is another tea garden. At the church you follow the path, which is now becoming narrower again, contrary to the existing route signs. First, some loose stones serve as a climbing aid, later on, segments of wooden beams, which have been nailed onto the path. At the sign to the Kizil Cukur (Red Pit) Valley you have reached the lookout point, and therefore you now deserve a cold drink. Up here, you are again surprised by the much-loved souvenir stands with their variety of goods. The running time is circa 1 to 1,5 hours.

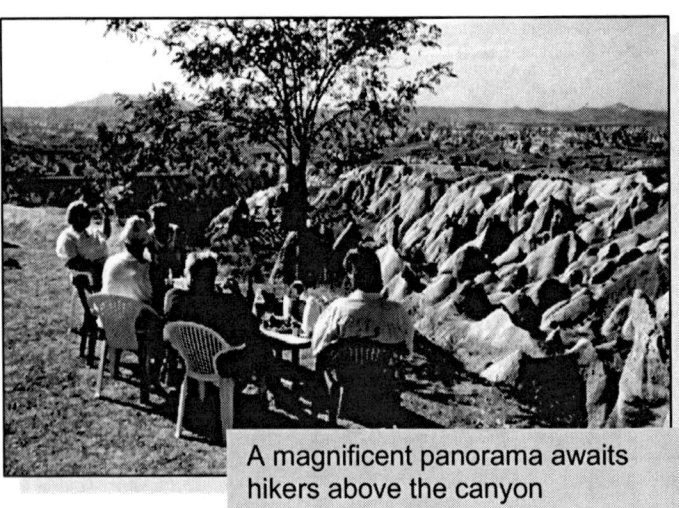

A magnificent panorama awaits hikers above the canyon

Tour 3 B:

Lookout point – Güllüdere - Çavuşin

This alternative return route from tour 3A belongs to the most interesting hiking routes in all Cappadocia, as several cave churches are situated by the roadside, and erosion has left an especially manifold variety of forms and colours behind. Most of the path is considerably simpler to go than tour 3C, and it leads through numerous rock cones at a medium height for quite some time. Tours 3B and 3C are only two options which you can choose between and which are situated between the rock wall on your right and the valley of tour 3A on your left. Numerous small paths cross the area from the lookout point towards Cavusin and beyond. Losing one's way is impossible here. But many paths take you back again to the initial dusty track of tour 3A very soon, following the diagonal valleys.

From the lookout point you follow the signs to the Güllüdere slightly uphill. But the path forks already after about 50 m. Tour 3C goes straight ahead, along the rock wall. Our path now first goes through tuff hills and then follows a water channel downhill on the left. Down in the valley on the left side are the Üzümlü Kilise and the path which brought us up here on tour 3A. On the right, there is a valley basin with many red rock cones. We continue along the mountain crest until the path takes a little turn and descends to a lower level. On the right are the remains of an old safety fence and the path is steep and slippery again. The rocks are particularly colourful here in this high valley: red, yellow and green are the predominant colours, and they are often combined in one and the same cone. The path divides after about 30 minutes. Straight on it leads deep down into a valley, into the Kizil Cukur (Red Pit), and our path continues at middle height around a rock cone to the right, and towards the Rose Valley. A short time later we reach a ruined cave church, which makes a nice place for a rest. Right next to it are two rather large dwelling cones. Now the path winds slightly up and down again, through tuff structures and past a rock on the left with particularly colourful stripes. In the valley on the right side some cave dwellings can be seen again, which the path leads to. In doing this, it first bypasses this small side valley. On the right hand side now appears the Flintstone Café with an attached souvenir shop. This is a good place for resting and for also visiting the Haclı-Kilise with its frescoes. The manager of the café is in charge of the key. If you are shocked by the high prices, you should remember that the good man has to haul everything up here on his back. There are some more open rooms above the church room, through which you can take a look into the neighbouring valley. The path winds on through the tuff hills, and after about 50 minutes of walking you reach another mountain ridge from where you can already see the old dwelling cone of Cavusin in the distance. We do not follow the path along the mountain, but make a 180° turn to the right and walk though a small gentle valley again. After an hour we are standing at the edge of the Rose Valley, which is deep below us. The path goes uphill close to the precipice of the valley for only about 20 m, when the steep way down into the valley begins. The place where this section, which is not easy to walk through, extends is marked with red arrows. Special attention is requested here in order not to begin to slide. Those who have reached the floor of the valley with great relief now walk through a vine orchard and towards the bed of the brook. Now and again it is rather moist here and very green, too. If you want to, you can visit another church now, the Ayvalı-Kilise, followed by another rest in the café attached to it. If you prefer not to do this, you walk slightly down the valley through the old irrigation system. After a short time you reach a brick archway, which in former times served as a viaduct for irrigation. The next tunnel shows excellently how a man-made canal has turned into a natural riverbed. The old rectangular shape has been preserved in the ceiling, whereas the brook has dug its wide and rugged bed in the lower part. Unfortunately we must pass by this tunnel, as its end is overgrown and the way down is a little too steep. The path widens, the first vehicle tracks become visible, and now it continues below the rock wall on the left.

In the rock wall on the right, another larger complex of cave dwellings with the remains of a church can be seen; it is accessible over a slippery rock. The valley widens after this, and isolated rock cones appear in the middle of it. After a good 1,5 hours, you reach the main path to Çavuşin again, and you keep to the right. This route also leads from the village to the lookout point on tour 3A.

The total walking time to the bus stop in the village is between 2 and 2,5 hours.

Tour 3 C:

Lookout Point – Çavuşin

This tour is another option of walking back from hike 3 A. As an alternative to this route, you can walk the 2 km of asphalt road to the crossroads above Ortahisar and stop the bus there. Those who have their lodgings in Ürgüp only need to follow the driveway on the other side of the lookout point and will reach the town automatically. This path is very easy to walk, but unfortunately also less interesting.
Walking route 3C requires a little more skill and, above all, being free from fear of heights, as it runs close to the escarpment for a long time. The path already has a rather Alpine character; it is crossed by dry water channels and often has a slight tilt towards the valleys. Although much surefootedness is necessary here, there are mountainbike tracks which facilitate orientation. It is simply inexplicable to us how anybody can ride a bicycle up here.
The route begins like route 3B, which means that you follow the signs to the Güllüdere slightly uphill. However, the path already divides after 50 m. We walk straight ahead, along the reddish eastern rock wall on the right. The path winds round some large protruding rock outcrops for some time, which have been visible since we left the lookout point. The first of them has a red and white windsleeve on its top and the path follows the slope down to the third one. There is no fork for a long time, and you keep following the narrow path which passes by the many little side valleys on the left. After about 30 minutes, the path forks almost unremarkably. Straight on, the route first runs across a little hilltop and then, after 50 m, to a half-collapsed cave complex. This is where the turnoff ends, but the caves make a nice shady resting place. Our path forks off slightly to the left a little earlier, following the rock wall on a lower level. A little deeper on the left there is an interesting rock formation, which shows well how the fairy chimneys and rock cones 'calve' out of the mountain. Next to it, two perforated dwelling cones rise in the valley. The first dovecotes can be seen again in the rock wall above the path, and after a little more than an hour the road forks. We now see Çavuşin down in the valley. On the right the path continues to Paşabağı, half-right there is a narrow path which leads to the village, and on the left you now follow the path towards another valley. Descending fast, the path winds through the relics of eroded rock cones of which only stumps have remained. After a

short time you reach the valley floor of the Calli Dere with its little dry brook bed. With the exception of the first tunnel, which must be bypassed, you now follow this little riverbed all the way down the valley through several tunnels. On your right is a steep white rock wall with many dovecotes in it, the path running along below it. The valley widens and the first tractor tracks are visible on the driveway, which has become wider. Then the last tunnel follows, and the driveway winds through the level mouth of the valley.

After about 1.5 hours and almost in front of the cemetery, we reach the main route to Çavuşin again. Here we keep to the right and reach the village.

This walk takes about 2 to 2,5 hours all the way up to the bus stop. The bus to Göreme leaves from it at 15 minutes past and the one to Avanos at 20 minutes past every full hour.

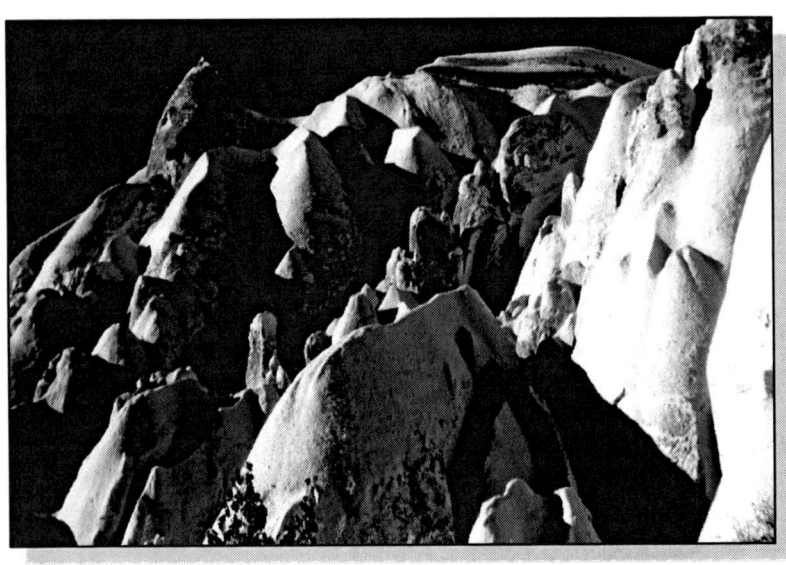

Tour 4:

Uçhisar – Aşkedere – Çavuşin

This route leads through the so-called 'Love Valley' (Aşk Dere), which begins below Uçhisar and ends a little west of the Çavuşin–Göreme road. You need about 1.5 to 2 hours for this tour. Some difficult sections have to be overcome, where one or other hikers will have to slide downhill on all fours. But basically, the path is easy to find, and it always goes downhill. The valley was probably named 'love valley' because there are numerous rock cones at its end whose shapes allow much room for speculation. The different layers of colour in the rocks can also be recognized quite easily in this valley. The attentive observer will also notice layers with sedimentary inclusions, which date back to a time when Cappadocia was still partly covered by a lakeland area.

The tour begins again at the Artisanal Center, where also tour 2 starts. But this time we turn to the north and first follow the dusty track for about 300 m. There, another rock path forks off left, which you leave again after a short time and turn right on a footpath. This now goes down into the valley and follows the steep western slope. Another valley joins from the right and the path forks after a few minutes. Walkers now keep left, climbing fans turn to the right, for it is the same thing with the valley as it is with Rome: all routes lead into it. But the hiking route, too, goes rather steeply downhill now, and the first possibility of a glissade comes along. On we go through overgrown gardens and through undergrowth. Just follow the valley from now on, with the frequent possibility of choosing between two paths. Again, a large valley comes from the right. If you have chosen the upper route, hikers now have a magnificent view over both valleys and the surrounding rock walls. Shortly after, you have to choose again, the lower path leading quite dangerously through a narrow and half-decayed, but very long system of canals. Part of the tunnel system can only be crossed in a duck-walk, as the sediments carried along by the little brook have been deposited on the bottom here. Some time later the path goes no further, and you have to follow the main path on the surface again. Another valley opens on the right side, bringing a very wide, but decayed canal system with it. Here, too, you can either follow the tunnel fragments again or choose the path above them through the gardens. After a rather long distance you arrive

322 Hiking Guide

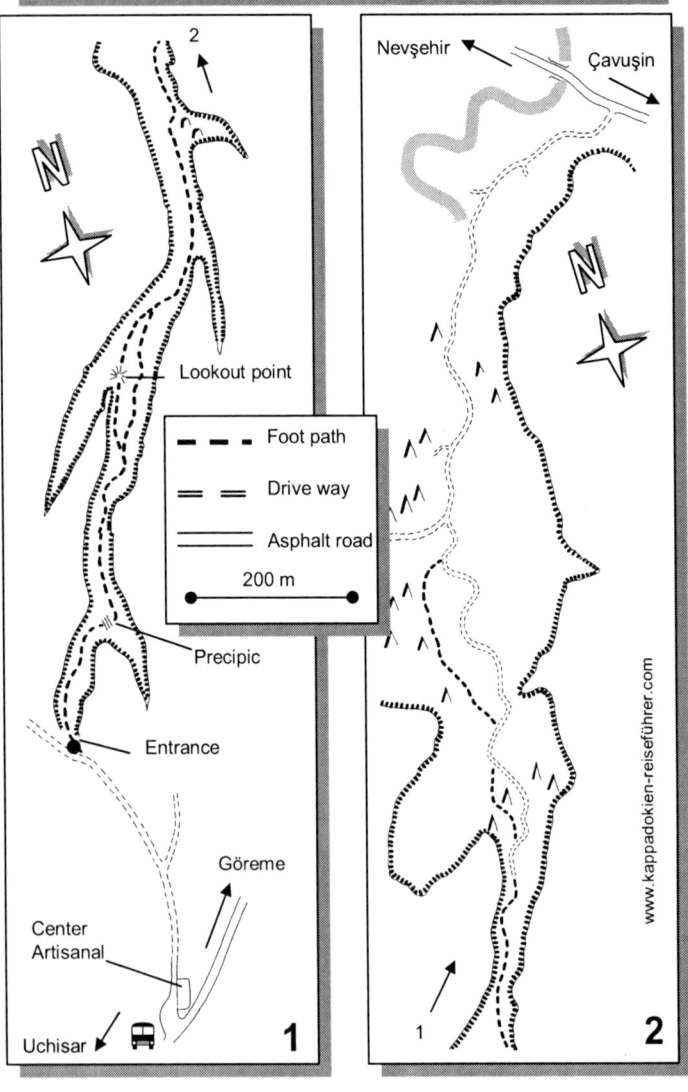

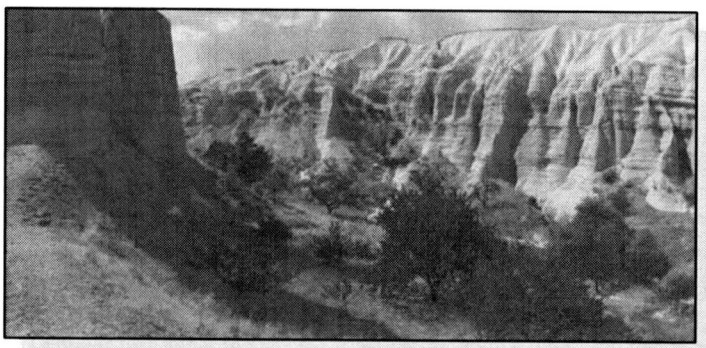

at an open, but very narrow canal. This must be walked through in order to reach the beginning of the driveway after a few meters. The gardens are in regular use again from here on, and there is also some garbage lying about. The valley gradually begins to widen, and for short parts of the route you can continue on footpaths above the driveway. In any case you should not miss the detour to the large fairy chimneys, which are said to have given the valley its name. The valley ends at the asphalt road which leads to the main road from Göreme to Çavuşin. Here you walk towards the right side for 100 m and then turn left again on a cart track that leads to the main road. Having arrived at the main road, you cross it and then choose between entering Çavuşin or taking the direct way to the bus stop. Straight ahead through the fields you enter the village, whereas on the left you follow the road directly to the bus stop. The bus from Avanos to Nevşehir stops at the beginning and at the end of this tour. Please tell the driver early enough where you want to get off, as otherwise he will drive right on, and then tour 4 will become a little longer for you.

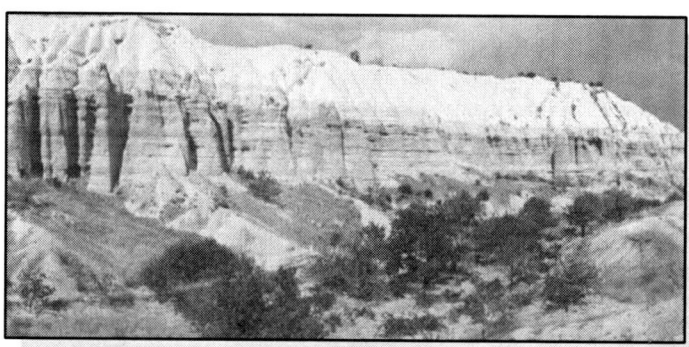

Tour 5:

Zemidere

This hike takes somewhat longer and requires more attention in terms of orientation. Besides, the way downhill though the valley is interspersed with some difficult passages. We would not recommend an uphill walk in this case, as some obstacles can only be overcome with a slide. The entrance to the valley is not so closely connected to the bus service system either this time. It can only be reached by taxi from Göreme or Uçhisar or by the Ürgüp – Nevşehir bus line. But all this should not deter you from a walk through one of the most impressive valleys of this region. However, a walking time of 2 to 3 hours on a partly narrow and bumpy path must be expected.

The entrance is about 750 m from the most eastern crossroads of Uçhisar in the direction to Ürgüp on the main road from Ürgüp to Nevşehir. When you see a souvenir stall in a left-hand bend of this road, you have found the entrance into the valley. The path initially runs swiftly down on stairs beaten into the rock. It winds narrowly through dry undergrowth and leads towards a first tunnel. You must turn left here, as there is a sheer drop behind the tunnel. Steep rock walls rise to the sky on both sides of the path. Soon a little riverbed with a tunnel system appears on the right, and on the left you can distinguish a rather large cave complex in the rock wall. The riverbed changes sides after about 10 minutes of walking time, and you reach a little spring which is enclosed in the mountain, with a twisted hollow willow tree next to it. The path continues through an old birch grove, in which you can find the first trail signs in the form of red dots, and then reaches an overhanging cliff on the left. The path now runs through here and follows the cliff along an old canal system and up to a tunnel with a rather low ceiling. But this can be bypassed on a little path, and the following tunnels are not so low any more. After a good half hour you reach a driveway which comes straight down from the plateau and even runs through another tunnel. Shortly behind this tunnel you leave the driveway again and keep right, following the rock wall. After some time another driveway crosses, which we follow only briefly towards the right.

Meanwhile the valley widens a little. Half hidden on the left, there is a watering place above the path, and here you follow the narrow footpath again. Soon the first slide follows: about 2 m steeply down the path, then the

Hiking Guide 325

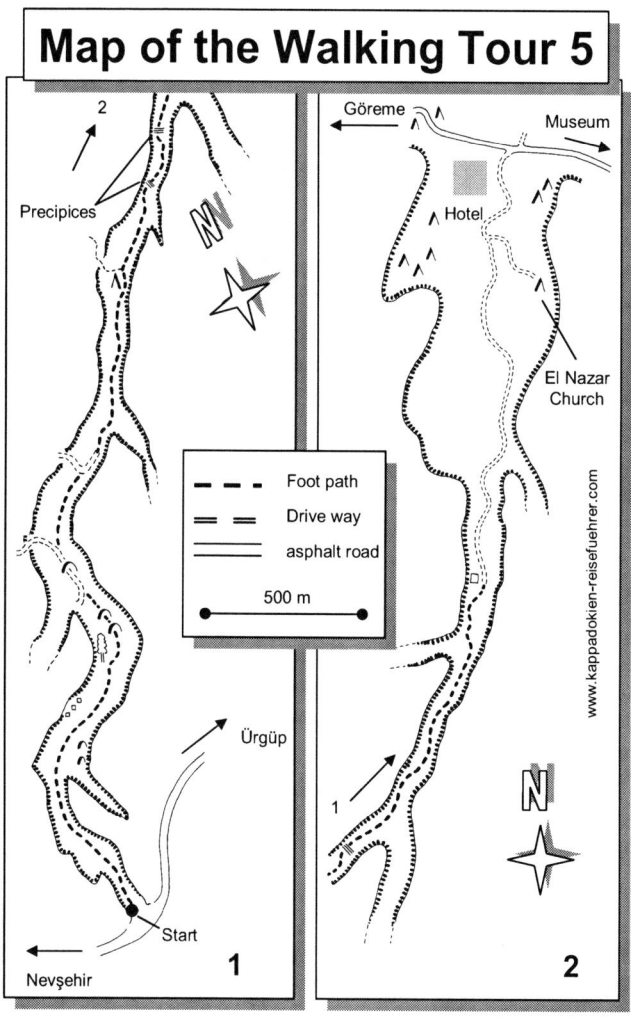

valley gets narrower again, and shortly after that you slide down again for about 3 m. Near an isolated medium-sized rock on the left side of the path, a walkway forks off in its direction. But this path leads out of the valley again, and so you have to follow the inconspicuous path straight ahead. If you happen to see a crossed-out red dot, you are wrong. You continue on narrow paths through overgrown gardens, and after circa 50 minutes you reach some large boulders that barricade the valley but can be passed. On stairs made of logs you walk deeper and deeper into the narrow and rather moist valley, which is covered with dense vegetation here. Shortly after this we reach the most difficult part of this tour: the path becomes very narrow, leads past a deep crevice and follows a dry water channel steeply down for about 5 m. Here at the very least, crawling on all fours becomes necessary, and extreme caution is required. But this has been the last obstacle to be overcome. The old wooden boardwalk construction which formerly used to secure the precipice has unfortunately been washed away. We continue our way through the very narrow, poplar-grown valley, and the first half of the route is behind us.

The path forks once again; we have to keep left again, and soon it traverses a collapsed tunnel with water in it. A valley comes from the right, and the path continues down the valley on the left side. A little hidden on the left side of the path, there is a rather large system of tunnels which after rains carries red ferruginous water. You reach a little rivulet, which you follow for some time and through several tunnels. After about 1 hour and 20 minutes, another small valley comes from the left, and you keep following the course of the brook. On both sides of the valley the cliffs now rise, both steeply and curved (reminding one of cream topping) and there follows another tunnel which has to be crossed. The path widens into a driveway, and on the left there is a garden fenced in with concrete posts. The valley generally widens, the gardens are cultivated again, and on the right some cave complexes can be seen in the cliff. Several picnic areas with old fireplaces are situated by the wayside, and a garden fenced in with stone walls appears on the left; it is accessible over a rickety wooden footbridge. The patterned arch stones are noteworthy here; but unfortunately, they have been distributed wildly, arbitrarily and crudely in the brickwork. After little more than 90 minutes, another large side valley joins our hiking route from the right. Soon after, the valley becomes very wide and open, and scattered rock cones can be seen far ahead in the distance. Almost at the end of the valley a driveway forks off right to the El Nazar Church, after which the valley is sometimes named. From here it is not far to the road which connects the Göreme museum with the town of Göreme. Having arrived at this road, you turn left and, having walked through rock cones for 500 m, you reach the terminal of the buses to Nevşehir, Ürgüp or Avanos.

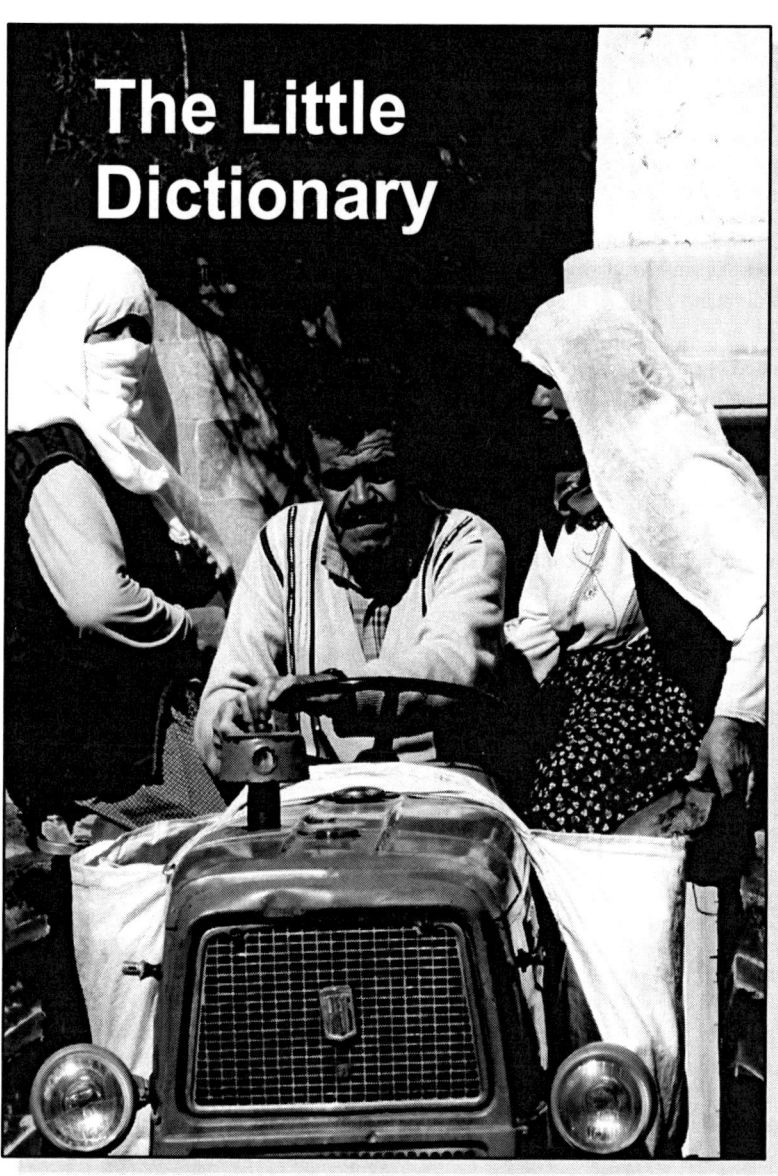

Foto: Johann Munker

At the end of this book we want to help you a little to cope verbally in Cappadocia. Turkish belongs to the Turkmen languages and is therefore significantly different from the Central European and Indogermanic / Romance languages. In Turkish grammar, all word forms are created by adding syllables, so-called suffixes, to the root word. If you studied Latin at school, you will know this type of word formation. The sentence structure is also completely different. This is especially noticeable when Turkish people have learned English words, but lack practical experience. In this case you understand them, but nevertheless the sentences sound rather strange. They just combine the English words the same way as they do in Turkish.

But do not worry, we do not want to dwell on Turkish grammar or sentence formation in detail, but only give you a little support in order to get along in the country.

The Letters

First, some Turkish letters that are different in English and their pronunciation:

Ç = CH   like in 'church'   (çorba - soup)

Ş = SH   as in 'show' or in 'fish'   (şehir – town)

I = [undotted i]   as in 'general'   (rakı – popular drink)

Ğ = **not** pronounced; lengthens preceding vowel
   slightly   as in 'pool'   (dağ – mountain)

C = J   as in 'jet' or 'Jimmy'   (cami – mosque)

H = initial and between two vowels:
   H   as in 'half'   (pastahane – pastry shop)
   after dark vowels: as in 'rachitis'   (kahvaltı – breakfast)
   after bright vowels: as in 'kitchen'   (tarih – story)

V = U if a 'A' before as in Mountain   (tavşan – rabbit)

Y = if a vowel before as in 'sister'   (kaytan – string)

Ü = like in french - 'musée'   (üç – three)

Ö = like in french - 'couleur' (dört - four)

The letters **X** and **W** do not exist in Turkish words.
There are **no 'silent' letters** in Turkish (except G, see above); also digraphs (sh, th, gh) are always pronounced as **two** consonants.

Numbers

1	bir	156	yüz elli altı
2	iki	200	iki yüz
3	üç	300	üç yüz
4	dört	400	dört yüz
5	beş	546	beş yüz kırk altı
6	altı	951	dokuz yüz elli bir
7	yedi	1.000	bin
8	sekiz	2.000	iki bin
9	dokuz	3.000	üç bin
10	on	5.800	beş bin sekiz yüz
11	on bir	10.000	on bin
12	on iki	100.000	yüz bin
20	yirmi	1.000.000	bir milyon
21	yirmi bir	1.000.000.000	bir milyar
22	yirmi iki		
30	otuz	½	yarım
40	kırk	1½	bir buçuk
50	elli	¼	Çeyrek
60	altmış		
70	yetmiş		
80	seksen	**first(ly)**	ilk olarak
90	doksan	**second(ly)**	ikince olarak
100	yüz	**last(ly)**	son

Weights and measures

liter	litre	second	saniye
gram(me)	gram	minute	dakika
kilogram(me)	kilo	hour	saat
metre	metre	day	gün
kilometer	kilometre	week	hafta
inch	inc	month	ay
foot	ayak	year	yıl / sene
mile	mil	century	yüzyıl

Days of the Week

Monday	pazartesi
Tuesday	salı
Wednesday	çarşamba
Thursday	perşembe
Friday	cuma
Saturday	cumartesi
Sunday	pazar

Months

January	ocak
February	şubat
March	mart
April	nisan
May	mayıs
June	haziran
July	temmuz
August	ağustos
September	eylül
Oktober	ekim
November	kasım
December	aralık

Other Time Expressions

today	bugün	later	sonra
yesterday	dün	erlier	önce
tomorrow	yarın	1 day later	bir gün sonra
before noon	sabah	all-day	bütün gün
at noon	öğleyin	daily	her gün
in the afternoon	öğleden sonra	during the day	gündüz
in the evening	akşamleyin	first	ilk
at night	gecede	last	son
		next	bir sonraki

Dimensions

little	az	much	çok
far	geniş	near	yakın
long	uzun	short	kısa
high	yüksek	low	alçak
broad, wide	enli	narrow	dar
thick	kalın	Thin	ince
tall	büyük	small	küçük

Colours

black	kara / siyah	red	kırmızı / kızıl
white	beyaz / ak	blue	mavi
green	yeşil	yellow	sarı

Question words

where	nerede	who	kim
when	ne zaman	from where	nereden
how much	kaç	where to	nereye
why	niçin	how	nasıl

Travelling

bus	otobüs	car	araba
minibus	minibüs /dolmuş	motorcycle	motosiklet
bus terminal	otogar/terminal	scooter	skuter
platform	peron	bicycle	bisiklet
non-smoker	sigara içmeyen	helmet	miğfer
seat	koltuk	horsecart	at arabası
stop	durak	lorry/truck	kamyon
ticket	bilet	filling station	petrol istasyonu
train	tren	full	full / doldurmak
station	tren istasyonu	tyres	lastik
sleeper car	yataklı vagon	air	hava
restaurant car	yemekli vagon	coolant	soğutma suyu
luggage	bagaj	oil	yağ

plane	uçak	battery	akü
airport	havaalanı	gas, fuel	petrol
tramway	tramvay	diesel	motorin
taxi	taksi	automechanic	oto tamircisi
entry	giriş	road map	yol haritası
departure	çıkış	crossroads	dörtyol
passport	pasaport	driver's licence	sürücü belgesi

Directions

straight on	dosdoğru	here	burada
right	sağda	there	orada
left	sol	this direction	bu yönde
back	geri	other direction	başka yönde
to the west	batıya	to the east	doğuya
to the north	kuzeye	to the south	güneye

Accommodation and Camping

hotel	otel	camping ground	kamp yeri
inn	pansiyon	tent	çadır
room	oda	camper van	karavan
single room	tek yataklı oda	drinking water	içme suyu
cave room	mağara odası	washing machine	çamaşır makinesi
shower	duş	cooker	ocak
bed	yatak	kitchen	mutfak
door	kapı	garbage	çöp
refrigerator	buzdolabı	electricity	elektrik
heating	kalorifer	shade	gölge
lighting/lamp	lamba	swimming pool	yüzme havuzu
telephone	telefon	TV set	televizyon
vermin	haşarat	breakfast	kahvaltı
bedclothes	yatak çarşafı	toilet	tuvalet
towel	havlu	toilet paper	tuvalet kağıdı
hot water	sıcak su	key	anahtar

Bank and Post Office

bank	banka	letter	mektup
money	para	stamp	posta pulu
exchange	değiştirmek	postcard	kartpostal
check	çek	packet/parcel	paket
exchange rate	kambiyo kuru	telegram	telgraf
dollar	dolari	telephone card	telefon kartı

Eat and Drink

eat	yemek	vegetables	sebze
drink / smoke	içmek	salad	salata
restaurant	restoran/lokanta	sweets	tatlı
waiter	garson	ice cream	dondurma
tip	bahşiş	fruit	meyve
breakfast	kahvaltı	sugar	şeker
lunch	öğle yemeği	salt	tuz
supper	akşam yemeği	pepper	biber
bread	ekmek	vinegar	sirke
butter	tereyağı	olive oil	zeytin yağı
honey	bal	toothpick	kürdan
jam	reçel	napkin	peçete
egg	yumurta	coffee	kahve
cheese	peynir	tea	çay
soup	çorba	milk	süt
starter	meze	water	su
meat	et	mineral water	maden suyu
chicken	tavuk	Fruit juice	meyve suyu
fish	balık	Yogurt drink	ayran
rice	pilav	beer	bira
potatoes	patates	red wine	kırımızı şarap
wheat semolina	bulgur	white wine	beyaz şarap
garlic	sarmısak	aniseed brandy	rakı
warm	sıcak	sweet	şekerli / tatlı
cold	soğuk	sour	ekşi
hot	açık	very delicious	çok lezzetli

Countryside and Buildings

mountain	dağ	canyon	boğaz
valley	dere	rock	kaya
river	ırmak	stone	taş
hill	tepe	cave	mağara
lake	göl	forest	orman
tree	ağaç	spring	çeşme
castle	kale	house	ev
palace	saray	old town	eski şehir
monument	anıt	bridge	köprü
fort	hisar	town	şehir
village	köy	church	kilise
market	pazar	mosque	cami
square	meydan	town hall	belediye
ruin	harabe	school	okul
borough	mahalle	town centre	şehir merkezi
street	cadde / sokak	way	yol
monastery	manastır	undergr. town	yeraltı şehri

Weather

sky	gök	snow	kar
clouds	bulut	ice	buz
sun	güneş	dust	toz
moon	ay	wind	rüzgar
star	yıdız	storm	fırtına
rain	yağmur	heat	sıcaklık

Animals

dog	köpek	scorpion	akrep
cat	kedi	moscito	sivrisinek
bird	kuş	fly	sinek
horse	at	wasp	yabanarısı
donkey	eşek	roach	hamamböceği
sheep	koyun	mouse	fare
goat	keçi	chicken	tavuk

Emergencies

hospital	hastane	police	polis
ambulance	hastane araba	theft	hırsızlık
doctor	doktor	fraud	dolandırıcılık
dentist	diş hekimi	accident	kaza
pain	acı	fire	yangın
anaesthesia	anestezi	fire service	itfaiye
medicine	ilaç	lost	kayıp
stitch	sokma	passport	pasaport
wound, injury	yara	drivers licence	sürücü belgesi
ointment	merhem	registration	taşıt belgeleri
bandage	pansuman	consulate	konsolosluğu
plaster	plaster	help	yardım

Common Signs

open	açık	closed	kapalı
entrance	giriş	exit	çıkış
attention	dikkat	slow	yavaş
stop	dur	prohibited	yasak
dangerous	tehlikeli		

Polite Phrases

thank you	teşekkür ederim	hello	iyi günler
please	lütfen	good evening	iyi akşamlar
hello	merhaba	good night	iyi geceler
good morning	gün aydın	good bye	Allaha ısmarladık
bon voyage	iyi yolculuklar	alright	tamam
yes	evet	no	hayır
sorry	pardon		

Welcome Ritual:

welcome	hoş geldiniz
answer:	hoş bulduk
how are you?	nasılsınız
answer: fine, thank you	teşekkür ederim, iyiyim

At Table:

Bon appetit	afiyet olsunuz
answer: thank you, same to you	mersi, size de
cheers!	şerefe
the bill, please	hesap lütfen

Permission to Take Photos:

may I take a photo of you ?	foto çekebilir miyim acaba ?
repeated request	çekmek ?
positive answer	çek ! çek !

Meeting your host (or others) at work:

may it be easy for you	kolay gelsin
answer: thank you	teşekkür ederim

Wishing a Speedy Recovery:

may it blow over soon	geçmiş olsun

Saying Farewell:

good bye (when leaving)	iyi günler *or* Allaha ısmarladık *or* görüşürüz
good bye (staying behind)	güle güle

Some Simple Sentences

Shopping:

How much is the Cola Turka ?	Cola turka kaça ?
Two, please !	Iki tane lütfen !
How much is it ?	Ne kadar ?
Is there bread ?	Ekmek var mı ?
Is there no bread ?	Ekmek yok mu ?
very expensive / inexpensive	Çok pahalı / Çok ucuz

At a Restaurant:

How many persons ?	Kac kişi ?
2 persons !	Iki Kişi !
Is there a menu ?	Mönünüz var mı ?
2 (pieces of) beer, please !	Iki tane bira lütfen !
One glass of wine, please !	Bir bardak sarap lütfen !
A small bottle of water, please !	Bir küçük şişe su lütfen !
Two Güveç (meat stew), please !	Iki tane güveç lütfen !
I don't want any tea.	Çay istimiyorum !
Where is the toilet ?	Tuvalet nerede ?
The bill / check, please !	Hesap lütfen !

Travelling:

How do we get to Göreme ?	Göreme nasil gidiler ?
When does the bus to G. Leave ?	Göreme otobüsü ne zaman kalkar ?
Where is the Sofa Hotel ?	Otel Sofa nerede ?
What time is it ?	Saat kaç ?
How many clocks (have you got) ?	Kaç saat ?
I'm sorry….	Affedersiniz….
I need information !	Bilgi larsım !
Cappadocia is very beautiful !	Kapadokya çok güzel !

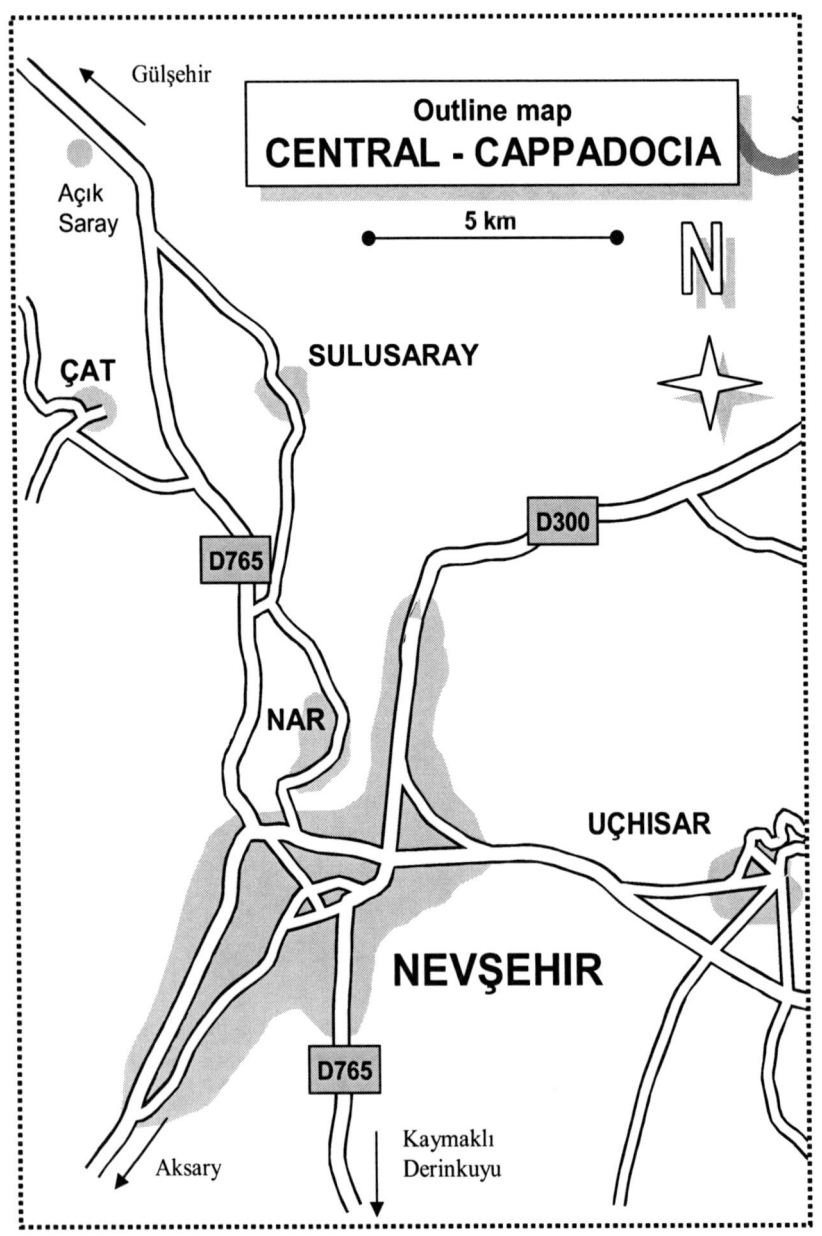

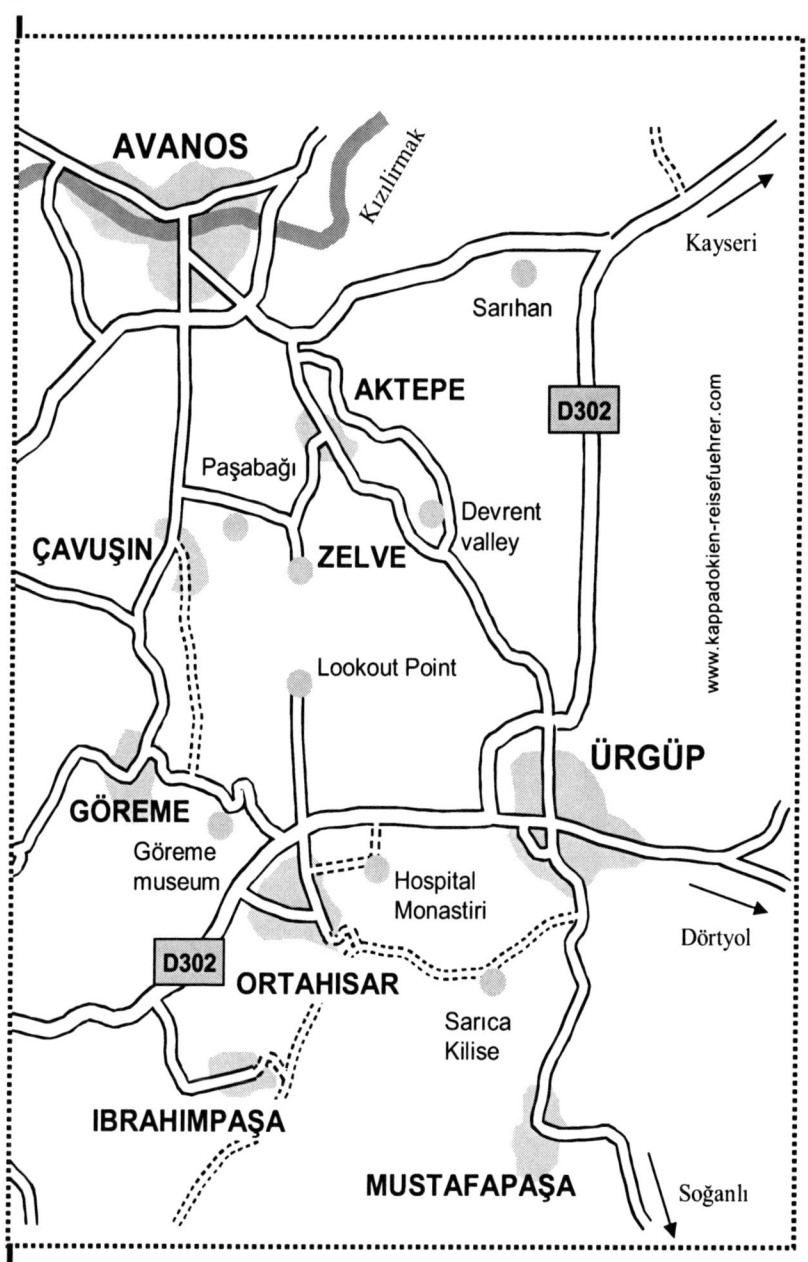

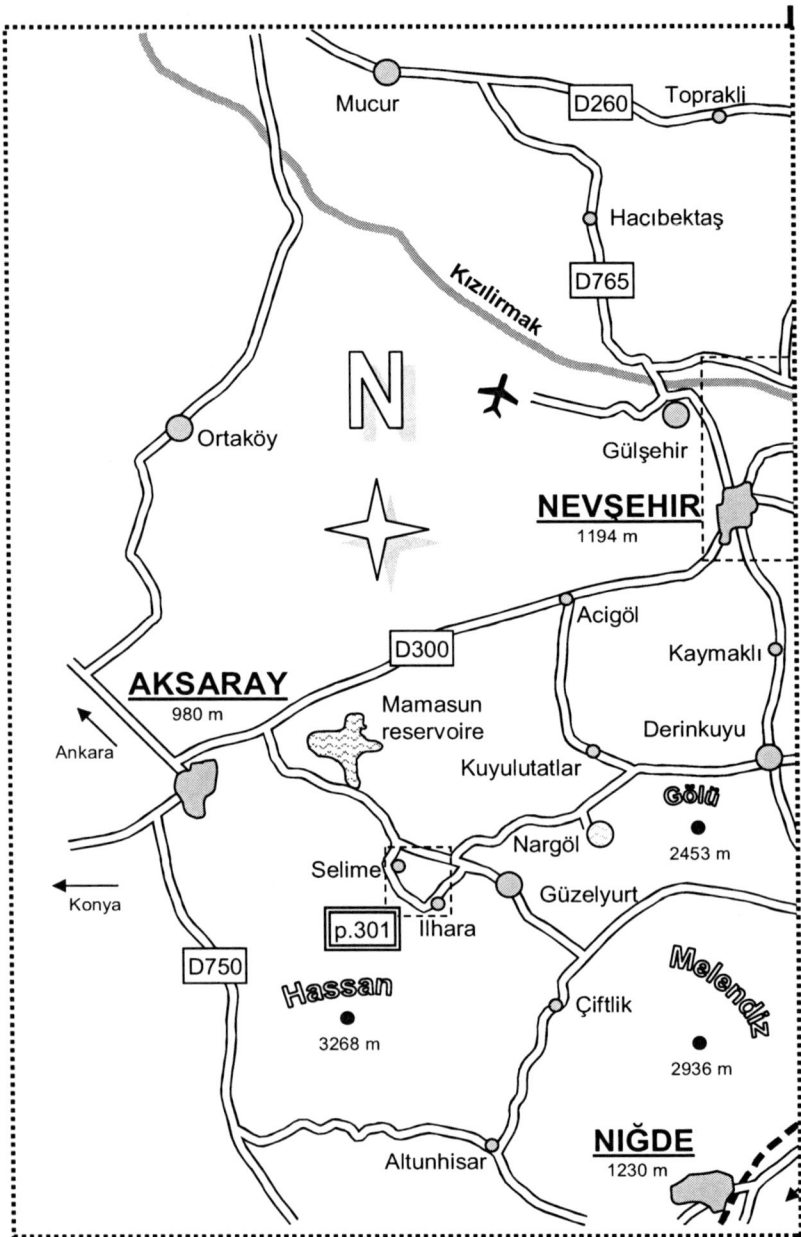

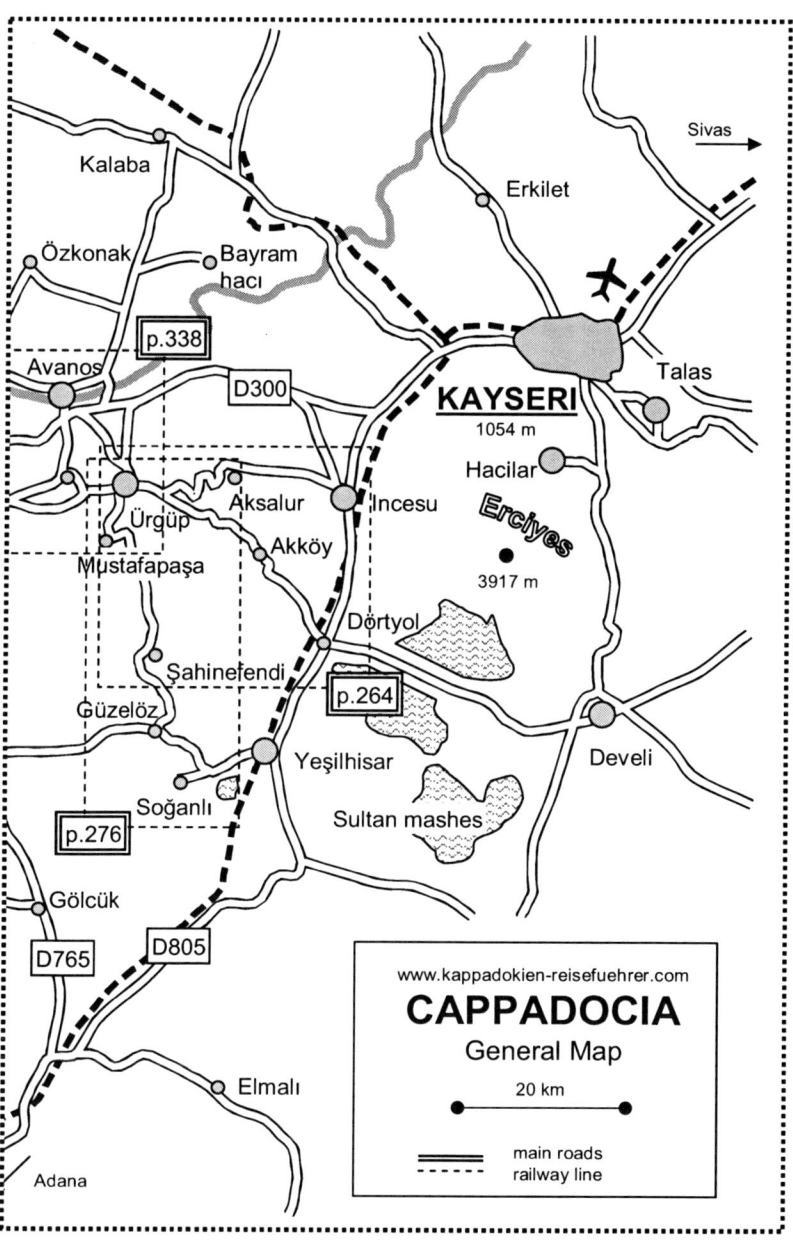

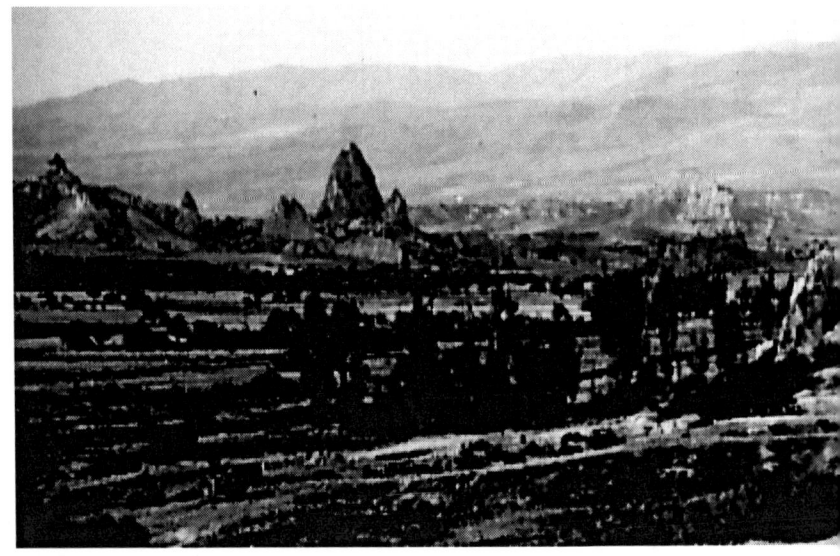

We wish you nice and exciting holidays in Cappadocia

Please visit our travel guide's website:

www.cappadocia-guidebook.com

For any suggestions or questions please contact us under: **avanos@gmx.de**

- or just come and see us in

Cappadocia…!

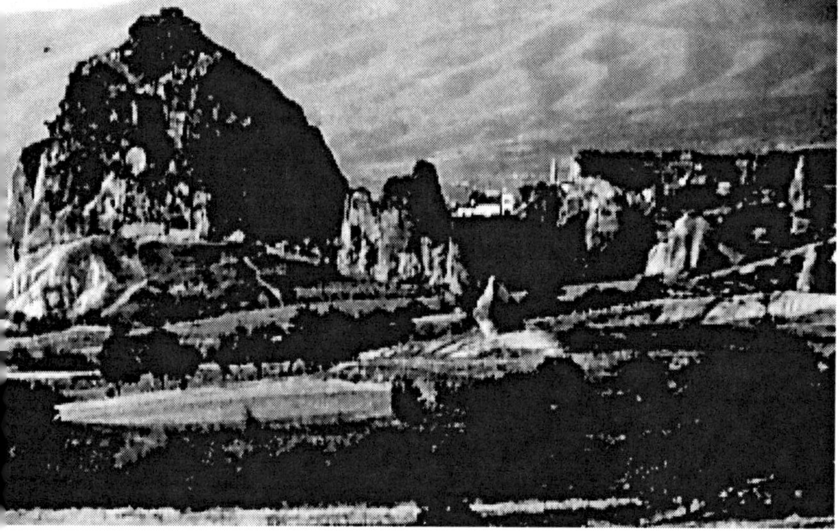

Travel with the authors
Susanne Oberheu and Michael Wadenpohl

Custom tours with **Kappadokya Travel**

www.kappadokya-travel.com

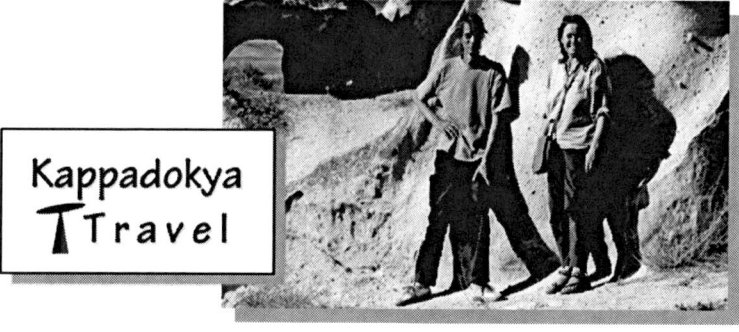

Acknowledgements

Finally, on this page we want to thank all those in Cappadocia who have actively and encouragingly supported us:

We thank **Andus Emge, Bernd Junghans, Ali Fuat Illleez** and **Ines Rebentrost** for their expert text articles;
Lars Eric Möre and **Kaili Kidner**, the operators of Kapadokya Balloons, for showing us Cappadocia from a different perspective;
Roman and **Ayşe Neumüller** for their substancial assistance and information – and of course for their good cuisine.

In Germany, we like to thank for their help:

Uwe Schmitz and **Angelika Baumann** for photos and maps;
Johann Munker, who also supplied photos;
Hendrik Finke, who regularly revises our websites;
and **Siegfried Heppner**, who translated all this into English.

Our gratitude also goes to Melbourne to **William Burlace** and **Lisa van Gaardner** for their proofreading.

And of course, a big thank-you goes to the many little helpers who are not specifically mentioned here.

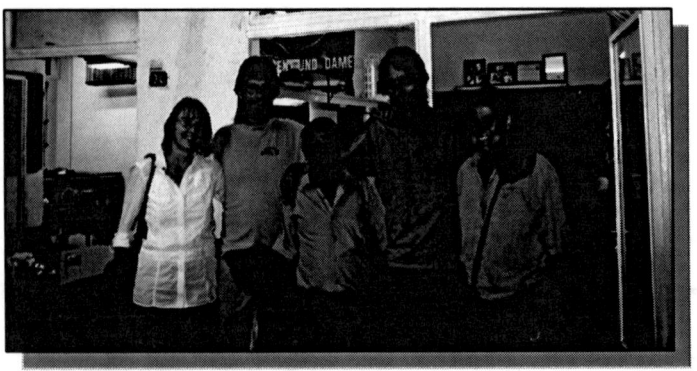

The Parable of the Elephant

Once a king had given the order to call all people of the capital who were blind from birth together in one place. He then ordered them to touch an elephant and then describe the appearance and condition of the animal. As expected, the answers were very different, depending on what body part the blind man had got hold of: the elephant was like a pillar...like an armchair...like a fan.... But each of the blind could hear what was said by his neighbour and was appalled by the false opinions of the others. The result was a heated argument among the blind, with each trying to drown out the other, about the real nature of an elephant.

This parable of Buddha finally migrated from India through the East and to Anatolia, where the dervish mystic Jalal ad-Din Rumi explains that many roads lead to God and that there is no objective truth. He also states that dogmas are a threat to religion and that everything divisive must be overcome; only love is a true religious feeling – and here he means also sexual love. This distinguishes Islamic mystics, called dervishes or Sufis, radically from the Christian monks and mystics, for whom celibacy is one of the highest Christian virtues. Muhammad had condemned abstinence: every good Muslim should have a family, have a job, participate in social life and lead a sensuous life. Once a year, in the fasting month of Ramasan, a believer should remember the deprivations of the poor and also practice sexual abstinence, but then the Muslim should celebrate and live joyfully again. But centuries after Buddha, Jesus and Muhammad, dogmas have established new rules for people which again emphasize what divides rather than what unites us, making life harder instead of easier. Only a few centuries after Jesus, the Christian church declared those heretics who did not believe in its God of the Trinity or in the two natures of Jesus. Only decades after Muhammad, the Sunni among the Muslims declared the Koran the ultimate and absolutely valid truth, to which nothing more could be added. Here, too, thousands of dissenters ended up in the torture chambers and on the pyre. Christian dogmas as well as the Sunnah of the Muslims, the so-called "true tradition", were not made by poor believers, but by powerful men, by caliphs and popes. The landscape must be the reason that it was on the barren plateau of Central Anatolia and in the hidden caves of Cappadocia where people were found who thought very differently and set the standards for a common life of all believers that have applied until today. Jalal ad-Din Rumi, founder of the

Mevlevi Order in nearby Konya, lived 800 years ago and is still one of the greatest mystics of Islam. Yunus Emre from the order of Bektaşı in the identically named Hacıbektaş in Cappadocia is still honoured and celebrated not only by the Turks. He preached the same thing over 700 years ago: "Find God in your heart, not in Jerusalem or Mecca," and "Whoever feels love, has God in his heart," and, "Many paths lead to God!"

While the Sunni in Islam regard the existing Koran as an unchangeable truth, the Shiites believe that the Koran can be interpreted again and again and must be read according to the time. But only the descendants of Muhammmad, that is, his son-in-law, Ali, and his sons, are divinely legitimized for that. These were, however, never recognized by the Sunni. The last descendant of Muhammad already died childless more than 1100 years ago. Since then, the Shiites have been in a waiting state for the so-called "Hidden Imam". And until he will appear as a saviour again, nobody has the sovereignty of interpretation, neither of the Koran nor the Sharia, which governs the laws and regulations in Islam. The Shiites now live as in a legal vacuum, which creates opportunities for a creative and flexible attitude to Islam, as an opportunity or a disaster. For this reason, almost all Shiites are dervishes. In times of great tyranny, they led the rebels in their fight against social evils and oppression, as clerics and scholars, but also with the sword. They were the philosophers of Islam, sometimes also warriors, but above all, they were free thinkers and social revolutionaries. The unworldliness of the Christian monks was not their business: "To be in the world but not to fall for it!", as Sufyan at-Tauri formulated it in 770.

The most famous dervishes were

in 880:	Al Hallaj:	"There are no eternally valid ideas, but there is only permanent change!"
in 900:	Hamdan Qarmat:	"No one must rule over the other!"
in 1090:	Al Ghazali:	"Where reasoning reaches its limits, the truth begins!"
in 1150:	Ibn Rushd (Averroes):	"Where does reason end, where does faith begin?"
in 1190:	Fariduddin Attar:	"Do you love gold more than sin? Why then do you take the sin with you to the afterlife, and leave the gold here?"

in 1200: Ibn Al Arabi explained, like almost all dervishes:
"No religion can claim the only revelation!"

They were scholars and philosophers, visionaries, theologians and scientists. They criticized the existing order and were persecuted and executed for it.
Their works have so far not lost their relevance. Through them, Europe was carried into the modern era. Only by them did Europe become acquainted with Aristotle and humanism. Without them, the so-called Western world would have remained frozen in the dark ages of misery and ignorance for many more centuries, by order of a jealous Christian Church, which forbade its followers to read. At the same time, Islamic mystics and dervishes were thinking beyond the limits of reason."If you want to get to the core, you need to break the shell!" – This was what all dervishes were convinced of. Clinging to externals, whether or not to material things or to religious rituals and rules, would make people unhappy and unfree. People were to understand themselves as part of the whole, as part of God, as a "wave in the sea", as Jalal ad-Din Rumi put it.
Hacı Bektaş was a Shiite itinerant dervish just like the humanist Yunus Emre. Jalal ad-Din Rumi is considered a Sunni dervish with Shiite roots. From him comes the spectacular statement: "Go the way of Muhammad, but if you cannot do that, then go the Christian way. Many paths lead to God!"
These dervishes from the vicinity of Cappadocia, whose ecstatic dance and meditation we marvel at today, whose Sufi music we admire, thought beyond all boundaries of religious pettiness. For them, God or Allah was personally perceptible in ecstasy. But no rule, neither the Koran nor the Bible, nor any human sense perception could make God visible, but one was close to God in love.
As in the parable of the elephant, we are all like blind people who can perceive only a part of the whole great idea. But, like lovers, we should turn to each other rather than exclude each other.
Let us sit in a Cappadocian cave, all alone and quiet, and listen into ourselves: then we are Jews, Christians, Muslims and Buddhists at the same time, and perhaps we sense something of the great mystery that surrounds us and unites us with the world and with nature. - This is what the Islamic dervishes of a bygone era teach us.

Place for your own notices ....